Advances in Experimental Medicine and Biology

More information about this series at http://www.springer.com/series/5584

Erica A. Fortson • Steven R. Feldman
Lindsay C. Strowd
Editors

Management of Atopic Dermatitis

Methods and Challenges

Springer

Editors
Erica A. Fortson
Department of Dermatology
Wake Forest University School of Medicine
Winston Salem, NC, USA

Steven R. Feldman
Department of Dermatology
Wake Forest University School of Medicine
Winston Salem, NC, USA

Lindsay C. Strowd
Department of Dermatology
Wake Forest University School of Medicine
Winston Salem, NC, USA

ISSN 0065-2598 ISSN 2214-8019 (electronic)
Advances in Experimental Medicine and Biology
ISBN 978-3-319-87876-8 ISBN 978-3-319-64804-0 (eBook)
DOI 10.1007/978-3-319-64804-0

Printed on acid-free paper

This Springer imprint is published by Springer Nature
The registered company is Springer International Publishing AG
The registered company address is: Gewerbestrasse 11, 6330 Cham, Switzerland

Foreword

This book has been a collaborative effort between many leading experts in the field of dermatology. This book is designed to serve as a resource to various practitioners to provide insight into the complex nature of atopic dermatitis and its treatment. Despite the field of atopic dermatitis therapeutics rapidly expanding and evolving, many "tried and true" therapies and tips can provide immediate and significant improvement in atopic dermatitis patient care. The editors thank all the contributing authors for their time and devotion to making this book a reality.

Acknowledgements

The editors of this book thank all the contributing authors, including dermatologists, dermatology residents, fellows, and medical students who contributed to this work. We also wish to thank Springer Publishing and the help and guidance of their staff in the publishing process. We also wish to thank the thousands of patients with atopic dermatitis who have agreed to participate in research studies which have led to a better understanding of this disease process and potential treatments.

Contents

Contributors

Brad Ackerson, B.S. Department of Dermatology, Duke University Hospital, Durham, NC, USA

Adewole S. Adamson, M.D., M.P.P. Department of Dermatology, University of North Carolina School of Medicine, Chapel Hill, NC, USA

Christine Ahn, M.D. Wake Forest School of Medicine, Medical Center Boulevard, Winston Salem, NC, USA

Rachel B. Anolik, M.D. Section of Dermatology, Reading Health Physician Network, Wyomissing, PA, USA

Alyssa G. Ashbaugh, B.A. Department of Dermatology, Johns Hopkins University School of Medicine, Baltimore, MD, USA

Steven Barilla, B.S. B.A. Department of Dermatology, Wake Forest University School of Medicine, Winston Salem, NC, USA

Mahima Bhayana, B.S. Department of Dermatology, Howard University School of Medicine, Washington, DC, USA

W. David Boothe, M.D. Department of Dermatology, Texas Tech University Health Sciences Center, Lubbock, TX, USA

Leah Cardwell, M.D. Department of Dermatology, Wake Forest University School of Medicine, Winston Salem, NC, USA

Taylor Edwards, B.S. Ohio University Heritage College of Osteopathic Medicine, Athens, OH, USA

William S. Farmer, B.S. Georgetown University School of Medicine, Washington, DC, USA

Steven R. Feldman, M.D., Ph.D. Department of Dermatology, Wake Forest University School of Medicine, Winston Salem, NC, USA

Kayla Felix, B.S. Department of Dermatology, Wake Forest University School of Medicine, Winston Salem, NC, USA

Erica A. Forston, B.S. Department of Dermatology, Wake Forest University School of Medicine, Winston Salem, NC, USA

Sandy François, B.S., M.Sc. Department of Dermatology, Emory School of Medicine, Atlanta, GA, USA

Zelma C. Chiesa Fuxench, M.D., M.S.C.E. Department of Dermatology, University of Pennsylvania Perelman School of Medicine, Philadelphia, PA, USA

Heather Gochnauer, B.S. Section of Dermatology, Reading Health Physician Network, Wyomissing, PA, USA

Department of Dermatology, Lewis Katz School of Medicine at Temple University, Philadelphia, PA, USA

William Huang, M.D. Wake Forest School of Medicine, Medical Center Boulevard, Winston Salem, NC, USA

Joseph L. Jorizzo, M.D. Department of Dermatology, Wake Forest University School of Medicine, Winston Salem, NC, USA

Shawn G. Kwatra, M.D. Department of Dermatology, Johns Hopkins University School of Medicine, Baltimore, MD, USA

Mary Laird, B.A. The Ronald O. Perelman Department of Dermatology, New York University Langone Health, New York, NY, USA

Angela J. Lamb, M.D. Department of Dermatology, The Mount Sinai Hospital, New York, NY, USA

Becky Li, B.S. Department of Dermatology, Howard University School of Medicine, Washington, DC, USA

Kalyani S. Marathe, M.D., M.P.H. Department of Dermatology, George Washington University, Washington, DC, USA

Department of Dermatology, Children's National Medical Center, Washington, DC, USA

Matilda W. Nicholas, M.D., Ph.D. Department of Dermatology, Duke University Hospital, Durham, NC, USA

Nupur Patel, M.S. Department of Dermatology, Wake Forest University School of Medicine, Winston Salem, NC, USA

Zakiya Rice, M.D. Department of Dermatology, Emory School of Medicine, Atlanta, GA, USA

Kristen Lo Sicco, M.D. The Ronald O. Perelman Department of Dermatology, New York University Langone Health, New York, NY, USA

Lindsay C. Strowd, M.D. Department of Dermatology, Wake Forest University School of Medicine, Winston Salem, NC, USA

Wayne Sy, M.S., M.P.H. Department of Dermatology, The Mount Sinai Hospital, New York, NY, USA

James A. Tarbox, M.D. Department of Internal Medicine, Texas Tech University Health Sciences Center, Lubbock, TX, USA

Michelle B. Tarbox, M.D. Department of Dermatology, Texas Tech University Health Sciences Center, Lubbock, TX, USA

Ryan Thorpe, M.D. Department of Dermatology, Duke University Hospital, Durham, NC, USA

Rodrigo Valdes-Rodriguez, M.D. Section of Dermatology, Reading Health Physician Network, Wyomissing, PA, USA

Department of Dermatology, Lewis Katz School of Medicine at Temple University, Philadelphia, PA, USA

Chapter 1
Introduction

Erica A. Fortson, Becky Li, and Mahima Bhayana

Abstract Atopic dermatitis (AD) is a chronic relapsing condition that is characterized by itching and redness of the skin. Our modern usage of atopic dermatitis dates back to 1933, when Wise and Sulzberger first coined the term to signify the disease's close association with other respiratory atopy, such as bronchial asthma and allergic rhinitis. A recent systematic review of 69 cross-sectional and cohort studies has confirmed that AD is now a worldwide phenomenon with lifetime AD prevalences of well over 20% in many affluent country settings. Although there is no obvious consistent overall global trend in the prevalence of AD, studies have shown that climate, urbanization, lifestyle, and socioeconomic class influence the prevalence of atopic dermatitis. Despite the pervasiveness of the disease, an understanding of atopic dermatitis has been hampered by a number of factors. Data suggests that extrinsic environmental factors work in concert with intrinsic immune mechanism and genetic factors to drive disease progression. With such a complex etiology, management of atopic dermatitis currently at best achieves symptomatic control rather than cure. This approach poses a significant burden on healthcare resources, as well as patients' quality of life. Current management methods of AD often involves a combination of non-pharmacologic modalities and prescription medications. Though they can be effective when employed, there are significant barriers to treatment for patients including time, costs, and medication side effects. Our aim, throughout this text, is to explore the complexities of AD, providing the healthcare provider with tips and tricks to improve patient care and satisfaction and the most current trends and treatment approaches on the horizon.

Keywords Atopic dermatitis • Besnier's prurigo • Atopic eczema • Intrinsic allergic dermatitis • Neurodermitis constitutionalis • Endogenous eczema • Eczema flexurarum • Asthma-eczema • Hay fever-eczema

E.A. Fortson, B.S. (✉)
Department of Dermatology, Wake Forest University School of Medicine,
Winston Salem, NC, USA
e-mail: efortson@wakehealth.edu

B. Li, B.S. • M. Bhayana, B.S.
Department of Dermatology, Howard University School of Medicine, Washington, DC, USA

E.A. Fortson et al. (eds.), *Management of Atopic Dermatitis*, Advances in Experimental Medicine and Biology 1027, DOI 10.1007/978-3-319-64804-0_1

1.1 Overview and History

Atopic dermatitis (AD) is a chronic relapsing condition that is characterized by itching and redness of the skin. It is primarily a disease of infancy and early childhood. In general, one third of children will present during the first year of life, another third during the second year, and the remaining one third during later childhood. Eighty percent of children have clinical symptoms by 5 years of age [1]. Patients usually outgrow the disease before adolescence. However, AD is often the first step in the so-called "atopic march" [2]. Therefore, the onset of atopic dermatitis in childhood often foreshadows the later development of asthma and/or allergic rhinitis.

Symptoms of AD include patches of skin that are red or brownish, cracked or scaly, dry, and itchy, especially at night. In infants, AD usually appears as tiny bumps on the cheeks. Older children and adults, on the other hand, often experience rashes on the knees or elbows (often in the folds of the joints), on the backs of the hands, or on the scalp [3].

Our modern usage of atopic dermatitis dates back to 1933, when Wise and Sulzberger first coined the term to signify the disease's close association with other respiratory atopy, such as bronchial asthma and allergic rhinitis [4]. Initially, atopic dermatitis was described as a form of "prurigo diasthesique" by Ernest Besnier in 1892 [5]. Since the inception of Besnier's prurigo, AD has had many other names, including atopic eczema, intrinsic allergic dermatitis, neurodermitis constitutionalis, endogenous eczema, eczema flexurarum, asthma-eczema, and hay fever-eczema [6].

1.2 Epidemiology

The prevalence of atopic dermatitis has risen dramatically since these initial descriptions. Seven decades ago, estimates of prevalence in Scandinavia revealed that 1.3% of patients suffered from AD [7]. By 1993, the prevalence of atopic dermatitis in Scandinavia had increased more than 20-fold to 23% [8].

Some of the most valuable AD prevalence and trend data have come from the International Study of Asthma and Allergies in Childhood (ISAAC). With close to two million children from 106 countries, ISAAC is the biggest and only allergy study that has taken a truly global approach. The study revealed that over 20% of children are affected by AD in some countries, but that the prevalence varies greatly throughout the world. For 6–7 year olds, data showed that the prevalence of AD ranged from 0.9% in India to 22.5% in Ecuador. New data showed high values in Asia and Latin America. For 13–14 year olds, data showed that the prevalence of AD ranged from 0.2% in China to 24.6% in Columbia. Prevalence over 15% was found in 4 of 9 regions studied, including Africa, Latin America, Europe, and Oceania [9]. In Phase Three of the ISAAC study, the latest available data set, results showed that AD reached a plateau in countries with the highest prevalence, such as the UK. However, AD continues to increase in prevalence in young children (age 6–7 vs. age 13–14) and in low-income countries, such as Latin America and Southeast Asia [10, 11].

In addition, a recent systematic review of 69 cross-sectional and cohort studies has confirmed that AD is now a worldwide phenomenon with lifetime AD prevalences of well over 20% in many affluent country settings [12].

Although there is no obvious consistent overall global trend in the prevalence of AD, studies have shown that climate, urbanization, lifestyle, and socioeconomic class influence the prevalence of atopic dermatitis.

Living in lower, more tropical latitudes and rural areas have been shown to correlate with a lower prevalence of atopic dermatitis [13, 14]. For example, Finnish children living in the eastern, more rural areas of the country showed a lower prevalence than those living in the southern, more industrialized areas [15]. Likewise, those living in rural areas of China near Hong Kong had a much lower prevalence (7.2%) than those living in the city of Hong Kong (20.1%) [16]. Lower outdoor temperatures also increase the risk of AD development. UV light exposure has an influence on AD prevalence as well, as demonstrated by a recent ecological analysis in a US cohort [17]. UV light has a well-established immunosuppressive effect. It helps convert the breakdown product of filaggrin, trans-urocanic acid, into its cis-urocanic acid isoform, which is immunosuppressive [18].

Higher prevalence of atopic dermatitis has been shown to be associated with areas of industrialization and urbanization. In Nigeria, rates of atopic dermatitis have increased with increasing urbanization, rising from 0.3% in the 1960s, to 2.6% in the 1970s, and to 6.1% in the 1980s [19]. This association may be explained by increased levels of air pollution, urban lifestyle, dietary modifications, and other alterations in behavior and environment [1]. Another example is the sharp increase of AD in 5–6 year olds in East Germany from 9.6% in 1991 to 23.4% in 1997 after adoption of a more Western lifestyle [20]. All the while, the prevalence of AD remained stable at approximately 12% in West Germany from 1991 to 1997. The adoption of a Western lifestyle and the sharp increase in AD prevalence may be explained by the increase in proinflammatory n-6 polyunsaturated fatty acid content in Western diets over the years [21]. In ISAAC Phase Three, a consistent protective effect was found between frequent consumption of fresh fruits (1–29/week) and AD risk (adjusted OR = 0.81, 0.67–0.97), whereas the opposite was true for fast-food consumption ($\geq$39/week, adjusted OR = 1.70, 1.48–1.95) [22].

Socioeconomic class has been shown to impact the prevalence of AD, with higher socioeconomic class correlating with increased prevalence. In a British study, the point-prevalence of atopic dermatitis at age seven in the highest socioeconomic class was twice that in the lowest socioeconomic class. An increase in prevalence was also seen in those families who owned their residences as compared to families who rented. Reasons for this disparity may be attributed to increased exposure to medical care, increased immunizations, a more allergenic home environment, and smaller family size [23, 24]. Larger family sizes have been associated with a decreased prevalence of atopic dermatitis and may confer protection through increased exposures to infections at an early age [24].

1.3 Complexity of Atopic Dermatitis Etiology

Despite the pervasiveness of the disease, an understanding of atopic dermatitis has been hampered by a number of factors. Data suggests that extrinsic environmental factors work in concert with intrinsic immune mechanism and genetic factors to drive disease progression.

The immune response observed during the course of AD is characterized by a biphasic inflammation. A Th2-dominant immune response occurs in the initial and acute phase of AD, while a Th1-dominant immune response ensues in chronic AD [25]. Studies have shown that microbial exposure may influence the balance of Th1 and Th2 immune responses. Microbial exposure promotes Th1 responses and down-regulates Th2 responses. Th1 cells are associated with responses to infection and the production of interferon-γ, whereas Th2 cells induce the production of IgE and the maturation of mast cells, basophils, and eosinophils. Th2 cells are therefore generally associated with "atopic" immune responses [3].

Genetics also influences the manifestations of the disease. In twin studies, there was a higher concordance rate in monozygotic twins compared to dizygotic twins [26]. Skin barrier function plays a role in the development of atopic dermatitis as well. Mutations in the FLG gene, encoding the epidermal barrier protein filaggrin, have a strong correlation with AD development [27]. It has been established that genetically determined alterations of the epidermis or lipid composition contribute to skin barrier dysfunction, which leads to inflammation. Furthermore, the defective epidermal barrier allows for easier and enhanced environmental allergen penetration through the skin, facilitating the interaction of the allergens with the local antigen-presenting cells and immune effector cells. This leads to systemic IgE sensitization and transition from the non-atopic state to the atopic state of the disease. The skin barrier defect in AD also predisposes patients to colonization or infection by pathogenic microbes, i.e., *Staphylococcus aureus*, whose exogenous proteases can also further damage the skin barrier.

Environmental factors that impact the development of AD include breastfeeding and time of weaning, obesity and physical exercise, and pollution and tobacco smoke. Breastfeeding is a protective factor up until 3 months of age [28]. Delayed weaning has also been shown to increase the risk of AD [29–32]. Based on the ISAAC Phase Three data, AD was found to have an association with obesity [33, 34]. The study also revealed that increased TV viewing (<5 h) positively correlated with AD risk [35]. We also mentioned previously: low outdoor temperature, UV light exposure, urbanization, and diet.

Environmental factors linked to microbial exposure also affect the manifestation of the disease. These factors include day care, farm environment and animals, pets, endotoxin exposure, antibiotic usage, and the composition of gut microbiome. The revised hygiene hypothesis states that decreased early childhood exposure to infections (i.e., any microbial exposure) increases the susceptibility to allergic diseases [36]. Therefore, AD risk is decreased in infants who attend day care during their first year of life. Farm environments and animals are also protective. However, rather than living in farm environments being protective, study results revealed that the consumption of unpasteurized farm milk during the first 2 years of life and the direct contact of pregnant mothers with farm animals are the protective factors [37]. Exposure to dogs are protective as well [38]. Also protective is exposure to endotoxins in early childhood. Endotoxin, a component of the outer membrane of gram-negative bacteria, promotes the maturation of naïve T cells into Th1 cells, instead of Th2 cells. Antibiotics (rather than the infection itself) appear to increase the risk of AD [39, 40]. This may be explained by the changes in microbiota, which is known to influence the immune response. There is actually evidence showing that the early gut microbiota of children who develop AD later in life is different from that of children who do not develop AD, both in terms of composition and diversity [41].

1.4 Disease Costs and Burden on Society

With such a complex etiology, management of atopic dermatitis currently at best achieves symptomatic control rather than cure. This approach poses a significant burden on healthcare resources, as well as patients' quality of life.

It is well established that atopic dermatitis has large cost implications. In 1995–1996, the total annual cost of AD in children age five or younger was estimated to be 47 million British pounds in the UK [42]. Looking at a broader age range, the total annual cost was estimated to be around 465 million British pounds [43]. In 2008, according to a systematic literature review of 418 atopic dermatitis articles, the total annual costs of AD ranged from 364 million to 3.8 billion US dollars in the United States [44]. In 2015, Chulmin and colleagues estimated the total annual cost of AD to be 5.8 trillion KRW in Korea [45]. In another US study, estimated annual national costs were $364 million, with hospitalizations totaling $49 million, office visits $107 million, emergency department visits $87 million, and outpatient prescriptions $121 million [46]. Atopic dermatitis clearly causes a major financial burden to both individual families and national healthcare systems.

Besides its economic cost, atopic dermatitis bears a significant burden to society. The Global Burden of Diseases Study recently demonstrated that skin diseases were the fourth leading cause of nonfatal disease burden [47]. AD patients often complain of sleep disturbance associated with aggravated symptoms and have significantly reduced sleep efficiency, longer sleep-onset latency, a greater degree of sleep fragmentation, and less nonrapid eye movement sleep [48–52]. This may be explained by the lower levels of nocturnal melatonin secretion associated with higher total and/or allergen-specific immunoglobulin E (IgE) levels [49]. Substance P and brain-derived neurotrophic factor (BDNF) are also released in atopic dermatitis and can interfere with skin barrier function, exacerbating nocturnal pruritis [53,

54]. Some studies have even shown that pro-inflammatory cytokines, secreted by eczematous inflammation, may penetrate the blood-brain barrier and activate neuropathogenic mechanisms related to emotional control [55–57]. Furthermore, the negative cosmetic effects of AD affect self-esteem and impair interpersonal relationships. AD is commonly associated with high levels of stigmatization, social withdrawal, anxiety, and depression among patients and may affect their careers. In fact, children and adolescents with atopic dermatitis repeatedly experience feelings of social isolation, peer-group rejection, teasing, and bullying, which may lead to a loss of confidence, mood changes, and/or depression [58]. This may lead to poor school performance because these kinds of emotional experiences impair concentration [59]. Children may also become withdrawn [60]. These behaviors increase the risk of developing pediatric and adolescent psychiatric disorders.

1.5 Atopic Dermatitis Treatment and Patient Barriers

Current management methods of AD often involve a combination of non-pharmacologic modalities to maximize overall skin barrier integrity and prescription medications to address chronic, active disease and flares. Though they can be effective when employed, there are significant barriers to treatment for patients. Daily preventive care is essential to skin barrier maintenance and thus long-term management of AD. Patients are instructed to take brief, luke-warm baths or showers using mild, hypoallergenic cleansing agents, and followed by liberal application of ceramide-rich moisturizers and hydrophilic emollients and ointments [61]. Many patients, however, tend towards long, hot showers/baths and find adherence to routines involving thick creams and emollients cumbersome and unappealing under clothing. Wet wraps or dressings may be applied to more severe or chronic lesions for immediate relief and as a temporary, protective barrier from further scratching behavior [61]. This technique can be complicated to execute and often time consuming for patients and caregivers. Topical prescription creams, gels or foams, including corticosteroids and calcineurin inhibitors are considered first-line prescription topical therapy [62]. Side effects, including skin atrophy, telangiectasias and striae limit topical steroid site and frequency of application. Misunderstanding regarding topical steroids in the lay community often results in noncompliance due to patient or caregiver concerns [63]. Phototherapy is an option for patients in which topical medications alone cannot achieve adequate control [63]. Often requiring several, short visits per week to the clinic, patients can find this approach time consuming and costly if insurance co-payments are a consideration. Oral steroids, cyclosporine, mycophenolate mofetil, methotrexate, azathioprine, and interferon gamma are systemic immunomodulators have become more commonly used, particularly in instances of severe refractory disease [62]. The more significant side effect profile of systemic medications in addition to increased costs can be an additional challenge for patients. Adjunct therapies such as brief courses of topical and systemic anti-infectives for bacterial, fungal and viral skin infections and antihistamines are occasionally required [61]. The sedating effects of antihistamines limit use to instances of sleep disturbance in AD patients and the risk of resistance limits the duration of antibiotic use [61]. Though choices abound for the provider in creating an effective management strategy for the AD patient, the importance of these barriers to patient treatment access and compliance to treatment cannot be ignored if optimal outcomes to therapy are to be accomplished.

1.6 Goals of Text

AD is a complicated, chronic condition that for many patients can require extensive, long-term care. The understanding and management of AD on the part of providers is equally challenging and ever evolving. Our aim, throughout this text, is to explore the complexities of AD, providing the healthcare provider with tips and tricks to improve patient care and satisfaction and the most current trends and treatment approaches on the horizon.

References

1. Levy RM, Gelfand JM, Yan AC. The epidemiology of atopic dermatitis. Clin Dermatol. 2003;21(2):109–15.
2. Spergel JM. From atopic dermatitis to asthma: the atopic march. Ann Allergy Asthma Immunol. 2010;105:99–106.
3. Nutten S. Atopic dermatitis: global epidemiology and risk factors. Ann Nutr Metab. 2015;66:8–16.
4. Hill LW, Sulzberger MB. Yearbook of dermatology and syphilology. Chicago: Year Book Medical Publishers; 1933. p. 1–70.
5. Besnier EH. Annals of dermatology and syphilography 1892;3:634–648.
6. Sulzberger M. Historical notes on atopic dermatitis: its names and nature. Semin Dermatol. 1983;2:1–4.
7. Nexmand PH. Clinical studies of Besnier's prurigo. Cophenhagen: Rosenkilde and Bagger; 1948.
8. Larsen FS, Diepgen T, Svensson A. The occurrence of atopic dermatitis in north Europe: an international questionnaire study. J Am Acad Dermatol. 1996;34:760–4.
9. Odhiambo JA, Williams HC, Clayton TO, Robertson CF, Asher MI, Group IPTS. Global variations in prevalence of eczema symptoms in children from ISAAC phase three. J Allergy Clin Immunol. 2009;124:1251–1258.e23.
10. Mallol J, Crane J, von Mutius E, Odhiambo J, Keil U, Stewart A. ISAAC phase three study group: the international study of asthma and allergies in childhood (ISAAC) phase three: a global synthesis. Allergol Immunopathol. 2013;41:73–85.
11. Williams H, Stewart A, von Mutius E, Cookson W, Anderson HR. International study of asthma and allergies in childhood (ISAAC) phase one and three study groups: is eczema really on the increase worldwide? J Allergy Clin Immunol. 2008;121:947–954.e15.
12. Deckers IA, McLean S, Linssen S, Mommers M, van Schayck CP, Sheikh A. Investigating international time trends in the incidence and prevalence of atopic eczema 1990–2010: a systematic review of epidemiological studies. PLoS One. 2012;7(7):e39803.

13. Williams HC. Epidemiology of atopic dermatitis. Clin Exp Dermatol. 2000;25:522–9.
14. Agata H, Kondo N, Fukutomi O, Hayashi T, Shinoda S, Nishida T, Yomo A, Suzuki Y, Shimozawa N, Tomatsu S. Comparison of allergic diseases and specific IgE antibodies in different parts of Japan. Ann Allergy. 1994;72:447–51.
15. Pöysä L, Korppi M, Pietikäinen M, Remes K, Juntunen-Backman K. Asthma, allergic rhinitis and atopic eczema in Finnish children and adolescents. Allergy. 1991;46:161–5.
16. Leung R, Ho P. Asthma, allergy and atopy in three south-east Asian populations. Thorax. 1994;49:1205–10.
17. Silverberg JI, Hanifin J, Simpson EL. Climatic factors are associated with childhood eczema prevalence in the United States. J Investig Dermatol. 2013;133:1752–9.
18. Miajlovic H, Fallon PG, Irvine AD, Foster TJ. Effect of filaggrin breakdown products on growth of and protein expression by Staphylococcus aureus. J Allergy Clin Immunol. 2010;126:1184–1190.e3.
19. George AO. Atopic dermatitis in Nigeria. Int J Dermatol. 1989;28:237–9.
20. Schafer T, Kramer U, Vieluf D, Abeck D, Behrendt H, Ring J. The excess of atopic eczema in East Germany is related to the intrinsic type. Br J Dermatol. 2000;143:992–8.
21. Sausenthaler S, Kompauer I, Borte M, Herbarth O, Schaaf B, Von Berg A, Zutavern A, Heinrich J. Margarine and butter consumption, eczema and allergic sensitization in children. Pediatr Allergy Immunol. 2006;17:85–93.
22. Ellwood P, Asher MI, Garcia-Marcos L, Williams H, Keil U, Robertson C, Nagel G. Do fast foods cause asthma, rhinoconjunctivitis and eczema? Global findings from the international study of asthma and allergies in childhood (ISAAC) phase three. Thorax. 2013;68:351–60.
23. McNally N, Phillips D. Social factors and atopic dermatitis. In: Williams HC, editor. Atopic dermatitis. Cambridge: Cambridge University Press; 2000. p. 139–47.
24. Strachan DP. Hay fever, hygiene and household size. Br Med J. 1989;299:1259–60.
25. Fiset PO, Leung DY, Hamid Q. Immunopathology of atopic dermatitis. J Allergy Clin Immunol. 2006;118:287–90.
26. Larsen FS, Holm NV. Atopic dermatitis in a population based twin series. Concordance rates and heritability estimation. Acta Dermato Venereologica. 1985;114:159.
27. Palmer CN, Irvine AD, Terron-Kwiatkowski A, Zhao Y, Liao H, Lee SP, Goudie DR, Sandilands A, Campbell LE, Smith FJ, O'Regan GM, Watson RM, Cecil JE, Bale SJ, Compton JG, JJ DG, Fleckman P, Lewis-Jones S, Arseculeratne G, Sergeant A, Munro CS, El Houate B, McElreavey K, Halkjaer LB, Bisgaard H, Mukhopadhyay S, WH ML. Common loss-of-function variants of the epidermal barrier protein filaggrin are a major predisposing factor for atopic dermatitis. Nat Genet. 2006;38:441–6.
28. Flohr C, Nagel G, Weinmayr G, Kleiner A, Strachan DP, Williams HC. Lack of evidence for a protective effect of prolonged breast-feeding on childhood eczema: lessons from the international study of asthma and allergies in childhood (ISAAC) phase two. Br J Dermatol. 2011;165:1280–9.
29. Sariachvili M, Droste J, Dom S, Wieringa M, Hagendorens M, Stevens W, van Sprundel M, Desager K, Weyler J. Early exposure to solid foods and the development of eczema in children up to 4 years of age. Pediatr Allergy Immunol. 2010;21:74–81.
30. Snijders BE, Thijs C, van Ree R, van den Brandt PA. Age at first introduction of cow milk products and other food products in relation to infant atopic manifestations in the first 2 years of life: the KOALA birth cohort study. Pediatrics. 2008;122:e115–22.
31. Zutavern A, Brockow I, Schaaf B, von Berg A, Diez U, Borte M, Kraemer U, Herbarth O, Behrendt H, Wichmann HE, Heinrich J. Timing of solid food introduction in relation to eczema, asthma, allergic rhinitis, and food and inhalant sensitization at the age of 6 years: results from the prospective birth cohort study LISA. Pediatrics. 2008;121:e44–52.
32. Filipiak B, Zutavern A, Koletzko S, von Berg A, Brockow I, Grubl A, Berdel D, Reinhardt D, Bauer CP, Wichmann HE, Heinrich J. Solid food introduction in relation to eczema: results from a four-year prospective birth cohort study. J Pediatr. 2007;151:352–8.

33. Murray CS, Canoy D, Buchan I, Woodcock A, Simpson A, Custovic A. Body mass index in young children and allergic disease: gender differences in a longitudinal study. Clin Exp Allergy. 2011;41:78–85.
34. Yao TC, Ou LS, Yeh KW, Lee WI, Chen LC, Huang JL. Associations of age, gender, and BMI with prevalence of allergic diseases in children: PATCH study. J Asthma. 2011;48:503–10.
35. Mitchell EA, Beasley R, Bjorksten B, Crane J, Garcia-Marcos L, Keil U. The association between BMI, vigorous physical activity and television viewing and the risk of symptoms of asthma, rhinoconjunctivitis and eczema in children and adolescents: ISAAC phase three. Clin Exp Allergy. 2013;43:73–84.
36. Flohr C, Yeo L. Atopic dermatitis and the hygiene hypothesis revisited. Curr Probl Dermatol. 2011;41:1–34.
37. von Mutius E. Maternal farm exposure/ingestion of unpasteurized cow's milk and allergic disease. Curr Opin Gastroenterol. 2012;28:570–6.
38. Langan SM, Flohr C, Williams HC. The role of furry pets in eczema: a systematic review. Arch Dermatol. 2007;143:1570–7.
39. Dom S, Droste JH, Sariachvili MA, Hagendorens MM, Oostveen E, Bridts CH, Stevens WJ, Wieringa MH, Weyler JJ. Pre- and post-natal exposure to antibiotics and the development of eczema, recurrent wheezing and atopic sensitization in children up to the age of 4 years. Clin Exp Allergy. 2010;40:1378–87.
40. Tsakok T, McKeever TM, Yeo L, Flohr C. Does early life exposure to antibiotics increase the risk of eczema? A systematic review. Br J Dermatol. 2013;169:983–91.
41. Wang M, Karlsson C, Olsson C, Adlerberth I, Wold AE, Strachan DP, Martricardi PM, Aberg N, Perkin MR, Tripodi S, Coates AR, Hesselmar B, Saalman R, Molin G, Ahrne S. Reduced diversity in the early fecal microbiota of infants with atopic eczema. J Allergy Clin Immunol. 2008;121:129–34.
42. Emerson RM, Williams HC, Allen BR. What is the cost of atopic dermatitis in preschool children? Br J Dermatol. 2001;144:514–22.
43. Herd RM, Tidman MJ, Prescott RJ, Hunter JAA. The cost of atopic eczema. Br J Dermatol. 1996;135:20–3.
44. Mancini AJ, Kaulback K, Chamlin SL. The socioeconomic impact of atopic dermatitis in the United States: a systematic review. Pediatr Dermatol. 2008;25:1–6.
45. Kim C, Park KY, Ahn S, Kim DH, Li K, Kim DW, Kim M, Jo S, Yim HW, Seo SJ. Economic impact of atopic dermatitis in Korean patients. Ann Dermatol. 2015;27(3):298–305.
46. Lapidus CS, Schwarz DF, Honig PJ. Atopic dermatitis in children: who cares? Who pays? J Am Acad Dermatol. 1993;29:699–703.
47. Hay RJ, Johns NE, Williams HC, Bollinger IW, Dellavalle RP, Margolis DJ, Marks R, Naldi L, Weinstock MA, Wulf SK, Michaud C, Murray CJ, Maghavi M. The global burden of skin disease in 2010: an analysis of the prevalence and impact of skin conditions. J Investig Dermatol Symp Proc. 2014;134:1527–34.
48. Senra MS, Wollenberg A. Psychodermatological aspects of atopic dermatitis. Br J Dermatol. 2014;170:38–43.
49. Chang YS, Chou YT, Lee JH, Lee PL, Yang-Shia D, Sun C, Lin YT, Wang LC, Yu H, Yang YH, Chen CA, Wan KS, Chiang BL. Atopic dermatitis, melatonin, and sleep disturbance. Pediatrics. 2014;134:e397–405.
50. Arndt J, Smith N, Tausk F. Stress and atopic dermatitis. Curr Allergy Asthma Rep. 2008;8:312–7.
51. Spergel JM, Paller AS. Atopic dermatitis and the atopic march. J Allergy Clin Immunol. 2003;112:S118–27.
52. Bender BG, Leung SB, Leung DY. Actigraphy assessment of sleep disturbance in patients with atopic dermatitis: an objective life quality measure. J Allergy Clin Immunol. 2003;111:598–602.
53. Hon KL, Lam MC, Wong KY, Leung TF, Ng PC. Pathophysiology of nocturnal scratching in childhood atopic dermatitis: the role of brain-derived neurotrophic factor and substance P. Br J Dermatol. 2007;157:922–5.

54. Oh SH, Bae BG, Park CO, Noh JY, Park IH, Wu WH, Lee KH. Association of stress with symptoms of atopic dermatitis. Acta Derm Venereol. 2010;90:582–8.
55. Denda M, Takei K, Denda S. How does epidermal pathology interact with mental state? Med Hypotheses. 2013;80:194–6.
56. Miller AH, Haroon E, Raison CL, Felger JC. Cytokine targets in the brain: impact on neurotransmitters and neurocircuits. Depress Anxiety. 2013;30:297–306.
57. Yarlagadda A, Alfson E, Clayton AH. The blood brain barrier and the role of cytokines in neuropsychiatry. Psychiatry. 2009;6:18–22.
58. Salek MS, Jung S, Brincat-Ruffini LA, MacFarlane L, Lewis-Jones MS, Basra MK, Finlay AY. Clinical experience and psychometric properties of the Children's dermatology life quality index (CDLQI), 1995–2012. Br J Dermatol. 2013;169:734–59.
59. Brenninkmeijer EE, Legierse CM, Sillevis Smitt JH, Last BF, Grootenhuis MA, Bos JD. The course of life of patients with childhood atopic dermatitis. Pediatr Dermatol. 2009;26:14–22.
60. LeBovidge JS, Elverson W, Timmons KG, Hawryluk EB, Rea C, Lee M, Schneider LC. Multidisciplinary interventions in the management of atopic dermatitis. J Allergy Clin Immunol. 2016;138:325–34.
61. Levy ML. Atopic dermatitis: understanding the disease and its management. Curr Med Res Opin. 2007;23(12):3091–103.
62. Gelbard CM, Hebert AA. New and emerging trends in the treatment of atopic dermatitis. Patient Pref Adherence. 2008;2:387–92.
63. Weidinger S, Novak N. Atopic dermatitis. Lancet. 2016;387(10023):1109–22.

Chapter 2
Atopic Dermatitis: Disease Background and Risk Factors

Zelma C. Chiesa Fuxench

Abstract Multiple risk factors have been associated with the development of atopic dermatitis (AD). Recent advances in understanding the role of genetics in this disease have been made, with discovery of the filaggrin (FLG) gene as the most notable so far. In addition to FLG gene mutations as a risk factor for AD, a positive family history of atopic or allergic disease in either parent, has been shown to confer a greater risk of developing AD. Atopic dermatitis usually presents early in life and is thought to represent the initial-step in the *"atopic march"* which is characterized by the development of other atopic diseases later in life such as asthma, allergic rhinitis and/or rhinoconjunctivitis, food allergies and hay fever. Other comorbid diseases that have been associated with AD include increase risk of viral and bacterial skin infections, neuropsychiatric diseases such as attention-deficit hyperactivity disorders (ADHD) and autistic spectrum disorder (ASD). Patients with AD, have also been found to have worse sleep quality overall compared to patients without AD. In this chapter, we will discuss the risk factors associated with development of atopic dermatitis as well as the most commonly reported comorbidities in patients with this disease.

Keywords Atopic dermatitis • Disease background • Risk factors • Comorbidities

2.1 Genetics of Atopic Dermatitis

Recent advances in understanding the role of genetics in atopic dermatitis have been made, with discovery of the filaggrin (FLG) gene as the most notable so far [1, 2]. Identification of the FLG gene, which codes for filaggrin, an important structural component of the epidermis, as the cause of ichthyosis vulgaris resulted in a significant breakthrough in increasing our understanding of the pathogenesis of atopic

Z.C. Chiesa Fuxench, M.D., M.S.C.E. (✉)
Department of Dermatology, University of Pennsylvania Perelman School of Medicine, Philadelphia, PA, USA
e-mail: zelma.chiesafuxench@uphs.upenn.edu

E.A. Fortson et al. (eds.), *Management of Atopic Dermatitis*, Advances in Experimental Medicine and Biology 1027, DOI 10.1007/978-3-319-64804-0_2

dermatitis (AD) [3]. Filaggrin is an integral part of the Epidermal Differentiation Complex (EDC), a group of proteins responsible for maintaining skin barrier function [4]. The EDC is located on chromosome 1 and consists of a series of genes which code for: (1) proteins of the cornified envelope (i.e., *loricrin, involucrin and 'late, cornified envelope proteins'*); (2) calcium-binding proteins (*S100 proteins*); and (3) 'fused gene proteins' (i.e., *filaggrin, filaggrin-2, trichohyalin, trichohyalin-like protein, hornerin, repetin, and cornulin*) [4].

Mutations in the FLG gene have been associated with skin barrier impairment and the *"outside-in-hypothesis"* [5]. In this hypothesis, a defect in the epidermal barrier results in increased transepidermal water loss, or TEWL, which explains the associated dryness or xerosis seen in patients with AD, as well as allows greater penetration of allergens, irritants, and skin colonizing organisms that can result in infection [5–7]. Defects in skin barrier function can also result in an increased Th-2 inflammatory response with increased production of pro-inflammatory cytokines such as IL-4 and IL-13 thus perpetuating the inflammatory cycle seen in AD [6].

The FLG gene codes for profilaggrin the main component of keratohyalin granules. The profilaggrin molecule is composed of an N-terminal domain, followed by multiple filaggrin repeats with keratin-binding properties, and a C-terminal domain [3]. As keratinocytes differentiate in the epidermis, profilaggrin is cleaved into filaggrin proteins, which then aggregate in the keratin cytoskeleton to form a dense protein-lipid matrix and results in a fully differentiated epidermal barrier [8]. Filaggrin is then further degraded into a group of proteins or amino acids known as natural moisturizing factors, which have an important role in maintaining skin hydration and barrier function [8]. The main breakdown products of filaggrin are *trans*-urocanic acid and pyrrolidone-5-carboxylic acid. These organic compounds are responsible for maintaining a physiologic, acidic pH and have also been shown to have an inhibitory effect on the growth of *Staphylococcus aureus* on the skin [3, 9]. Conversion of *trans*-urocanic acid to *cis*-urocanic acid, a molecule with an action spectrum of 280–310 nm, has been suggested to have a possible photoprotective role [10, 11].

Loss-of function (LOF) mutations in the FLG gene are considered the strongest known genetic risk factor for AD and the presence of 2 homozygous mutations has been associated with more persistent disease [12, 13]. The FLG gene mutations most strongly associated with an increased risk for AD include R501x and 2282del4, both located on exon 3, with one study showing a higher risk for R501x compared to 2282del4 [14]. The prevalence of FLG gene mutations varies widely. It is estimated that approximately 20–50% of patients with AD and 8–10% of the normal population carry a FLG mutation [15, 16]. Filaggrin mutations have been more frequently described in Caucasian populations particularly those of Eastern Europe as well as various Asian populations [3]. However, although R501x and 2282del4 are frequently identified in populations of European descent, these have not been consistently observed in Asian and African populations [17–19]. While other LOF mutations in the FLG gene have been identified in Asian populations [20], these have not been observed in those of African ancestry. On the contrary, mutations in filaggrin-2 (FLG2), which is has been shown to have a similar skin barrier function as FLG, have been found to be more prevalent in AD patients of African ancestry and have also been associated with more persistent disease in this population [21, 22].

While specific mutations in the FLG gene have been well established as a risk factor for a subset of patients with AD, it has also been shown that down-regulation of filaggrin gene expression can be induced by active inflammation independent of the presence or absence of FLG gene mutations [3, 23, 24].

2.2 Familial and Environmental Risk Factors in Atopic Dermatitis

In addition to FLG gene mutations as a risk factor for atopic dermatitis, a positive family history of atopic or allergic disease in either parent has been shown to be a strong risk factor for the development of AD. It is estimated that approximately 70% of patients with AD have a positive family history for AD [25]. Children of one or two affected parents with AD are thought to have a two to threefold, or three to sixfold increased odds of developing atopic dermatitis, respectively [25–28]. Children whose mothers had atopic dermatitis are also thought to be at an increased risk for developing AD [27, 28]. One study showed having a mother with a FLG-mutation was associated with a 1.5-fold increased risk of developing AD independent from the patient's carrier status [29].

Populations at higher risk for developing AD include those with a strong family history of atopic diseases as well as the presence of FLG gene mutations in certain populations, particularly caucasians of Eastern European descent and Asian populations. There is increasing evidence to suggest that the prevalence of AD may be higher in populations who identify as black or of African ancestry compared to Caucasians [30–32]. Other factors including daycare exposure [33], level of parental education [34], socioeconomic status [35], place of residence (i.e., rural vs. urban setting) [36], smoking [37, 38], type of delivery during childbirth (i.e., vaginal vs. cesarean section) [25, 39], weight at birth [40], breast-feeding [28, 41], being overweight [42], exposure to hard water [43], pets [44–47] and/or dust mites [48], may influence the risk of developing AD, but the data is varied and inconclusive. Because the microbiota of patients with and without AD are known to be different, it has been suggested that exposure to antibiotics early in life leads to alteration in colonizing organisms, resulting in an increased risk of developing AD. Current data is insufficient to determine if early exposure to antibiotics is associated with an increased risk of developing AD [41].

2.3 The Role of Diet Atopic Dermatitis Development

The relationship between dietary intake and risk for developing atopic dermatitis is not fully understood. It is unclear if maternal dietary restriction, breastfeeding or timing of food introduction affects the risk of developing AD [25]. A systematic review of sixty studies confirmed the association between AD, food sensitization and food allergies (FA), with increased AD severity and duration of AD being more strongly associated with FA [49]. This study also found that the onset of AD usually preceded that of FA, thus suggesting a positive causal relationship [49]. Another study found evidence that dysfunction in the skin barrier as measured by increased TEWL during the neonatal period was a positive predictor for the development of FA at 2 years of age, thus supporting the role of transcutaneous sensitization in AD [50]. Care must be taken when considering strict elimination diets in these patients as there is evidence to support that avoidance may increase the likelihood of developing new, immediate, food reactions in the future [51].

2.4 Atopic Dermatitis: Comorbidities

Atopic dermatitis usually presents early in life and is thought to represent the initial-step in the *"atopic march"* which is characterized by the development of other atopic diseases later in life [52, 53]. Skin barrier defects in AD lead to the introduction of foreign antigens through the epidermis resulting in activation of the innate immune system and promotion of a Th2 inflammatory response which can lead to the development of other atopic diseases [52].

In patients with AD, the most commonly reported comorbidities include other *atopic diseases* such as asthma, allergic rhinitis and/or rhinoconjunctivitis, food allergies and hay fever [54]. The prevalence of these diseases varies by age [55]. In the case of asthma, a systematic review found the prevalence of asthma in AD varied between 20–45% [55, 56]. The prevalence of allergic rhinitis and food allergies varies between 33–45% and 13–47%, respectively. [57, 58] The occurrence of asthma, food allergies and allergic rhinitis in patients with AD can persist for several years, and in some cases resolve with increasing age [59]. The estimated prevalence of hay fever in patients with AD is approximately 30–47% [56]. Other atopic diseases that have been reported include contact dermatitis and hand dermatitis [60, 61].

Patients with AD are at an increased risk for infections, in particular skin infections with *Staphylococcus aureus*, eczema herpeticum, eczema vaccinatum, and eczema cocksackium [62]. It is estimated that *S. aureus* is present in nearly 90% of AD lesions and that MRSA colonization occurs in approximately 12% of patients with AD [62, 63]. *Streptococcus pyogenes* is also frequently identified in patients with AD [64]. Eczema herpeticum occurs as a result of herpes virus infection and is more frequently seen in patients with more severe atopic disease [65]. Eczema cocksackium is considered a newer recognized complication of AD and is oftentimes confused with eczema herpeticum [54, 66]. Eczema vaccinatum is a potentially life-threatening infection in AD which occurs as a result of vaccination with the smallpox vaccine in susceptible patients [62]. Warts and infection with molluscum contagiosum have also been reported as more prevalent in children with AD compared to children without atopic disease [67]. Other infectious diseases associated with AD include sinus infections, recurrent ear infections, strep throat, influenza, pneumonia, varicella zoster and urinary tract infections [67].

Higher rates of neuropsychiatric diseases have been reported in patients with AD including attention-deficit hyperactivity disorders (ADHD) and autistic spectrum disorder (ASD), depression, anxiety and somatization disorder [68–71]. A large population-based, longitudinal study found that children with early-onset AD had a greater risk of developing ADHD and ASD compared to children without AD. The risk was fourfold higher in those patients who also had other allergic diseases including asthma and allergic rhinitis [68].

Atopic dermatitis has also been demonstrated to have a negative impact on sleep, including decreased sleep duration and worse quality of sleep [72–74]. AD does not only impact sleep in patients but has also been shown to have a negative impact in patient's caregivers. Caregivers of patients with AD often report poorer quality of sleep, increased symptoms of insomnia and chronic sleep deprivation [75]. The mechanism of sleep disturbance in patients with AD is unclear and it is though that pruritus alone is not the sole cause [76]. Alterations in the circadian rhythm, immune dysregulation and increased TEWL are also thought to play a role [76].

Other diseases that have been reported to be more prevalent in adult patients with AD include cardiovascular disease (CVD). A study in the US adult population showed that patients with AD had higher odds of CVD, including coronary artery disease, myocardial infarction, and peripheral vascular disease [77]. Other studies have found marginal or no association between AD and CVD after adjustment for risk factors [78–80]. It is unclear if the association between AD and CVD is due to the chronic inflammatory state seen in patients with AD or if it is due to the presence of poor health behaviors (e.g., smoking, obesity) that are more prevalent in this population [38, 81].

The relationship between AD and cancer is complex [82] and remains to be clearly defined. Prior studies have shown inconsistent results and are difficult to interpret due to dissimilarities in study design, small sample sizes, and varying case definitions for AD [82–84]. Most studies failed to examine the impact of AD severity on cancer risk and did not control for confounding factors such as smoking. The risk of acute lymphoblastic leukemia, meningioma, and glioma have been shown to be lower in pediatric patients with a history of atopy [83]. [85] Legendre et al. [86] showed a slightly increased risk of lymphoma, particularly cutaneous T-cell lymphoma (CTCL), compared to an inverse or null association with solid-organ malignancies. Other studies show increased risk of non-melanoma skin cancer, however results are not consistent [83, 85, 87]. It is unclear if the increased risk for cancer seen in some studies is due to disease misclassification, persistent systemic inflammation, and/or exposure to multiple immune suppressive medications.

References

1. Palmer CN, Irvine AD, Terron-Kwiatkowski A, et al. Common loss-of-function variants of the epidermal barrier protein filaggrin are a major predisposing factor for atopic dermatitis. Nat Genet. 2006;38:441–6.
2. Fallon PG, Sasaki T, Sandilands A, et al. A homozygous frameshift mutation in the mouse Flg gene facilitates enhanced percutaneous allergen priming. Nat Genet. 2009;41:602–8.

3. Brown SJ, McLean WH. One remarkable molecule: filaggrin. J Invest Dermatol. 2012;132:751–62.
4. Kypriotou M, Huber M, Hohl D. The human epidermal differentiation complex: cornified envelope precursors, S100 proteins and the 'fused genes' family. Exp Dermatol. 2012;21:643–9.
5. Wang D, Beck LA. Immunologic targets in atopic dermatitis and emerging therapies: an update. Am J Clin Dermatol. 2016;17:425–43.
6. Elias PM, Steinhoff M. "outside-to-inside" (and now back to "outside") pathogenic mechanisms in atopic dermatitis. J Invest Dermatol. 2008;128:1067–70.
7. Proksch E, Folster-Holst R, Jensen JM. Skin barrier function, epidermal proliferation and differentiation in eczema. J Dermatol Sci. 2006;43:159–69.
8. McLean WH. Filaggrin failure—from ichthyosis vulgaris to atopic eczema and beyond. Br J Dermatol. 2016;175(Suppl 2):4–7.
9. Miajlovic H, Fallon PG, Irvine AD, Foster TJ. Effect of filaggrin breakdown products on growth of and protein expression by Staphylococcus aureus. J Allergy Clin Immunol. 2010;126:1184–1190.e3.
10. McLoone P, Simics E, Barton A, Norval M, Gibbs NK. An action spectrum for the production of cis-urocanic acid in human skin in vivo. J Invest Dermatol. 2005;124:1071–4.
11. Barresi C, Stremnitzer C, Mlitz V, et al. Increased sensitivity of histidinemic mice to UVB radiation suggests a crucial role of endogenous urocanic acid in photoprotection. J Invest Dermatol. 2011;131:188–94.
12. Irvine AD, McLean WH. Breaking the (un)sound barrier: filaggrin is a major gene for atopic dermatitis. J Invest Dermatol. 2006;126:1200–2.
13. Margolis DJ, Apter AJ, Gupta J, et al. The persistence of atopic dermatitis and filaggrin (FLG) mutations in a US longitudinal cohort. J Allergy Clin Immunol. 2012;130:912–7.
14. Rodriguez E, Baurecht H, Herberich E, et al. Meta-analysis of filaggrin polymorphisms in eczema and asthma: robust risk factors in atopic disease. J Allergy Clin Immunol. 2009;123:1361–1370.e7.
15. Visser MJ, Landeck L, Campbell LE, et al. Impact of atopic dermatitis and loss-of-function mutations in the filaggrin gene on the development of occupational irritant contact dermatitis. Br J Dermatol. 2013;168:326–32.
16. O'Regan GM, Irvine AD. The role of filaggrin in the atopic diathesis. Clin Exp Allergy. 2010;40:965–72.
17. Winge MC, Bilcha KD, Lieden A, et al. Novel filaggrin mutation but no other loss-of-function variants found in Ethiopian patients with atopic dermatitis. Br J Dermatol. 2011;165:1074–80.
18. Margolis DJ, Gupta J, Apter AJ, et al. Exome sequencing of filaggrin and related genes in African-American children with atopic dermatitis. J Invest Dermatol. 2014;134:2272–4.
19. Sun LD, Xiao FL, Li Y, et al. Genome-wide association study identifies two new susceptibility loci for atopic dermatitis in the Chinese Han population. Nat Genet. 2011;43:690–4.
20. Hsu CK, Akiyama M, Nemoto-Hasebe I, et al. Analysis of Taiwanese ichthyosis vulgaris families further demonstrates differences in FLG mutations between European and Asian populations. Br J Dermatol. 2009;161:448–51.
21. Makino T, Mizawa M, Yamakoshi T, Takaishi M, Shimizu T. Expression of filaggrin-2 protein in the epidermis of human skin diseases: a comparative analysis with filaggrin. Biochem Biophys Res Commun. 2014;449:100–6.
22. Margolis DJ, Gupta J, Apter AJ, et al. Filaggrin-2 variation is associated with more persistent atopic dermatitis in African American subjects. J Allergy Clin Immunol. 2014;133:784–9.
23. Pellerin L, Henry J, Hsu CY, et al. Defects of filaggrin-like proteins in both lesional and nonlesional atopic skin. J Allergy Clin Immunol. 2013;131:1094–102.
24. Thawer-Esmail F, Jakasa I, Todd G, et al. South African amaXhosa patients with atopic dermatitis have decreased levels of filaggrin breakdown products but no loss-of-function mutations in filaggrin. J Allergy Clin Immunol. 2014;133:280–282.e2.
25. Eichenfield LF, Tom WL, Chamlin SL, et al. Guidelines of care for the management of atopic dermatitis: section 1. Diagnosis and assessment of atopic dermatitis. J Am Acad Dermatol. 2014;70:338–51.

26. Schmitz R, Atzpodien K, Schlaud M. Prevalence and risk factors of atopic diseases in German children and adolescents. Pediatr Allergy Immunol. 2012;23:716–23.
27. Lee YL, Li CW, Sung FC, Yu HS, Sheu HM, Guo YL. Environmental factors, parental atopy and atopic eczema in primary-school children: a cross-sectional study in Taiwan. Br J Dermatol. 2007;157:1217–24.
28. Purvis DJ, Thompson JM, Clark PM, et al. Risk factors for atopic dermatitis in New Zealand children at 3.5 years of age. Br J Dermatol. 2005;152:742–9.
29. Esparza-Gordillo J, Matanovic A, Marenholz I, et al. Maternal filaggrin mutations increase the risk of atopic dermatitis in children: an effect independent of mutation inheritance. PLoS Genet. 2015;11:e1005076.
30. Shaw TE, Currie GP, Koudelka CW, Simpson EL. Eczema prevalence in the United States: data from the 2003 National Survey of Children's health. J Invest Dermatol. 2011;131:67–73.
31. Williams HC, Pembroke AC, Forsdyke H, Boodoo G, Hay RJ, Burney PG. London-born black Caribbean children are at increased risk of atopic dermatitis. J Am Acad Dermatol. 1995;32:212–7.
32. Wegienka G, Havstad S, Joseph CL, et al. Racial disparities in allergic outcomes in African Americans emerge as early as age 2 years. Clin Exp Allergy. 2012;42:909–17.
33. de Meer G, Janssen NA, Brunekreef B. Early childhood environment related to microbial exposure and the occurrence of atopic disease at school age. Allergy. 2005;60:619–25.
34. Wen HJ, Chen PC, Chiang TL, Lin SJ, Chuang YL, Guo YL. Predicting risk for early infantile atopic dermatitis by hereditary and environmental factors. Br J Dermatol. 2009;161:1166–72.
35. Uphoff E, Cabieses B, Pinart M, Valdes M, Anto JM, Wright J. A systematic review of socio-economic position in relation to asthma and allergic diseases. Eur Respir J. 2015;46:364–74.
36. Xu F, Yan S, Zheng Q, et al. Residential risk factors for atopic dermatitis in 3- to 6-year old children: a cross-sectional study in shanghai, China. Int J Environ Res Public Health. 2016;13(6):537.
37. Bohme M, Kull I, Bergstrom A, et al. Parental smoking increases the risk for eczema with sensitization in 4-year-old children. J Allergy Clin Immunol. 2010;125:941–3.
38. Kantor R, Kim A, Thyssen JP, Silverberg JI. Association of atopic dermatitis with smoking: a systematic review and meta-analysis. J Am Acad Dermatol. 2016;75:1119–1125.e1.
39. Papathoma E, Triga M, Fouzas S, Dimitriou G. Cesarean section delivery and development of food allergy and atopic dermatitis in early childhood. Pediatr Allergy Immunol. 2016;27:419–24.
40. Panduru M, Salavastru CM, Panduru NM, Tiplica GS. Birth weight and atopic dermatitis: systematic review and meta-analyis. Acta Dermatovenerol Croat. 2014;22:91–6.
41. Taylor-Robinson DC, Williams H, Pearce A, Law C, Hope S. Do early-life exposures explain why more advantaged children get eczema? Findings from the U.K. millennium cohort study. Br J Dermatol. 2016;174:569–78.
42. Sybilski AJ, Raciborski F, Lipiec A, et al. Obesity—a risk factor for asthma, but not for atopic dermatitis, allergic rhinitis and sensitization. Public Health Nutr. 2015;18:530–6.
43. Perkin MR, Craven J, Logan K, et al. Association between domestic water hardness, chlorine, and atopic dermatitis risk in early life: a population-based cross-sectional study. J Allergy Clin Immunol. 2016;138:509–16.
44. Pelucchi C, Galeone C, Bach JF, La Vecchia C, Chatenoud L. Pet exposure and risk of atopic dermatitis at the pediatric age: a meta-analysis of birth cohort studies. J Allergy Clin Immunol. 2013;132:616–622.e7.
45. Zirngibl A, Franke K, Gehring U, et al. Exposure to pets and atopic dermatitis during the first two years of life. A cohort study. Pediatr Allergy Immunol. 2002;13:394–401.
46. Epstein TG, Bernstein DI, Levin L, et al. Opposing effects of cat and dog ownership and allergic sensitization on eczema in an atopic birth cohort. J Pediatr. 2011;158:265–271.e5.
47. Schuttelaar ML, Kerkhof M, Jonkman MF, et al. Filaggrin mutations in the onset of eczema, sensitization, asthma, hay fever and the interaction with cat exposure. Allergy. 2009;64:1758–65.
48. Ricci G, Patrizi A, Bellini F, Medri M. Use of textiles in atopic dermatitis: care of atopic dermatitis. Curr Probl Dermatol. 2006;33:127–43.

49. Tsakok T, Marrs T, Mohsin M, et al. Does atopic dermatitis cause food allergy? A systematic review. J Allergy Clin Immunol. 2016;137:1071–8.
50. Kelleher MM, Dunn-Galvin A, Gray C, et al. Skin barrier impairment at birth predicts food allergy at 2 years of age. J Allergy Clin Immunol. 2016;137:1111–1116.e8.
51. Chang A, Robison R, Cai M, Singh AM. Natural history of food-triggered atopic dermatitis and development of immediate reactions in children. J Allergy Clinical Immunol Pract. 2016;4:229–236.e1.
52. Egawa G, Kabashima K. Multifactorial skin barrier deficiency and atopic dermatitis: essential topics to prevent the atopic march. J Allergy Clin Immunol. 2016;138:350–358.e1.
53. Spergel JM, Paller AS. Atopic dermatitis and the atopic march. J Allergy Clin Immunol. 2003;112:S118–27.
54. Brunner PM, Silverberg JI, Guttman-Yassky E, et al. Increasing comorbidities suggest that atopic dermatitis is a systemic disorder. J Invest Dermatol. 2017;137:18–25.
55. van der Hulst AE, Klip H, Brand PL. Risk of developing asthma in young children with atopic eczema: a systematic review. J Allergy Clin Immunol. 2007;120:565–9.
56. Silverberg JI, Simpson EL. Association between severe eczema in children and multiple comorbid conditions and increased healthcare utilization. Pediatr Allergy Immunol. 2013;24:476–86.
57. Gustafsson D, Sjoberg O, Foucard T. Development of allergies and asthma in infants and young children with atopic dermatitis—a prospective follow-up to 7 years of age. Allergy. 2000;55:240–5.
58. Eigenmann PA, Sicherer SH, Borkowski TA, Cohen BA, Sampson HA. Prevalence of IgE-mediated food allergy among children with atopic dermatitis. Pediatrics. 1998;101:E8.
59. Spergel JM. Epidemiology of atopic dermatitis and atopic march in children. Immunol Allergy Clin North Am. 2010;30:269–80.
60. Gittler JK, Krueger JG, Guttman-Yassky E. Atopic dermatitis results in intrinsic barrier and immune abnormalities: implications for contact dermatitis. J Allergy Clin Immunol. 2013;131:300–13.
61. Thyssen JP, McFadden JP, Kimber I. The multiple factors affecting the association between atopic dermatitis and contact sensitization. Allergy. 2014;69:28–36.
62. Ong PY, Leung DY. Bacterial and viral infections in atopic dermatitis: a comprehensive review. Clin Rev Allergy Immunol. 2016;51:329–37.
63. Leyden JJ, Marples RR, Kligman AM. Staphylococcus Aureus in the lesions of atopic dermatitis. Br J Dermatol. 1974;90:525–30.
64. Hayakawa K, Hirahara K, Fukuda T, Okazaki M, Shiohara T. Risk factors for severe impetiginized atopic dermatitis in Japan and assessment of its microbiological features. Clin Exp Dermatol. 2009;34:e63–5.
65. Beck LA, Boguniewicz M, Hata T, et al. Phenotype of atopic dermatitis subjects with a history of eczema herpeticum. J Allergy Clin Immunol. 2009;124:260–269.e7. 9.e1–7
66. Mathes EF, Oza V, Frieden IJ, et al. "eczema coxsackium" and unusual cutaneous findings in an enterovirus outbreak. Pediatrics. 2013;132:e149–57.
67. Silverberg JI, Silverberg NB. Childhood atopic dermatitis and warts are associated with increased risk of infection: a US population-based study. J Allergy Clin Immunol. 2014;133:1041–7.
68. Lee CY, Chen MH, Jeng MJ, et al. Longitudinal association between early atopic dermatitis and subsequent attention-deficit or autistic disorder: a population-based case-control study. Medicine. 2016;95:e5005.
69. Kim SH, Hur J, Jang JY, et al. Psychological distress in young adult males with atopic dermatitis: a cross-sectional study. Medicine. 2015;94:e949.
70. Liao TC, Lien YT, Wang S, Huang SL, Chen CY. Comorbidity of atopic disorders with autism spectrum disorder and attention deficit/hyperactivity disorder. J Pediatr. 2016;171:248–55.
71. Strom MA, Fishbein AB, Paller AS, Silverberg JI. Association between atopic dermatitis and attention deficit hyperactivity disorder in U.S. children and adults. Br J Dermatol. 2016;175:920–9.

72. Yu SH, Attarian H, Zee P, Silverberg JI. Burden of sleep and fatigue in US adults with atopic dermatitis. Dermatitis. 2016;27:50–8.
73. Choi JH, Nam GE, Kim DH, Lee JY, Han KD, Cho JH. Association between sleep duration and the prevalence of atopic dermatitis and asthma in young adults. Asian Pacific J Allergy Immunol. 2016;34:265. doi:10.12932/AP0772.
74. Kong TS, Han TY, Lee JH, Son SJ. Correlation between severity of atopic dermatitis and sleep quality in children and adults. Ann Dermatol. 2016;28:321–6.
75. Meltzer LJ, Booster GD. Sleep disturbance in caregivers of children with respiratory and atopic disease. J Pediatr Psychol. 2016;41:643–50.
76. Chang YS, Chiang BL. Mechanism of sleep disturbance in children with atopic dermatitis and the role of the circadian rhythm and melatonin. Int J Mol Sci. 2016;17:462.
77. Silverberg JI. Association between adult atopic dermatitis, cardiovascular disease, and increased heart attacks in three population-based studies. Allergy. 2015;70:1300–8.
78. Drucker AM, Li WQ, Cho E, et al. Atopic dermatitis is not independently associated with nonfatal myocardial infarction or stroke among US women. Allergy. 2016;71:1496–500.
79. Standl M, Tesch F, Baurecht H, et al. Association of atopic dermatitis with cardiovascular risk factors and diseases. J Invest Dermatol. 2017;137:1074–81.
80. Egeberg A, Andersen YM, Gislason GH, Skov L, Thyssen JP. Prevalence of comorbidity and associated risk factors in adults with atopic dermatitis. Allergy. 2017;72(5):783–91.
81. Silverberg JI, Becker L, Kwasny M, Menter A, Cordoro KM, Paller AS. Central obesity and high blood pressure in pediatric patients with atopic dermatitis. JAMA Dermatol. 2015;151:144–52.
82. Wang H, Rothenbacher D, Low M, Stegmaier C, Brenner H, Diepgen TL. Atopic diseases, immunoglobulin E and risk of cancer of the prostate, breast, lung and colorectum. Int J Cancer. 2006;119:695–701.
83. Wang H, Diepgen TL. Is atopy a protective or a risk factor for cancer? A review of epidemiological studies. Allergy. 2005;60:1098–111.
84. Wang H, Diepgen TL. Atopic dermatitis and cancer risk. Br J Dermatol. 2006;154:205–10.
85. Deckert S, Kopkow C, Schmitt J. Nonallergic comorbidities of atopic eczema: an overview of systematic reviews. Allergy. 2014;69:37–45.
86. Legendre L, Barnetche T, Mazereeuw-Hautier J, Meyer N, Murrell D, Paul C. Risk of lymphoma in patients with atopic dermatitis and the role of topical treatment: a systematic review and meta-analysis. J Am Acad Dermatol. 2015;72:992–1002.
87. Margolis DJ, Abuabara K, Hoffstad OJ, Wan J, Raimondo D, Bilker WB. Association between malignancy and topical use of pimecrolimus. JAMA Dermatol. 2015;151:594–9.

Chapter 3
Atopic Dermatitis: Pathophysiology

W. David Boothe, James A. Tarbox, and Michelle B. Tarbox

Abstract The pathophysiology of atopic dermatitis is complex and multifactorial, involving elements of barrier dysfunction, alterations in cell mediated immune responses, IgE mediated hypersensitivity, and environmental factors. Loss of function mutations in filaggrin have been implicated in severe atopic dermatitis due to a potential increase in trans-epidermal water loss, pH alterations, and dehydration. Other genetic changes have also been identified which may alter the skin's barrier function, resulting in an atopic dermatitis phenotype. The imbalance of Th2 to Th1 cytokines observed in atopic dermatitis can create alterations in the cell mediated immune responses and can promote IgE mediated hypersensitivity, both of which appear to play a role in the development of atopic dermatitis. One must additionally take into consideration the role of the environment on the causation of atopic dermatitis and the impact of chemicals such as airborne formaldehyde, harsh detergents, fragrances, and preservatives. Use of harsh alkaline detergents in skin care products may also unfavorably alter the skin's pH causing downstream changes in enzyme activity and triggering inflammation. Environmental pollutants can trigger responses from both the innate and adaptive immune pathways. This chapter will discuss the multifaceted etiology of atopic dermatitis which will help us to elucidate potential therapeutic targets. We will also review existing treatment options and their interaction with the complex inflammatory and molecular triggers of atopic dermatitis.

Keywords Atopic dermatitis • Pathophysiology • Barrier • Hypersensitivity • Environment

---

W. David Boothe, M.D. • M.B. Tarbox, M.D. (✉)
Department of Dermatology, Texas Tech University Health Sciences Center, Lubbock, TX, USA
e-mail: michelle.tarbox@ttuhsc.edu

J.A. Tarbox, M.D.
Department of Internal Medicine, Texas Tech University Health Sciences Center, Lubbock, TX, USA

E.A. Fortson et al. (eds.), *Management of Atopic Dermatitis*, Advances in Experimental Medicine and Biology 1027, DOI 10.1007/978-3-319-64804-0_3

3.1 Introduction

The exact etiology of atopic dermatitis (AD) is still under investigation. Both genetic and environmental factors have been implicated as risk factors for the development of AD and the pathogenesis of the disease is clearly multifactorial involving immunologic processes including type 1 IgE dysfunction, defects in cell-mediated immune responses, and changes related to barrier dysfunction. Below the contributing factors to the etiology of AD will be discussed in detail including intrinsic and extrinsic causes of barrier dysfunction and the role of inflammatory cascade in AD.

3.2 Skin Barrier Dysfunction in Atopic Dermatitis

One of the main pathophysiologic theories regarding atopic dermatitis involves dysfunction of the natural skin barrier. A foundational concept in the current understanding of AD is the premise that barrier abnormalities are a driver of AD rather than a consequence. Proof for such a theory broadly comes from the fact that clinically uninvolved skin in patients suffering from AD, or skin that has been clear of inflammation for a short period of time, shows continuing barrier dysfunction [1]. Intrinsic causes of such dysfunction are one major component of skin barrier issues. It is important to discuss the genetic, cell mediated, and other processes implicated in skin barrier dysfunction to fully understand the pathogenesis of AD.

The foundation of a normally functioning skin barrier begins with the stratum corneum (SC), a tissue layer consisting of anucleate corneocytes supported in a lamellar matrix. The basic functions of the SC include acting as a permeable barrier that prevents transcutaneous evaporative water loss and provides an antimicrobial barrier, as well as encouraging colonization by nonpathogenic bacteria flora [2]. Lamellar sheets, a supporting matrix in the SC, are composed of high concentrations of ceramides, cholesterol, and free fatty acids. These extra cellular hydrophobic molecules are a major component of water loss prevention in the skin. The precursors of the hydrophobic matrix are delivered by lamellar bodies in the form of phospholipids, cholesterol sulfates, and other molecules. Likewise, enzymes required for lamellar matrix synthesis are also carried by lamellar bodies [3]. The interaction between precursors and enzymes create molecules such as ceramides that are necessary for the above components to self-organize into the matrix. Proteases and antimicrobial particles are simultaneously generated by lamellar bodies as well. Several antimicrobial molecules including human β-defensin 2 and the carboxyterminal cathelicidin peptide are delivered to the SC intercellular matrix through lamellar body excretions [4, 5].

3.3 Genetics and Skin Barrier Dysfunction in Atopic Dermatitis

Genetics play a significant role in the proper functioning of the skin barrier. Many genetic mutations have been studied in relation to atopic dermatitis; however, the filaggrin (FLG) mutation currently stands out as a primary driver of atopic change [3, 6, 7]. Multiple FLG mutations are possible and have been discovered through detailed research. Most predominantly, the R501X and 2282del4 FLG mutations have been found to lead to complete loss of FLG products [7]. Up to 60% of Europeans affected with atopic dermatitis show an FLG mutation of some kind [3]. Finding decreased FLG expression, and thus low F type keratohyalin, can result in a paucity of keratohyalin granules [8]. This paucity of keratohyalin granules causes disruption of the stratum granulosum. Such a disruption has many effects, and greatly influences the differentiation and growth of a normal SC. The FLG pre-product, pro-FLG, is a highly cationic phospho-protein that is composed of a large amount of hydrophobic amino acids [9]. During normal processing from pro-FLG to FLG, these amino acids are removed from the protein as corneocytes mature and are then deaminated into polycarboxylic acids also known as natural moisturizing factors (NMF). Recent studies have suggested that an increase of pro-FLG could interfere with lamellar body secretions [9]. Similarly, the disruption of the pro-FLG to FLG processing that normally occurs during the transition from stratum granulosum to SC, leads to the loss of all byproducts including natural moisturizing factors (NMF). This disruption decreases the osmotic draw, due to lower solutes creating pull, which normally hydrates corneocytes. An immediate effect from such a decrease is the creation of a large water gradient across the SC layer which is likely to increase cutaneous water loss from normal levels [3]. The loss of NMFs also affects the skin biome. NMFs have been shown to favor adhesion of non-pathogenic bacteria preventing the aggregation of *S. aureus* often preventing infections [10].

The increase in antigen presentation found due to atopic dermatitis can also be explained by FLG mutation changes. Lack of downstream acid metabolites, such as trans-urocanic acid, lead to a pH increase found in the SC [3] resulting in a less acidic surface pH. The normal acidic pH of the SC serves many roles in maintaining a healthy skin barrier, including discouraging the growth of pathogenic bacteria, encouraging the growth of normal skin flora, and maintaining skin surface serine proteases in an inactive state. The less acidic pH produced in AD allows for these serine proteases to become activated leading to further barrier dysfunction through the degradation of corneodesmosomes and enzymes important in lipid metabolism [11].

In addition to FLG mutations, there are other genetic pathways implicated in the pathogenesis of atopic dermatitis. An inherited loss of function mutation in the *SPINK5* gene encoding the serine peptidase inhibitor lymphoepithelial Kazal-type trypsin inhibitor (LEKTI), results in a cluster of clinical symptoms known as Netherton Syndrome which prominently features relatively severe AD, helping to create a case for the role of serine protease imbalance in the pathogenesis of AD [12, 13]. This syndrome involves unrestricted serine protease mediated degradation of lipid processing enzymes and corneodesmosome proteins due to loss of function of the typical inhibitor of these enzymes. Major thinning of the SC follows the degradation of these vital components of the epidermal barrier leading to the classic findings of AD along with mucosal thinning. While not all genetic studies agree on the subject, animal experiments conducted with an increase of serine protease caused corneodesmosome degradation and failure of ceramide generation in AD models. It has been suggested that serine protease elevations may provoke a secondary mechanism of dysfunction in plasminogen activating type 2 receptor (PAR2). This type of receptor activation down regulates lamellar body secretions causing a further down regulation of SC lipid production. These results correlate with the decrease of extracellular products from lamellar bodies seen in AD.

3.4 Abnormal Protein and Enzyme Processing in Atopic Dermatitis

Another possible cause for direct barrier failure comes from abnormal protein and enzyme processing when optimal SC characteristics are disrupted. Changes in skin pH, calcium gradient, and other factors can all alter the expression of proteins and enzymes necessary for proper barrier function [10]. Disruption of lamellar bodies in atopic skin can result in deficits of acids, lipids, and enzymes needed for normal barrier function [10]. Structural proteins such as FLG, loricrin, and involucrin all need proper functioning skin based enzymes to fully form. FLG, for instance, is specifically deaminated by peptidyl deiminase. Normally, FLG is then broken down into smaller peptides and free amino acids finally creating natural moisturizing factors (NMF) such as carboxylic acid or urocanic acid at the end of the process [14]. These factors help to avoid gaps between corneocytes thus improving the integrity of the SC.

For many years, skin has been known to have a naturally occurring acidic pH that helps in proper barrier function. The average surface pH of skin in a healthy male is between 5.4 and 5.9 [15]. Newer studies have shown many endogenous paths that help to maintain such an acidic state. Byproducts of free fatty acid synthesis, the sodium-proton exchange, and keratinization pathways have all been found as sources of skin acidity [16, 17]. This acidic pH normally allows favorable non-pathogenic bacteria to adhere to skin over invasive bacteria. Disruption of the skin's natural pH allows infections to take hold in an easier fashion opening up the possibility for secondary infections.

Serine proteases, such as KLK5 or KLK7, have a pH optimum near the neutral range. pH changes causing skin acidity to near 7 can increase the activity of these enzymes by up to 50% in some cases [18]. Since KLK5 and KLK7 are involved in desquamation, their over activation can thin the skin barrier. Some beneficial enzymes require an acidic environment for optimal function; Beta-glucocerebrosidase and sphingomyelinase normally generate lipids. Their preferred pH levels are much nearer the skin's normal pH. Taken in combination, the normal range of skin's pH is very important for proper barrier function. It has been shown in studies that atopic dermatitis patients have significantly elevated skin pH levels [19]. This change in skin pH level is also found in uninvolved skin and is found, to a greater extent, when active lesions are present [1]. Epidermal abnormalities can be easily noticed when blocking secretory phospholipase A2 or the sodium-proton exchanger. Delay in epidermal barrier rejuvenation is also noticed when the skin's pH is increased by these mechanisms [20].

The calcium gradient is another important component of epidermal homeostasis that is relevant. This gradient is important in maintaining proper cell differentiation, and can be disrupted easily with a simple tape striping test [21]. In normal function, skin barrier repair is initiated by the secretion of lamellar bodies and thus the delivery of their products. The loss of a normal calcium gradient stops this process, by stopping the proper creation of lamellar bodies. Interestingly, this problem can be counteracted by pH changes in a normal individual [10].

3.5 Tight Junction Dysfunction in Atopic Dermatitis

Impaired tight junction function in atopic dermatitis is another mechanism supporting an "outside in" hypothesis of intrinsic barrier dysfunction. Tight junction dysfunction in the stratum granulosum leads to improper barrier function in the SC. Normally, tight junctions mediate one type of cell-cell adhesion. These junctions are considered to be a network of strands that provide a primary barrier to diffusion of solutes in-between cells. Each strand is comprised of trans-membrane proteins, occludins and claudins [22]. These transmembrane proteins, along with zonula occludens form a cytosolic structure and regulate the assembly of tight junctions. The SC, the major external barrier of the body, is backed by these tight junctions found in the granular cell layer. Infiltration of pathogens into the epidermis immediately up regulates the tight junction function via toll-like receptor signaling indicating tight junctions are a fundamental part of the innate immune system in preventing further invasion [23]. From this relationship, it would seem likely that the junctions also help maintain barrier homeostasis. Indeed, one study exposed skin with damaged tight junctions to *Clostridium perfringens* enterotoxin and identified a pro-filaggrin processing issue that greatly affected the skin barrier [24]. Likewise, the same effects where seen in claudin-1 knockout mice. It follows that tight junctions play a major role in the function and formation of the SC and that abnormal claudin-1 function in atopic dermatitis can contribute to the dysfunction of the SC barrier. Studies have shown, through western blot analysis, that atopic dermatitis skin has lower amounts of claudin-1 compared to normal skin, supporting the tight junction hypothesis [23]. ZO-1 protein found in zonula occludens was also found to be abnormally low in skin affected with atopic dermatitis.

The tight junction failure may also be related to immunological abnormalities commonly found in atopic dermatitis. It is well known that Th2 and Th17 cells are implicated in the pathogenesis of AD. This principle inspired studies designed to assess the effects of Th2 and Th17 cytokines, IL-4, IL-17, IL-22, and tumor necrosis factor alpha, on the tight junctions. These studies showed that IL-17 in particular could affect the skin in doses as low as 1 ng/mL [23]. In skin model specimens exposed to 10 and 100 ng/mL of IL-17, tracers reached upper granular layers in an unrestricted fashion in areas of tight junctions. The other cytokines appeared to have little effect on tracer diffusion, thus tracers did not reach the granular layers. Consequently, it was decided that IL-17 attenuated the tight junction barrier in the skin models. Further investigation showed that claudin-1 and claudin-4, key components of tight junctions, where degraded in a dose dependent manner when exposed to IL-17 [23]. Impairment of tight junctions leads to disruption of the SC and also a disruption of the FLG processing. More investigation into IL-17 showed an effect on the processing of FLG itself. Skin models treated with 100 ng/mL of IL-17 showed thickening of the SC, but all FLG granules had disappeared. Epidermal thickness was also reduced in treatment with IL-17. Oddly, the overall signal of FLG was increased by IL-17, therefore; it is theorized that degradation of FLG to amino acids may be what is impaired by the IL-17. FLG monomers were greatly increased, but the amino acids extracted where decreased in the SC with further research supporting the theory of breakdown impairment.

3.6 Antimicrobial Barrier Dysfunction in Atopic Dermatitis

A less physical but equally important barrier that is disrupted in atopic dermatitis is the antimicrobial barrier. The antimicrobial effect of the epidermal barrier and the physical characteristics of the barrier are directly linked; therefore, the disruption of the physical barrier causes water egress and allows for ingress of infection. This commonly leads to colonization of the skin by *S. aureus*. Such colonization of the skin can lead to AD exacerbation due to increased IgE production as well as increasing IgE targeted specially at *S. aureus* toxins [25, 26]. The disruption of the physical skin barrier can lead to increased infection rates that can further disrupt both the antimicrobial function of the skin and the skin's physical barrier. Prevention of additional infections is also compromised due to the increase of SC pH along with the loss of free fatty acids, ceramide metabolites, and other normally functioning molecules that all have antimicrobial effects. Surface proteins that exist on *S. aureus* itself can also down regulate free fatty acid production [27]. Barrier function can also be damaged by Th2 mediated down regulation of several cyclic AMP processes. Human cathelicidin product, cathelicidin, and human β -defensins 2 and 3 are all down regulated in the Th2 dominated environment found in AD. Several of these molecules are normally active against *S. aureus* and their down regulation leads to easier infection of the skin from the resulting barrier disruption. Likewise, cathelicidin is directly involved in extra cutaneous epithelia integrity and its decrease disrupts the skin barrier.

3.7 Environmental Factors of Skin Barrier Dysfunction

Environmental factors may also play a meaningful part in the intrinsic failure of the skin barrier. Prolonged exposure to reduced environmental humidity accelerates transepidermal water loss (TEWL) in atopic dermatitis, and amplifies the barrier defects allowing more cytokine signaling of inflammatory molecules [3, 28]. Outside psychological stress can also cause the skin barrier issues commonly seen in atopic dermatitis [29, 30]. Stress induced changes in glucocorticoids can inhibit the synthesis of ceramides, cholesterols, and free fatty acids normally found in healthy skin. This inhibition of molecules disrupts the hydrophobic barrier allowing even more water loss from the skin worsening AD and other inflammatory skin conditions.

3.8 External Factors in Atopic Dermatitis Development

External factors and stimuli are also major components in the development of AD. A number of stimuli have been studied and shown to increase the risk of AD or atopic dermatitis like symptoms due to exposure. One external factor recognized as the molecule necessary for base survival and directly related to the development of AD is water. Water hardness, which is the amount of calcium carbonate ($CaCO_3$) dissolved in water, and water chlorine concentration have both been shown to have a correlation with AD [31]. One study conducted in the United Kingdom explored the effects of both $CaCO_3$ and chlorine in water in 317 infants diagnosed with atopic dermatitis. In this study, atopic dermatitis was more common in the subgroup of infants exposed to elevated $CaCO_3$ and chlorine when compared to the baseline hard water and chlorine infant groups [31]. Estimations of TEWL where increased in FLG mutation positive groups that were also exposed to high amounts of $CaCO_3$ in their water. This positive association was not found in children without the FLG mutations. The final findings of the study led the authors to conclude that high levels of water hardness lead to a statistically significant increase of visible instances of AD in the infants studied. Exposure to the chlorine in water suggested an increased instance of visible atopic dermatitis, but it missed the threshold necessary to be considered significant by the study's standards [31]. A proposed influence on gene expression with $CaCO_3$ levels was discussed but not confirmed.

Other studies have looked at the effect of common industrial pollutants as an external factor related to the health of skin both with and without AD. One study in particular examined airborne formaldehyde's effect on skin. Two groups of children, one with AD and one without, were exposed to either a placebo or aerosolized formaldehyde [32]. Large increases in trans-epidermal water loss were noticed in both groups exposed to formaldehyde, with the effects having a greater magnitude in AD sufferers. The AD groups also demonstrated changes in skin pH towards a neutral pH. The possible effects of such a change have been discussed above. Similar studies have shown that substances such as carbon monoxide, nitrogen dioxide, benzene, toluene, and volatile organics have important effects on skin health; however the study focusing on formaldehyde was the first to confirm a direct link between worsening AD and airborne exposure to such chemicals [32]. Several mechanisms have been proposed to explain the relationship between airborne chemicals and skin health, but the exact answer remains under study. The induction of cell death, increased expression of IL-4 and other Th2 cytokines, or increased mRNA expression leading to an increase in pro-inflammatory cytokines have all been suggested as possible mechanisms [32]. In a mouse model, formaldehyde solution increased expression of IL-4, IL-13, and IFN-γ. The effect of environmental pollution in skin health may explain some disparities in prevalence of AD in children raised in urban environments and will likely present a meaningful area of research in the future.

An increase in air pollutants has been associated with a rise in allergic type diseases in general and some epidemiologic studies suggested that this also holds true specifically for AD [33]. These air pollutants may directly modify the immune response and increase risk of atopic disease. Studies have shown a correlation between the expression of atopic dermatitis and the proximity of their place of residence with respect to major road ways [33, 34]. Pollutants of all kinds, it seems, may be responsible for either causing or worsening atopic dermatitis. In studies it can be shown that eczema symptoms were significantly associated with the presence of benzene, Particulate Matter 10 (PM10), nitrogen oxide compounds, and carbon monoxide. Benzene and its metabolites in particular have been shown to actually affect the immunologic cascade [35]. Mast cells, basophils, and a combination of T-cells and macrophages where all implicated, leading to increases in atopic dermatitis symptoms. One study of 3 year-old children showed exposure to benzene and other chemicals increased numbers of IL-4 producing CD3+ T cells possibly providing a mechanism for the type 2 allergic response leading to AD [36]. German studies have shown that simple activities such as painting or obtaining new furniture in the first year of a child's life are associated with the development of AD.

Prenatal and childhood exposure to environmental stimuli has also been linked to AD. For example, exposure to environmental tobacco smoke is thought to induce a Th2 dominant state after birth [37]. This change to a Th2 dominant state increases the chances of developing AD. Contact allergens may also exacerbate AD and increase the chances of its development. More than 3700 compounds have been identified as possible contact allergens in the environment [38]. Metals such as nickel, cobalt, and chromium are considered very common sources of hypersensitivity reactions that may mimic AD [39]. Stimulation of skin with nickel and other metals leads to a specific pattern of cytokine secretion that involves both Th1- and Th2-type cytokines [40, 41]. This release of immune factors is very similar to the cytokines found in cases of AD; based on a blood analysis, IFN-γ and IL-5 seem to play an important role in metal exposure disease activation [42].

3.9 The Role of Personal Care Products and Food in the Development of Atopic Dermatitis

Other common things encountered in daily life can also contain a myriad of possible skin barrier disruptors. Personal care products very often have fragrances and other compounds that may cause an allergic reaction. Likewise, preservatives found in everything from nail polishes to certain foods may be implicated in the atopic march and may influence the development of AD. The use of soap has greatly increased across the industrialized world since 1981 starting from 76 million and soaring to 453 million pounds in more recent years [10]. The use of soap products is important because the use of soaps on skin, particularly alkaline soaps, has been shown to significantly increase the pH of skin while simultaneously decreasing the skin's fat content [43]. Similarly concerning, the use of soap caused thinning of the SC in both normal and non-lesion atopic skin. Both of the change in the skin's pH and the thinning of the SC can cause or worsen atopic dermatitis. Detergent use has been shown to both increase the release of cytokines and change the release of degradative enzymes [44, 45]. It is likely that the PAR2 pathway in skin, which is involved in itch and is regulated by pH dependent serine proteases, responds to soap and detergent use [10, 46]. Such an increase in usage may, by itself, contribute to the pathogenesis of AD.

Ingredients in cosmetics and food are often implicated in the atopic pathway. Methyldibromo-glutaronitrile, a commonly used preservative in cosmetics and other chemicals commonly used in toiletries, cosmetics, and nail polishes have a clear association with contact dermatitis [47]. The contact dermatitis pathway is similar to the inflammatory cascade seen in AD and therefore positive associations between such chemical and AD should be suspected. Similarly, it is now generally accepted that food allergens have an effect on atopic dermatitis though the level of this effect is still under investigation [48, 49]. The five common food allergens recognized as possibly participating in the pathogenesis of AD are eggs, milk, soy, peanuts, and wheat with eggs and milk demonstrating the tightest correlative link [50]. Older studies likely overestimated the importance of food allergy in the causation and exacerbation of AD; however, there is likely a subpopulation of patients in whom food allergy plays an important stimulatory role. It is important to note that randomly or blindly eliminating food groups from the diets of patients afflicted with AD has not proven effective in improving disease course and may create nutritional deficiencies in developing children. Patients with moderate to severe AD with a history of worsening clinical symptoms following intake of certain foods, or patients with recalcitrant disease may benefit from screening by an allergist.

Topical steroids, a long-term treatment for atopic dermatitis, may also increase the risk of recurrence. Studies have suggested that barrier defects are not repaired by steroid use and that skin is up to 70% thinner in areas where the steroids are used [10, 51]. There is a decrease in the lipid lamellae and lower numbers of granules found at the SC and the stratum granulosum junction when steroids are used [52]. The rebound flare often seen after topical steroid use is discontinued stopped suggests responses similar to tape stripping [10]. Similarly, steroids have been shown to increase expression of desquamatory protease KLK7 [53]. This increase has been positively associated with increasing atopic dermatitis lesions. A complete strategy for the treatment of atopic dermatitis must address both controlling inflammation with judicious use of topical steroids, along with barrier repair utilizing nutritive moisturizers and substituting gentle cleansers in the place of harsher detergents.

3.10 The Inflammatory Cascade in Atopic Dermatitis

Any discussion of AD must include a review of the inflammatory cascade and its effects. Recent genome-wide studies have emphasized Th2 cytokines such as KIF3A, IL-4, and IL 13 as major molecules involved in atopic dermatitis [54, 55].

Likewise, IL-1 receptors have also been implicated. The basic understanding of the inflammatory cascade in AD is described as a biphasic T cell disease. Th2 signals dominate the early phases of the disease process, where a switch from Th2 to Th1 seems to promote chronicity of the disease [56, 57]. Newer studies have also implicated IL-22 producing T cells and IL-17 producing T cells in both the initiation and maintenance of AD. Infiltrations of CD3+ T cells, CD1c+ dendritic cells, and CD1c+ dendritic cells are also found in acute atopic dermatitis [57].

Histologically, cells expressing mRNA for Th2 cytokines, such as IL-4 and IL-13, are greatly expressed in acute lesions during atopic dermatitis while chronic lesions have a larger number of cells expressing mRNA for INF-γ [58]. House dust mite antigen has been used in patch testing to confirm the switch between mRNA types from IL-4 to INF-γ [59]. The importance of Th2 to Th1 deviation cannot be ignored; IL-4 and IL-13 related molecules such as CCL17 and galectin-9 directly correlate with atopic dermatitis disease severity. Recent studies have also indicated a unique role for IL-22 producing T22 cells in atopic dermatitis. Human T22 cells produce IL-22 without the IL-17 seen coproduced in murine cells. These infiltrated cells include CD4+ Th22 helper cells and CD8+ Tc22 cytotoxic cells [60]. Disease severity correlated much more closely with the Tc22 cells instead of the Th22 cells. Flow cytometry was used to prove childhood atopic dermatitis lacked the typical Th1 cells while adult atopic dermatitis, generally more chronic in nature, was high in Th22 cell types [61].

In addition Th2 and Th22 cytokines also regulate the proteins needed in the epidermal barrier during normal function. Th2 cytokines IL-4 and IL-13 were both shown to inhibit FLG function as well as to inhibit the necessary mRNAs for proper FLG production [62, 63]. This effect was strong enough in some patients to simulate a loss of function mutation in FLG already discussed above. In contrast to these changes, skin with active atopic dermatitis lesions had upregulated S100A7, a gene also located in the locus for FLG.

Dendritic cells play a key role in AD as well. Dendritic cells are a cell subset that specializes in antigen uptake and presentation. When these cells are found in the epidermis they are called Langerhans cells and generally contain Birbeck granules. Langerhans cells are found in lesional and non-lesional skin in atopic dermatitis patients. They have very high affinity for IgE receptors and are required for immune responses to protein antigen penetration of the epidermis [64]. Another dendritic cell subset involved in inflammatory processes infiltrates atopic skin very early in the process [65]. This subset of cells has high levels of CD11b and CD11c instead of the normal Birbeck granules. Because the high levels of CD11b and CD11c is a significant difference, these molecules have been suggested as targets for treatment and further study [66, 67].

A generally acceptable definition of atopy is the overproduction of IgE antibodies or a personal history of asthma, allergic rhinitis, AD, or other allergic diseases [58]. The function of IgE must therefore be explained in relation to AD. Th2 cytokines help to activate B cells into the IgE production pathway [68]. This is congruent with the Th2 deviation seen in childhood AD. Specific studies have confirmed that Th2 related cytokines CCL17 and CCL22 are correlated directly with serum levels of IgE for wheat and mite allergens. Plausible self-antigens such as profilin 1, cyclophilin B, and ribosomal P2 protein have all been suggested as potential targets of IgE in AD. Auto reactive CD8+ T cells have been found in studies of such auto antigens highlighting the possible role of autoreactive IgE in exacerbating or perpetuating AD severity [69]. Due to the interaction between T cells and IgE, auto reactive T cells must also be considered in atopic pathogenesis. A transcriptional coactivator alpha-NAC is normally involved in sorting newly synthesized polypeptides without any homology with environmental known allergens [70]. Atopic dermatitis patients with anti-alpha-NAC IgE antibodies produced much larger amounts of IL-17, IL-22, and INF-γ [70]. Very recently, auto reactivity between CD8+ T cells and alpha-NAC has been found specifically in AD [71]. These mechanisms of self-antigen recognition may provide a rational for the role of autoreactive IgE and T cells in the exacerbation and continuation of AD.

Cell death also plays a role in worsening AD. Keratinocytes of patients with AD show an increase in IFN-γ mediated apoptosis when compared to healthy skin. Apoptosis related genes *NOD2*, *DUSP1*, and *ADM* were all induced by the IFN-γ process in primary keratinocytes found in AD patients [72]. The loss of skin cells due to apoptosis may cause gaps in the skin barrier allowing increased water loss and antigen penetration. It would be reasonable to assume that such cell death would also decrease the number of molecules, such as free fatty acids and NMF, required for proper barrier maintenance.

Colonization of AD lesions with *S. aureus* in can also affect immune function. Such bacterial stimulus leads to predominance of the Toll-like receptor 2 ligands [66, 73]. Other factors cause epithelial IL-25, IL-33, and thymic stromal lymphopoietin to be upregulated in the lesions. The interaction of these inflammatory mediators drives an accumulation of type 2 innate lymphoid cells which are theorized to take part in atopic dermatitis. The type 2 innate lymphoid cells are believed to cause dendritic cells to foster a Th2 phenotype found in T cells [74]. The immunochemical disruption further impacts the skin's barrier possibly leading to prolonged flares of AD [66].

3.11 Emerging Therapies

The vast avenues of study for AD and the pathways producing this condition afford a multitude of targets for potential treatment. Many new medications are under phase 2 trials and several other mechanisms are under study for advancing the treatment of AD. The ongoing studies of the pathways involved in AD leave room for the development of many new treatments. Novel therapeutic agents for atopic dermatitis will be further discussed in a later chapter.

Out of all of the new treatments, the most promising drug for AD treatment still under study is dupilumab. A fully human monoclonal antibody directed at the alpha subunit of IL-4 receptors, Dupilumab was approved by the Food and Drug Administration in early 2017 [71, 75]. Dupilumab blocks signals from both IL-4 and IL-13 causing significant improvement in inflammation and pruritus with no dose limiting toxicity [76, 77]. Decreases in mRNA expression genes associated with Th2 chemokines were also detected with the drug's use. Little to no Th1 modulation was found. The Eczema Area and Severity Index (EASI) was assessed at 16 weeks during phase II trials, and a 73% improvement during treatment vs an 18% improvement in the placebo group was found [78]. Similar results were found in phase III trials with adverse effects as low as 1%, which was lower than the 5% found in the placebo group. Dupilumab is a very bright spot in the research of treatment for AD and represents a large step forward for any patients who suffer from AD.

Another area under study for atopic dermatitis treatment is anti-IL-31 alpha receptor antibodies, Nemolizumab (CIM331). In studies involving humans and mice, IL-31 is produced by Th2 cells; and injection of IL-31 causes pruritus such as that found in AD [79]. Treatments with CIM331 inhibited pruritus and improved sleep in short trials [80]. Likewise, the study of Janus kinase inhibitors has yielded several possible treatments for atopic dermatitis. Tofacitinib, as an additional treatment option, showed EASI improvement in phase IIa studies. It is a pan-JAK inhibitor that mostly affects JAK1 and JAK3, with a lesser effect in JAK2 [71]. Both oral and topical Tofacitinib are under study and show promising results. Unfortunately, potential immune suppression has been noticed as a side effect in current studies and must be very carefully investigated before the drug can be considered for widespread use. Similarly, histamine H4's roll in pruritus and inflammation has made it a target for study as well. One study in Japan found significant improvement in the pruritus in both daytime and nighttime symptoms. The possibility of agranulocytosis with such treatment has raised red flags [71].

Another area under serious investigation in the research for AD treatments is Phosphodiesterase 4 (PDE-4) inhibitors. Apremilast, an oral PDE-4 inhibitor, is currently in use for psoriasis and is being researched for AD. An uncontrolled study showed improvement in AD symptoms equal to that seen in patients treated with cyclosporine and similar drugs based on EASI scores and quality of life indices [81-83]. Several topical PDE-4 inhibitors are also being studied. Crisaborole 2% ointment was approved for the treatment of AD by the FDA in December 2016 and when used twice daily showed a 71% improvement based on Atopic Dermatitis Severity Index (ADSI) [81]. The most common side effect with crisaborole is application site stinging. Other PDE-4 inhibitors under investigation include E6005 and OPA-15406 [69, 74].

Omalizumab is a humanized monoclonal antibody that binds to IgE antibodies. It is approved for treatment in severe allergic asthma and chronic uticaria. Use of omalizumab has been studied in AD, but the results are mixed [84]. One double blinded study showed improvement versus placebo; however, a 2014 study showed patients with FLG mutations did not respond at all to its use as a treatment [85]. The role of IgE in the atopic march is important, so other medications targeting this area may soon emerge.

Vitamin D has been suggested by several studies to have a significant role in the pathogenesis of atopic dermatitis [86, 87]. Evidence suggests that vitamin D supplementation may help ease the symptoms of atopic dermatitis. A small 2008 study showed that 4 out of 5 children had symptom relief on 1000 IU of vitamin D. Sadly, larger studies have shown mixed results related to this effect, and the target dosage is also unclear [88].

Thymic stromal lymphopoietin (TSLP), previously discussed above, may be another good target for future treatment options. This epithelial derived cytokine is implicated in triggering T cell switching into the Th2 phenotype. AMG 157, the first TSLP drug tested, has shown good results in the control of allergen based asthma. In a phase I study, AMG 157 proved effective in attenuating most measures in allergy-induced early and late asthmatic response, lessening decrease of FEV 1 upon allergen exposure and decreasing serum and sputum eosinophilia [89] This research provides a promising start for investigation toward TSLP in atopic dermatitis treatment.

Several publications have called atopic dermatitis the "itch that rashes;" therefore, stopping the itch that occurs with atopic dermatitis with a successful treatment option would be an obvious high priority for research studies. CT327 and tradipitant are two medications in trails that aim to address this itching sensation. They seek to antagonize the tropomyosin-receptor kinase A (trkA) for CT327 and neurokinin 1 receptors (NK-1Rs) for tradipitant. This neuronal approach to itch has shown some benefit in studies [90]. Further study into the direct effect of these drugs on atopic dermatitis may provide exciting new options for patient relief.

3.12 Conclusion

AD is a complex and multifactorial disease with a significant impact on the quality of life of afflicted patients and their families. As physicians come to better understand the pathogenesis of this challenging condition, modern medicine may be able to provide more comprehensive treatment regimens, novel therapeutic options, and insightful behavioral interventions to better address patients' needs. The role of environmental and airborne pollutants in the development of AD provides impetus for physicians to actively advocate for considerate utilization of resources and thoughtful environmental policies. Unfortunately, AD is not a simple condition with a straightforward, one-size-fits-all solution; however, as medicine embarks on this new era of genetic and molecular discovery, there will be better tools to address this condition on an individualized basis. The future may hold vast improvements in the lives of patients suffering from AD with personalized treatments based upon genetic and molecular testing, but this depends on the better understanding of the delicate interplay of genetics, environment, habit, and inflammation that create this difficult but fascinating condition. AD demonstrates how integral a role the skin barrier plays in overall health and highlights the magnificent complexity of the body's largest organ.

References

1. Seidenari S, Giusti G. Objective assessment of the skin of children affected by atopic dermatitis: a study of pH, capacitance and TEWL in eczematous and clinically uninvolved skin. Acta Derm Venereol. 1995;75(6):429–33.
2. Elias PM. Stratum corneum defensive functions: an integrated view. J Invest Dermatol. 2005;125(2):183–200.
3. Elias PM, Schmuth M. Abnormal skin barrier in the etiopathogenesis of atopic dermatitis. Curr Opin Allergy Clin Immunol. 2009;9(5):437–46.
4. Braff MH, Di Nardo A, Gallo RL. Keratinocytes store the antimicrobial peptide cathelicidin in lamellar bodies. J Invest Dermatol. 2005;124(2):394–400.
5. Oren A, et al. In human epidermis, beta-defensin 2 is packaged in lamellar bodies. Exp Mol Pathol. 2003;74(2):180–2.
6. McAleer MA, Irvine AD. The multifunctional role of filaggrin in allergic skin disease. J Allergy Clin Immunol. 2013;131(2):280–91.
7. Palmer CN, et al. Common loss-of-function variants of the epidermal barrier protein filaggrin are a major predisposing factor for atopic dermatitis. Nat Genet. 2006;38(4):441–6.
8. Fleckman P, Brumbaugh S. Absence of the granular layer and keratohyalin define a morphologically distinct subset of individuals with ichthyosis vulgaris. Exp Dermatol. 2002;11(4):327–36.
9. Scharschmidt TC, et al. Filaggrin deficiency confers a paracellular barrier abnormality that reduces inflammatory thresholds to irritants and haptens. J Allergy Clin Immunol. 2009;124(3):496–506.e6.
10. Cork MJ, et al. Epidermal barrier dysfunction in atopic dermatitis. J Invest Dermatol. 2009;129(8):1892–908.
11. Brattsand M, et al. A proteolytic cascade of kallikreins in the stratum corneum. J Invest Dermatol. 2005;124(1):198–203.
12. Kato A, et al. Association of SPINK5 gene polymorphisms with atopic dermatitis in the Japanese population. Br J Dermatol. 2003;148(4):665–9.
13. Walley AJ, et al. Gene polymorphism in Netherton and common atopic disease. Nat Genet. 2001;29(2):175–8.
14. Harding C, Rawlings A. Effects of natural moisturizing factor and lactic acid isomers on skin function. In: Dry skin and moisturizers. Boca Raton: CRC Press; 2005. p. 187–209.
15. Braun-Falco O, Korting HC. Normal pH value of human skin. Hautarzt. 1986;37(3):126–9.
16. Rippke F, Schreiner V, Schwanitz HJ. The acidic milieu of the horny layer: new findings on the physiology and pathophysiology of skin pH. Am J Clin Dermatol. 2002;3(4):261–72.
17. Fluhr JW, Elias PM. Stratum corneum pH: formation and function of the 'acid mantle'. Exog Dermatol. 2002;1(4):163–75.
18. Ekholm IE, Brattsand M, Egelrud T. Stratum corneum tryptic enzyme in normal epidermis: a missing link in the desquamation process? J Invest Dermatol. 2000;114(1):56–63.
19. Anderson DS. The acid-base balance of the skin. Br J Dermatol. 1951;63(8–9):283–95.
20. Lee H-J, Lee S-H. Epidermal permeability barrier defects and barrier repair therapy in atopic dermatitis. Allergy Asthma Immunol Res. 2014;6(4):276–87.
21. Elias PM, et al. Modulations in epidermal calcium regulate the expression of differentiation-specific markers. J Invest Dermatol. 2002;119(5):1128–36.
22. Sugawara T, et al. Tight junction dysfunction in the stratum granulosum leads to aberrant stratum corneum barrier function in claudin-1-deficient mice. J Dermatol Sci. 2013;70(1):12–8.
23. Yuki T, et al. Impaired tight junctions in atopic dermatitis skin and in a skin-equivalent model treated with interleukin-17. PLoS One. 2016;11(9):e0161759.
24. Yuki T, et al. Impaired tight junctions obstruct stratum corneum formation by altering polar lipid and profilaggrin processing. J Dermatol Sci. 2013;69(2):148–58.
25. Gong JQ, et al. Skin colonization by Staphylococcus aureus in patients with eczema and atopic dermatitis and relevant combined topical therapy: a double-blind multicentre randomized controlled trial. Br J Dermatol. 2006;155(4):680–7.

26. Kobayashi T, et al. Dysbiosis and Staphylococcus aureus colonization drives inflammation in atopic dermatitis. Immunity. 2015;42(4):756–66.
27. Parsons JB, et al. Membrane disruption by antimicrobial fatty acids releases low-molecular-weight proteins from Staphylococcus aureus. J Bacteriol. 2012;194(19):5294–304.
28. Sato J, et al. Abrupt decreases in environmental humidity induce abnormalities in permeability barrier homeostasis. J Invest Dermatol. 2002;119(4):900–4.
29. Amano H, et al. Psychological stress can trigger atopic dermatitis in NC/Nga mice: an inhibitory effect of corticotropin-releasing factor. Neuropsychopharmacology. 2007;33(3):566–73.
30. SuÁRez AL, et al. Psychoneuroimmunology of psychological stress and atopic dermatitis: pathophysiologic and therapeutic updates. Acta Derm Venereol. 2012;92(1):7–15.
31. Perkin MR, et al. Association between domestic water hardness, chlorine, and atopic dermatitis risk in early life: A population-based cross-sectional study. J Allergy Clin Immunol. 2016;138(2):509–16.
32. Kim J, et al. Airborne formaldehyde causes skin barrier dysfunction in atopic dermatitis. Br J Dermatol. 2016;175(2):357–63.
33. Kim K. Influences of environmental chemicals on atopic dermatitis. Toxicol Res. 2015;31(2):89–96.
34. Montnemery P, et al. Prevalence of self-reported eczema in relation to living environment, socio-economic status and respiratory symptoms assessed in a questionnaire study. BMC Dermatol. 2003;3:4.
35. Penard-Morand C, et al. Long-term exposure to close-proximity air pollution and asthma and allergies in urban children. Eur Respir J. 2010;36(1):33–40.
36. Lehmann I, et al. Enhanced in vivo IgE production and T cell polarization toward the type 2 phenotype in association with indoor exposure to VOC: results of the LARS study. Int J Hyg Environ Health. 2001;204(4):211–21.
37. Wang IJ, et al. Prenatal smoke exposure, DNA methylation, and childhood atopic dermatitis. Clin Exp Allergy. 2013;43(5):535–43.
38. Thyssen JP, et al. The epidemiology of contact allergy in the general population—prevalence and main findings. Contact Dermatitis. 2007;57(5):287–99.
39. Yoshihisa Y, Shimizu T. Metal allergy and systemic contact dermatitis: an overview. Dermatol Res Pract. 2012;2012:749561.
40. Borg L, et al. Nickel-induced cytokine production from mononuclear cells in nickel-sensitive individuals and controls. Cytokine profiles in nickel-sensitive individuals with nickel allergy-related hand eczema before and after nickel challenge. Arch Dermatol Res. 2000;292(6):285–91.
41. Minang JT, et al. Nickel, cobalt, chromium, palladium and gold induce a mixed Th1- and Th2-type cytokine response in vitro in subjects with contact allergy to the respective metals. Clin Exp Immunol. 2006;146(3):417–26.
42. Thyssen JP, McFadden JP, Kimber I. The multiple factors affecting the association between atopic dermatitis and contact sensitization. Allergy. 2014;69(1):28–36.
43. Gfatter R, Hackl P, Braun F. Effects of soap and detergents on skin surface pH, stratum corneum hydration and fat content in infants. Dermatology. 1997;195(3):258–62.
44. Wood LC, et al. Barrier disruption stimulates interleukin-1 alpha expression and release from a pre-formed pool in murine epidermis. J Invest Dermatol. 1996;106(3):397–403.
45. Torma H, Lindberg M, Berne B. Skin barrier disruption by sodium lauryl sulfate-exposure alters the expressions of involucrin, transglutaminase 1, profilaggrin, and kallikreins during the repair phase in human skin in vivo. J Invest Dermatol. 2008;128(5):1212–9.
46. Steinhoff M, et al. Proteinase-activated receptor-2 mediates itch: a novel pathway for pruritus in human skin. J Neurosci. 2003;23(15):6176–80.
47. Yim E, Baquerizo Nole KL, Tosti A. Contact dermatitis caused by preservatives. Dermatitis. 2014;25(5):215–31.
48. Wuthrich B. Food-induced cutaneous adverse reactions. Allergy. 1998;53(46 Suppl):131–5.

49. Hanifin JM. Critical evaluation of food and mite allergy in the management of atopic dermatitis. J Dermatol. 1997;24(8):495–503.
50. Bjorksten B. Genetic and environmental risk factors for the development of food allergy. Curr Opin Allergy Clin Immunol. 2005;5(3):249–53.
51. Sheu HM, et al. Depletion of stratum corneum intercellular lipid lamellae and barrier function abnormalities after long-term topical corticosteroids. Br J Dermatol. 1997;136(6):884–90.
52. Kao JS, et al. Short-term glucocorticoid treatment compromises both permeability barrier homeostasis and stratum corneum integrity: inhibition of epidermal lipid synthesis accounts for functional abnormalities. J Invest Dermatol. 2003;120(3):456–64.
53. Yousef GM, et al. The KLK7 (PRSS6) gene, encoding for the stratum corneum chymotryptic enzyme is a new member of the human kallikrein gene family—genomic characterization, mapping, tissue expression and hormonal regulation. Gene. 2000;254(1–2):119–28.
54. Paternoster L, et al. Meta-analysis of genome-wide association studies identifies three new risk loci for atopic dermatitis. Nat Genet. 2011;44(2):187–92.
55. Tamari M, Hirota T. Genome-wide association studies of atopic dermatitis. J Dermatol. 2014;41(3):213–20.
56. Leung DY, et al. New insights into atopic dermatitis. J Clin Invest. 2004;113(5):651–7.
57. Gittler JK, et al. Progressive activation of T(H)2/T(H)22 cytokines and selective epidermal proteins characterizes acute and chronic atopic dermatitis. J Allergy Clin Immunol. 2012;130(6):1344–54.
58. Furue M, et al. Atopic dermatitis: immune deviation, barrier dysfunction, IgE autoreactivity and new therapies. Allergol Int. 2017;66(3):398–403.
59. Thepen T, et al. Biphasic response against aeroallergen in atopic dermatitis showing a switch from an initial TH2 response to a TH1 response in situ: an immunocytochemical study. J Allergy Clin Immunol. 1996;97(3):828–37.
60. Fujita H, et al. Human Langerhans cells induce distinct IL-22-producing CD4+ T cells lacking IL-17 production. Proc Natl Acad Sci U S A. 2009;106(51):21795–800.
61. Czarnowicki T, et al. Early pediatric atopic dermatitis shows only a cutaneous lymphocyte antigen (CLA)(+) TH2/TH1 cell imbalance, whereas adults acquire CLA(+) TH22/TC22 cell subsets. J Allergy Clin Immunol. 2015;136(4):941–951.e3.
62. Furue M, et al. Gene regulation of filaggrin and other skin barrier proteins via aryl hydrocarbon receptor. J Dermatol Sci. 2015;80(2):83–8.
63. Howell MD, et al. Cytokine modulation of atopic dermatitis filaggrin skin expression. J Allergy Clin Immunol. 2007;120(1):150–5.
64. Nakajima S, et al. Langerhans cells are critical in epicutaneous sensitization with protein antigen via thymic stromal lymphopoietin receptor signaling. J Allergy Clin Immunol. 2012;129(4):1048–55.e6.
65. Kerschenlohr K, et al. Atopy patch test reactions show a rapid influx of inflammatory dendritic epidermal cells in patients with extrinsic atopic dermatitis and patients with intrinsic atopic dermatitis. J Allergy Clin Immunol. 2003;111(4):869–74.
66. Werfel T, et al. Cellular and molecular immunologic mechanisms in patients with atopic dermatitis. J Allergy Clin Immunol. 2016;138(2):336–49.
67. Schuller E, et al. Tacrolimus ointment causes inflammatory dendritic epidermal cell depletion but no Langerhans cell apoptosis in patients with atopic dermatitis. J Allergy Clin Immunol. 2004;114(1):137–43.
68. Poulsen LK, Hummelshoj L. Triggers of IgE class switching and allergy development. Ann Med. 2007;39(6):440–56.
69. Heratizadeh A, et al. The role of T-cell reactivity towards the autoantigen alpha-NAC in atopic dermatitis. Br J Dermatol. 2011;164(2):316–24.
70. Hradetzky S, et al. Cytokine effects induced by the human autoallergen alpha-NAC. J Invest Dermatol. 2014;134(6):1570–8.
71. Roesner LM, et al. Alpha-NAC-specific autoreactive CD8+ T cells in atopic dermatitis are of an effector memory type and secrete IL-4 and IFN-gamma. J Immunol. 2016;196(8):3245–52.

72. Rebane A, et al. Mechanisms of IFN-gamma-induced apoptosis of human skin keratinocytes in patients with atopic dermatitis. J Allergy Clin Immunol. 2012;129(5):1297–306.
73. Travers JB, et al. Infected atopic dermatitis lesions contain pharmacologic amounts of lipoteichoic acid. J Allergy Clin Immunol. 2010;125(1):146–52.e1–2.
74. Hammad H, Lambrecht BN. Barrier epithelial cells and the control of type 2 immunity. Immunity. 2015;43(1):29–40.
75. Kraft M, Worm M. Dupilumab in the treatment of moderate-to-severe atopic dermatitis. Expert Rev Clin Immunol. 2017;13(4):301–10.
76. Wambre E, et al. Specific immunotherapy modifies allergen-specific CD4(+) T-cell responses in an epitope-dependent manner. J Allergy Clin Immunol. 2014;133(3):872–9.e7.
77. Tam H, et al. Specific allergen immunotherapy for the treatment of atopic eczema. Cochrane Database Syst Rev. 2016;2:Cd008774.
78. Eichenfield LFM, et al. Assessing the new and emerging treatments for atopic dermatitis. Semin Cutan Med Surg. 2016;35(5 Suppl):S92–6.
79. Hijnen D, et al. CD8(+) T cells in the lesional skin of atopic dermatitis and psoriasis patients are an important source of IFN-gamma, IL-13, IL-17, and IL-22. J Invest Dermatol. 2013;133(4):973–9.
80. Hennino A, et al. CD8+ T cells are recruited early to allergen exposure sites in atopy patch test reactions in human atopic dermatitis. J Allergy Clin Immunol. 2011;127(4):1064–7.
81. Barton M, Sidbury R. Advances in understanding and managing atopic dermatitis. F1000Res. 2015;4. doi:10.12688/f1000research.6972.1.
82. Volf EM, et al. A phase 2, open-label, investigator-initiated study to evaluate the safety and efficacy of apremilast in subjects with recalcitrant allergic contact or atopic dermatitis. J Drugs Dermatol. 2012;11(3):341–6.
83. Samrao A, et al. A pilot study of an oral phosphodiesterase inhibitor (apremilast) for atopic dermatitis in adults. Arch Dermatol. 2012;148(8):890–7.
84. El-Qutob D. Off-Label Uses of Omalizumab. Clin Rev Allergy Immunol. 2016;50(1):84–96.
85. Hotze M, et al. Increased efficacy of omalizumab in atopic dermatitis patients with wild-type filaggrin status and higher serum levels of phosphatidylcholines. Allergy. 2014;69(1):132–5.
86. Peroni DG, et al. Correlation between serum 25-hydroxyvitamin D levels and severity of atopic dermatitis in children. Br J Dermatol. 2011;164(5):1078–82.
87. Back O, et al. Does vitamin D intake during infancy promote the development of atopic allergy? Acta Derm Venereol. 2009;89(1):28–32.
88. Chiu YE, et al. Serum 25-hydroxyvitamin D concentration does not correlate with atopic dermatitis severity. J Am Acad Dermatol. 2013;69(1):40–6.
89. Gauvreau GM, et al. Effects of an anti-TSLP antibody on allergen-induced asthmatic responses. N Engl J Med. 2014 May 29;370(22):2102–10.
90. Roblin D, et al. Topical TrkA kinase inhibitor CT327 is an effective, novel therapy for the treatment of pruritus due to psoriasis: results from experimental studies, and efficacy and safety of CT327 in a phase 2b clinical trial in patients with psoriasis. Acta Derm Venereol. 2015;95(5):542–8.

Chapter 4
Clinical Presentation of Atopic Dermatitis

Christine Ahn and William Huang

Abstract Atopic dermatitis, commonly known as eczema, is a chronic inflammatory dermatosis that can affect individuals from infancy to adulthood. Also referred to as "the itch that rashes", atopic dermatitis is classically associated with significant pruritus that is accompanied by characteristic cutaneous and other clinical findings. The diagnosis of atopic dermatitis can be challenging due to the wide range of clinical presentations based on patient factors such as age, skin type, ethnicity, and other comorbid conditions. This chapter reviews the classical findings as well as the less common manifestations of atopic dermatitis.

Keywords Atopy • Eczema • Eczematous • Erythroderma • Lichenification • Pruritus • Rash

4.1 Introduction

Atopic dermatitis (AD) is a chronic and relapsing inflammatory dermatosis with an estimated prevalence of up to 20% in children and 5% in adults in the United States. Its peak prevalence is seen in early childhood, with 45% of affected individuals presenting within the first 6 months of life, 60% within the first 12 months of life, and 85% before the age of 5 years [1]. The term atopy refers to a tendency towards increased immunoglobulin E (IgE) production in response to certain allergens. Atopic diseases include atopic dermatitis, asthma, and rhinoconjunctivitis, and are frequently seen together in the classic "atopic triad" [2].

C. Ahn, M.D. (✉) • W. Huang, M.D.
Wake Forest School of Medicine, Medical Center Boulevard, Winston Salem, NC 27104, USA
e-mail: cahn@wakehealth.edu

E.A. Fortson et al. (eds.), *Management of Atopic Dermatitis*, Advances in Experimental Medicine and Biology 1027, DOI 10.1007/978-3-319-64804-0_4

4.2 Clinical Features

Atopic dermatitis is a clinical diagnosis made based on history, morphology, distribution of lesions, and associated clinical signs and symptoms. Due to its wide range of clinical presentations, diagnostic criteria have been developed to aid in the diagnosis and classification of atopic dermatitis [3]. Using revised criteria developed by a consensus conference in 2003, atopic dermatitis is defined by the presence of pruritus *and* at least three of the following criteria: personal or first-degree relative with a history of atopy such as allergic rhinitis or asthma, dry skin, history of flexural dermatitis, visible flexural dermatitis, and onset of rash before 2 years of age (unless currently under 4 years of age) [4].

4.2.1 Infantile AD

The infantile phase is defined as atopic dermatitis occurring before the age of 2 years. It usually begins between birth and 6 months of age and predominantly involves acute lesions of eczema, characterized by pruritic papules and vesicles with associated serous exudate or crusting. Lesions often involve the head and neck, starting as scaling and erythema on the cheeks and extending to the forehead, scalp, and neck. Crusting and lichenification are commonly present secondary to scratching and rubbing the areas involved. The distribution of infantile AD is distinct from the distribution in older children and adults, as it tends to involve the extensor surfaces of the extremities rather than flexural surfaces, although these sites can be affected as well. Infantile AD generally spares the groin and diaper area, likely due to increased hydration in this location and inaccessibility to scratching and rubbing, which can help distinguish it from other entities such as irritant or allergic contact dermatitis.

4.2.2 Childhood AD

The childhood phase of AD occurs from 2 years of age to puberty. In contrast to the acute lesions of the infantile phase, lesions of childhood AD are morphologically similar to those of the adult form of AD. Children present with dry, lichenified papules and plaques rather than exudative or crusted lesions, and the classic areas of involvement include the wrist, ankles, hands, feet, and antecubital and popliteal fossae (Fig. 4.1a, b, c). Facial involvement is less prominent in the childhood phase, but when involved, is typically observed in a perioral and periorbital distribution rather than the cheeks, chin, and forehead as in infantile AD (Fig. 4.1d). In some cases, childhood AD can demonstrate an inverse pattern with predominantly extensor involvement. In African American children, the morphology of AD can be more papular and follicular-based in appearance.

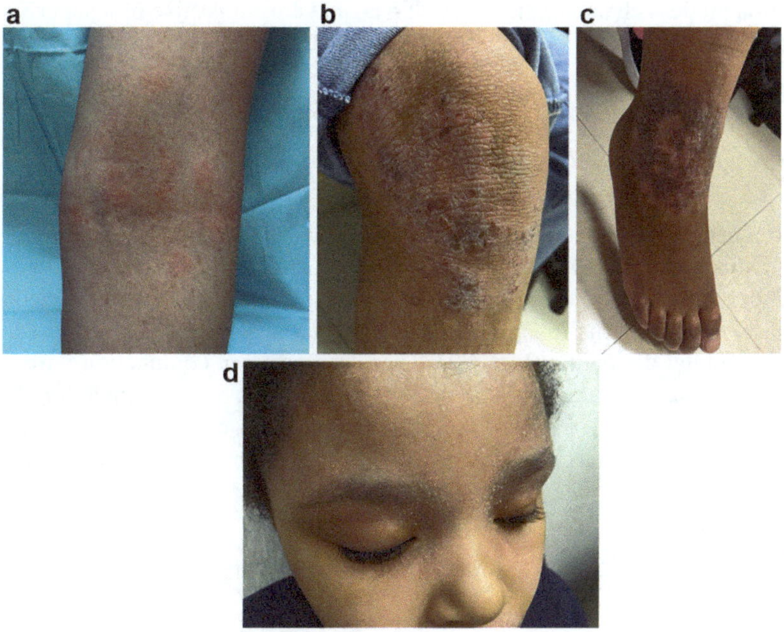

Fig. 4.1 (**a**) Erythematous papules in the antecubital fossa, (**b**) Hyperkeratotic, lichenified plaque on the knee with excoriations and heme-crust, representing a chronic lesion of AD, (**c**) Lichenified plaque with pigmentary alternations on the ankle, (**d**) Hypopigmented, erythematous, thin plaques with overlying scale affecting the forehead, eyelids, and cheeks of a child with severe AD

Pruritus is severe and secondary changes such as excoriations and lichenification due to the itch-scratch cycle are often seen. Scratching can occur during sleep, leading to poor sleep and chronic fatigue. There is a known association between childhood AD and an increased risk of attention deficit hyperactivity disorder (ADHD). Both severity of AD and sleep disturbance independently contribute to an increased risk of ADHD; these factors appear to act in a synergistic manner [12]. In addition, severity of atopic dermatitis is associated with a higher body mass index (BMI) percentile in children older than 2 years [5].

4.2.3 Adult AD

The adult phase of AD begins at puberty and continues into adulthood. The distribution in adults is predominantly flexural, in addition to the face, neck, and distal extremities. In older adults, the distribution can be less classic and may manifest in localized areas such as a hand, nipple, or eyelid dermatitis. In adult AD, characteristic lesions are symmetric, dry, scaly papules and plaques. Secondary changes of lichenification and excoriations are commonly seen. Prurigo nodularis in reponse to underlying AD is most commonly observed in adolescents and adults. Crusting and exudation are less characteristic of adult AD, and are suggestive of a superimposed infection when present.

4.2.4 Clinical Variations of AD

Less frequently, atopic dermatitis can manifest as localized or site-specific disease or as distinct morphologic variants. Localized variants include nipple dermatitis, fingertip or hand dermatitis, eyelid dermatitis, infraauricular, retroauricular, or infranasal fissuring, cheilitis, perioral involvement presenting as lip licker's dermatitis, and genital dermatitis (Fig. 4.2). These can occur in conjunction with classic lesions or as the sole manifestation of AD. Morphologic variants including follicular, papular-lichenoid, prurigo-like, nummular, and erythroderma have been described (Fig. 4.3). In a comparison study of the less common clinical variations of

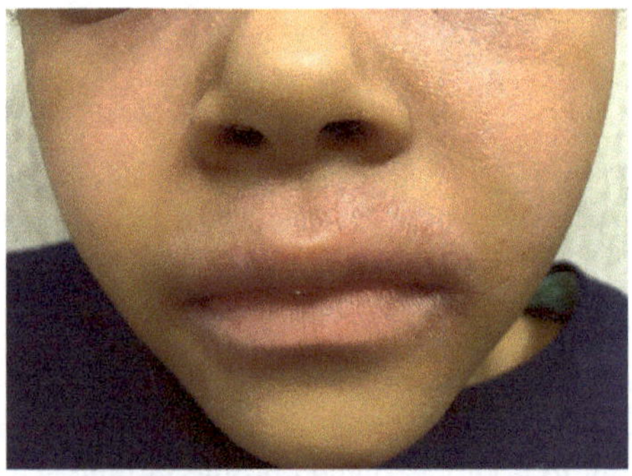

Fig. 4.2 Atopic dermatitis on the face with lip-licker's dermatitis manifesting as accentuated skin lines, lichenification, and hypopigmentation around the mouth

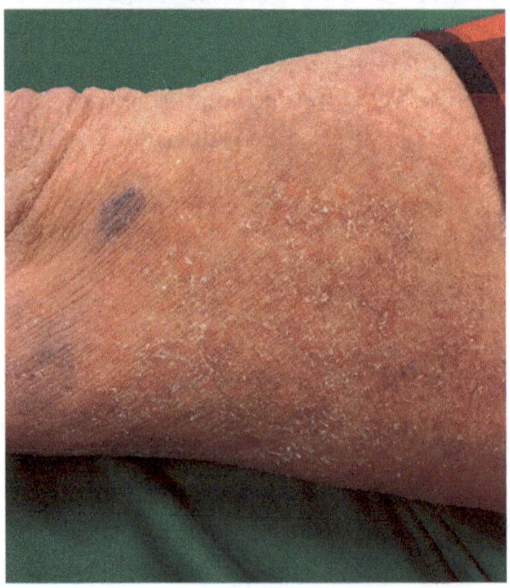

Fig. 4.3 Severe atopic dermatitis presenting as erythroderma in an adult. Diffuse erythema, fine scale, and eczema craquele appearance on the thigh

AD, genital dermatitis and papular-lichenoid AD were predominantly observed in infants, whereas eyelid and nipple dermatitis were observed in adolescents and adults. Nipple dermatitis was observed more frequently in girls whereas nummular dermatitis was seen more often in boys [6].

4.3 Associated Clinical Signs

Atopic dermatitis can be associated with a variety of clinical signs indicative of other atopic diseases such as allergic rhinitis or conjunctivitis. An exaggerated linear nasal crease from repeated rubbing of the nasal tip, also known as the *allergic salute*, is a frequent clinical finding in individuals with AD. *Dennie-Morgan lines*, also called *atopic pleats*, refer to dark lines beneath the lower eyelids, resulting from edema of the eyelids and lichenification. *Allergic shiners* describe gray or violaceous discoloration and swelling around the eyes, likely representing stasis changes as a result of edema causing increased pressure on the underlying venous plexuses [7]. In addition to skin findings, ocular pruritus and photophobia associated with allergic keratoconjunctivitis has been described concurrently in up to 30% of children with AD [8].

Postinflammatory pigmentation changes are frequently observed in AD, although these clinical findings are not specific to AD. In some individuals, postinflammatory hyperpigmentation is prominent and persists for months to years after lesions of AD clear. Pityriasis alba, which consists of asymptomatic hypopigmented patches often distributed on the face, neck, and upper trunk, is thought to represent postinflammatory hypopigmentation. It is observed more often in darker-skinned individuals and children, and is accentuated after sun exposure as areas of pityriasis alba do not show a pigmentary response to sunlight due to decreased epidermal melanosomes and melanocyte degeneration. The pigmentation changes associated with AD are temporary but may require more than 6 months to normalize.

White dermatographism is a blanching response to mechanical stimuli often seen in AD individuals. In contrast to red dermatographism, stroking the skin with a blunt instrument leads to a white line without an associated wheal. This reaction is thought to be the result of local edema and vasoconstriction. Although white dermatographism can be seen in other entities such as pityriasis rubra pilaris, erythrodermic psoriasis, and mycosis fungoides, this phenomenon is considered to be more characteristic of AD.

Ichthyosis vulgaris is a distinct dermatologic disease inherited in a semi-dominant manner that can occur concomitantly with AD. Ichthyosis vulgaris can be clinically diagnosed by the presence of hyperlinear palms and soles and general dry skin with fine scale. Historically, patients report worsening xerosis during cold weather months and more severe scaling on the legs. The close association with AD results from the role of filaggrin gene mutations in both conditions, which is responsible for ichthyosis vulgaris and is a predisposing factor for AD. In some studies, up to 37% of patients with AD have clinical evidence of ichthyosis vulgaris. The presence of ichthyosis vulgaris is clinically significant as affected AD patients tend to have a more severe dermatologic phenotype along with a higher risk of developing allergic respiratory disease [9]. Keratosis pilaris is another separate entity frequently seen in AD patients. It is characterized by hyperkeratosis and erythema around the follicles, which represents a cornified plug in the upper part of the hair follicle. It is most frequently found on the cheeks, extensor upper arms, and anterior thighs. The onset is typically during childhood and can persist into adulthood. Photosensitivity in the form of a polymorphous light eruption-type reaction or exacerbation of AD with ultraviolet (UV) exposure is observed in up to 3% of patients with atopic dermatitis. Although most patients demonstrate sensitivity to both UVA and UVB, a subset of patients are sensitive to only UVA or UVB.

Table 4.1 Differential diagnosis of atopic dermatitis

Infectious
Scabies
Molluscum contagiosum-associated dermatitis
Dermatophytosis (tinea capitis, corporis, incognito)
Syphilis
Impetigo
Viral exanthem
Candidiasis
Inflammatory
Seborrheic dermatitis
Irritant dermatitis
Allergic contact dermatitis
Psoriasis
Dermatomyositis
Neoplastic
Mycosis fungoides
Langerhans cell histiocytosis
Pityriasis lichenoides chronica
Photodermatoses
Polymorphous light eruption
Actinic prurigo
Other
Nutritional deficiency
Zinc deficiency
Graft-versus-host-disease
HIV/AIDS-related skin changes
Drug eruption

4.4 Differential Diagnosis

Given the morphologic variation and range of clinical manifestations of atopic dermatitis, the differential diagnosis can be broad and includes infectious, inflammatory, and neoplastic processes, among others (Table 4.1) [10]. Acute, exudative lesions of AD seen in infancy can resemble infectious etiologies such as scabies and impetigo. Molluscum contagiosum, often seen in higher burden in patients with AD, can present with lesions without the characteristic umbilication but a local inflammatory response that can mimic AD. In infants, seborrheic dermatitis is common and can appear in a similar distribution as AD or occur concurrently, making the diagnosis more challenging. Other inflammatory dermatoses that can mimic AD include psoriasis, dermatomyositis, irritant dermatitis, and allergic contact dermatitis. Several neoplastic processes may present with an eczematous morphology. Mycosis fungoides (MF), a primary cutaneous T-cell lymphoma, can resemble atopic dermatitis in both children and adults. In children, the hypopigmented clinical variant of MF, which occurs most often in darkly pigmented skin, can appear identical to pityriasis alba. In adults, patch- and plaque-stage classical MF presents as eczematous patches and plaques on the buttocks, trunk, and extremities. The possibility of this entity should always be considered in the setting of AD that is recalcitrant to therapy or presents later in life. Although tissue biopsy is necessary to distinguish MF from AD, serial biopsies are often required to establish this diagnosis [11].

In addition, severe AD in infants younger than 3 months should signal clinicians to consider primary immunodeficiency syndromes such as Omen syndrome, selective IgA-deficiency, hyper-IgE syndrome, and Wiskott Aldrich syndrome, genetic disorders with impaired barrier function such as Comel-Netherton syndrome, and metabolic disorders such as biotin deficiency and phenylketonuria [2].

References

1. Kay J, Gawkrodger DJ, Mortimer MJ, Jaron AG. The prevalence of childhood atopic eczema in a general population. J Am Acad Dermatol. 1994;30(1):35–9.
2. Wollenberg A, Oranje A, Deleuran M, et al. ETFAD/EADV eczema task force 2015 position paper on diagnosis and treatment of atopic dermatitis in adult and paediatric patients. J Eur Acad Dermatol Venereol. 2016;30(5):729–47.
3. Eichenfield LF, Tom WL, Chamlin SL, et al. Guidelines of care for the management of atopic dermatitis: section 1. Diagnosis and assessment of atopic dermatitis. J Am Acad Dermatol. 2014;70(2):338–51.
4. De D, Kanwar AJ, Handa S. Comparative efficacy of Hanifin and Rajka's criteria and the UK working party's diagnostic criteria in diagnosis of atopic dermatitis in a hospital setting in North India. J Eur Acad Dermatol Venereol. 2006;20(7):853–9.
5. Koutroulis I, Magnelli L, Gaughan J, et al. Atopic dermatitis is more severe in children over the age of two who have an increased body mass index. Acta Paediatr. 2015;104(7):713–7.
6. Julián-Gónzalez RE, Orozco-Covarrubias L, Durán-McKinster C, et al. Less common clinical manifestations of atopic dermatitis: prevalence by age. Pediatr Dermatol. 2012;29(5):580–3.

7. Bieber T, Bussmann C. Atopic dermatitis. In: Bolognia JL, Jorizzo JJ, Schaffer JV, editors. Dermatology. Philadelphia: Elsevier Saunders; 2012. p. 204–10.
8. Gelmetti C. Extracutaneous manifestations of atopic dermatitis. Pediatr Dermatol. 1992;9(4):380–2.
9. Bremmer SF, Hanifin JM, Simpson EL. Clinical detection of ichthyosis vulgaris in an atopic dermatitis clinic: implications for allergic respiratory disease and prognosis. J Am Acad Dermatol. 2008;59(1):72–8.
10. Siegfried EC, Hebert AA. Diagnosis of atopic dermatitis: mimics, overlaps, and complications. J Clin Forensic Med. 2015;4(5):884–917.
11. Barrett M, Luu M. Differential diagnosis of atopic dermatitis. Immunol Allergy Clin North Am. 2017;37(1):11–34.
12. Strom MA, Fishbein AB, Paller AS, Silverberg JI. Association between atopic dermatitis and attention deficit hyperactivity disorder in U.S. children and adults. Br J Dermatol. 2016;175(5):920–9.

Chapter 5
Atopic Dermatitis Disease Complications

Alyssa G. Ashbaugh and Shawn G. Kwatra

Abstract This chapter will describe infectious complications of atopic dermatitis, including bacterial, viral, and fungal infections and the evolving understanding of the relationship between atopic dermatitis and infectious disease. The underlying immunological dysregulation and poor skin barrier function associated with atopic dermatitis not only increases the likelihood of infectious complications, but also lends atopic dermatitis skin vulnerable to flares induced by environmental triggers. Thus, this chapter will also highlight the impact of common external environmental agents on precipitating flares of disease. Lastly, this chapter will discuss complications that can arise from treatments and the association of atopic dermatitis with more serious conditions such as lymphoma.

Keywords Complications • Infection • Immunological dysregulation • Environmental triggers • Treatment complications

5.1 Introduction

Until recently, the etiology of atopic dermatitis pathogenesis has been attributed to a dysregulated cutaneous immune response. Though the underlying immune dysregulation responsible for the pathogenesis of atopic dermatitis potentiates cutaneous infection [1], the field is beginning to appreciate how infection may also modulate disease pathogenesis. While viral infections have been viewed mostly as infectious complications rather than contributors to atopic dermatitis allergic inflammation, bacterial and, though less well-described, fungal infections, are now often considered causal factors of atopic dermatitis. Thus, there is a shifting paradigm in our understanding of the relationship between atopic dermatitis and cutaneous infections [2]: cutaneous infections can serve as both a cause and effect of the allergic skin inflammation associated with atopic dermatitis [3].

A.G. Ashbaugh, B.A. • S.G. Kwatra, M.D. (✉)
Department of Dermatology, Johns Hopkins University School of Medicine,
Baltimore, MD, USA
e-mail: shawn.kwatra@gmail.com

E.A. Fortson et al. (eds.), *Management of Atopic Dermatitis*, Advances in Experimental Medicine and Biology 1027, DOI 10.1007/978-3-319-64804-0_5

5.2 Infection and Atopic Dermatitis

Atopic dermatitis is marked by abnormal skin barrier function and chronic inflammation of the epidermis [4]. Both characteristics of the disease make the skin more susceptible to microbial colonization and infection. One established risk factor for atopic dermatitis is a loss-of-function filaggrin mutation [5]. In normal skin, filaggrin supports strong stratum corneum formation via natural breakdown products that promote skin moisture and lower skin pH [1]. This more acidic cutaneous pH confers antimicrobial resistance. A deficiency in filaggrin thus leads to reduced skin hydration and poor barrier function [6], increasing the risk for atopic disease and ultimately infection given that healthy skin is our bodies' first line of immune defense [1]. Furthermore, filaggrin deficiency also increases pH, yielding the skin more susceptible to microbial colonization [2]. The propensity towards colonization is further exacerbated in atopic dermatitis by the disease's underlying immune dysregulation. Patients with atopic dermatitis have both systemic and cutaneous immune abnormalities that contribute to a T_h2 immune phenotype [1, 2]. This T_h2 polarization manifests in increased serum IgE levels and increased cutaneous IL-4, IL-5 and IL-13 expression [4]. The resulting T_h2-skewed inflammatory microenvironment in the skin suppresses the normal innate TLR-mediated activation of epithelial cells [4], reducing antimicrobial peptide production and leaving the skin even more prone to infection.

In addition to abnormal skin barrier function and immune dysregulation, atopic dermatitis is also associated with microbiome changes. Natural resident flora, such as *Staphylococcus epidermidis* and *Propionibacterium acnes*, normally regulate the skin flora and prevent pathogenic bacteria growth without activating the immune system. However, in atopic dermatitis, the skin is more susceptible to pathogenic colonization and infection by microbes, such as *S. aureus* [1].

Infection with *S. aureus* is the most common skin infection in atopic dermatitis patients [1]. The skin of atopic dermatitis patients is more often colonized with *S. aureus* compared to the skin of healthy patients [7]. Though *S. aureus* colonizes atopic dermatitis skin at both lesional and nonlesional skin sites [3, 8, 9], higher bacteria counts are found in more severe lesions [7]. Thus, increased disease severity correlates with increased colonization [3].

This increased colonization is likely attributed to the underlying pathogenesis of atopic dermatitis. For example, increases in cutaneous pH promote *S. aureus* adhesion and proliferation [1]. Furthermore, immune defects, such as reduced antimicrobial peptide expression [10], increase bacterial adherence. There is also evidence that suggests that T_h2-mediated inflammatory skin sites have greater bacterial binding than T_h1-mediated inflammatory skin sites [8], making the skin of atopic dermatitis patients even more susceptible to colonization. This is likely due to T_h2-driven downregulation of antimicrobial peptides and increased production of extracellular matrix molecules that act as adhesions to *S. aureus* [11]. Once colonized, *S. aureus* can form a biofilm, which further promotes *S. aureus* adhesion and survival [12, 13]. In addition to immune deficiencies, barrier defects due to patient scratching also promote increased adherence given that physical injury of the stratum corneum promotes bacterial binding [3].

Just as the skin of atopic dermatitis patients is more likely to be colonized with *S. aureus*, the skin of atopic dermatitis patients is also more often infected with *S. aureus* [14]. Interestingly, anti-inflammatory drugs decrease patient *S. aureus* bacterial burden even though they have no antimicrobial activity [15, 16]. This suggests that the allergic skin inflammation of atopic dermatitis itself promotes bacterial colonization [3].

The virulence of *S. aureus*, which is often attributed to superantigen and α-toxin production, also contributes to the increased adherence and infection of atopic dermatitis patients. Atopic dermatitis patients are more likely to be colonized with superantigen-producing *S. aureus* [1]. This increased colonization of superantigen-producing *S. aureus* correlates with increased disease severity of atopic dermatitis [1]. α-toxin, a cytotoxic agent produced by *S. aureus* [17], directly exacerbates the pathogenesis of atopic dermatitis by promoting keratinocyte cytotoxicity [6]. Of note, methicillin-resistant *S. aureus* (MRSA) is increasingly more prevalent in atopic dermatitis patients [7], especially in more severe atopic dermatitis patients [6]. MRSA releases more superantigens than methicillin-sensitive *S. aureus*, leaving patients even more vulnerable to infection and cutaneous inflammation.

Though less common and less well-described, in addition to *S. aureus*, *Streptococcus pyogenes* can lead to systemic infections in patients with moderate to severe atopic dermatitis [6] and streptococcal impetigo due to infection with *β*-hemolytic streptococci is increasingly reported in patients with atopic dermatitis [13].

While viral skin infections are not as common as bacterial infections, atopic dermatitis patients are more susceptible to viral skin infections [1, 17]. These infections can be life-threatening [6]. An increased propensity for viral infections may be due to innate and adaptive immune dysfunction [17], with many contributing mechanisms similar to those that predispose atopic dermatitis patients to bacterial infections. For example, the T_h2 inflammatory milieu of atopic skin suppresses antiviral immune responses [1] such as antimicrobial peptide expression [6]. Immunosuppression from atopic dermatitis treatments could also potentially be responsible for making patients more susceptible to cutaneous viral infection, though causation versus correlation is difficult to distinguish given that patients with stronger treatment regimens likely have greater disease severity to begin with [13]. Similarly to bacterial infections, scratching promotes inoculation via skin barrier disruptions and contributes to viral complications [13].

Though herpes simplex virus Type 1 (HSV1) is commonly isolated from the general population [6], the spread of HSV in atopic dermatitis patients can lead to eczema herpeticum (EH) [13]. While only 3% of atopic dermatitis patients present with EH [6], patients oftentimes have recurrent infections [13] and the complication is often associated with earlier onset and more severe atopic dermatitis, along with an increased propensity to develop food allergies and asthma [1].

A few established predisposing factors for the development of EH have been identified. For example, decreased production of cathelicidin, which normally has antiviral activity but is downregulated by the T_h2 phenotype of atopic dermatitis [2], predisposes patients to EH [4, 6]. In addition, patients with filaggrin mutations have a higher risk for developing EH [14]. Interestingly, atopic dermatitis patients with a history of *S. aureus* infection are also more susceptible to EH development [6].

Another potential severe viral complication of atopic dermatitis is eczema vaccinatum (EV). EV is caused by the vaccinia virus (VV) contained in smallpox vaccines and occurs in atopic dermatitis patients upon smallpox vaccination or exposure to vaccinated individuals [8]. Filaggrin deficiency and downstream increased IL-17a expression increases viral replication of VV and contributes to infection [6]. Cathelicidin deficiency in atopic dermatitis skin confers decreased antimicrobial activity and could contribute to the defective innate and adaptive immune responses thought to be responsible for heightened EV in atopic dermatitis patients [17]. Other viral infections such as molluscum contagiosum are also believed to be more common [17] in both atopic and normal skin of atopic dermatitis patients [1].

Fungal infections are also common complications affecting patients with atopic dermatitis. Yeasts such as *Malassezia furfur* (*M. furfur*) are part of the normal skin flora [13], especially on the head and neck [17]. *M. furfur* is equally common among atopic dermatitis patients and healthy patients, yet more atopic dermatitis patients have IgE antibodies against *M. furfur* than healthy controls [17]. This is potentially due to the T_h2-skewed skin immunity of atopic dermatitis patients [17] and skin barrier defects associated with the disease [18]. Infections with *Trichophyton rubrum* and *Epidermophyton* are more likely in atopic dermatitis patients [17, 18], particularly in patients with head and scalp involvement [8]. Interestingly, antifungal therapies have been shown to improve atopic dermatitis [13].

The underlying cutaneous immune dysregulation responsible for the pathogenesis of atopic dermatitis has been known to potentiate infectious complications in atopic dermatitis. Recently, more research has revealed how infection may also contribute to atopic dermatitis pathogenesis. Thus, the relationship between atopic dermatitis and cutaneous infections is perhaps more complex than originally thought. A multifaceted therapeutic approach focused on addressing both skin barrier abnormalities and underlying immune dysregulation may help control disease in atopic dermatitis patients.

5.3 Impact of External Environmental Agents on Disease Flares

Given that atopic dermatitis has varied rates among similar ethnicities [19] and an increasing prevalence in industrialized societies [4], more research has recently been dedicated to examining the impact of environmental agents on precipitating flares of disease.

Atopic dermatitis is often associated with a personal or family history of type 1 hypersensitivity reactions and seasonal allergies [20]. Common allergens include house dust mite antigen, soaps, detergents [1], and aeroallergens [8], among others.

Though investigation into possible environmental triggers of atopic dermatitis is ongoing, results are conflicting and more research has yet to be done [20].

The epidermal abnormalities associated with atopic dermatitis facilitate environmental triggers of atopic dermatitis flares. Abnormal lipid composition of the stratum corneum in atopic dermatitis skin allows for greater allergen and irritant permeability [11]. This increased allergen penetration through the skin may further polarize atopic dermatitis skin towards T_h2 inflammation [14].

One well-established trigger of atopic dermatitis flares is aeroallergens [8, 11]. Inhalation and epicutaneous application of aeroallergens (e.g., house dust mites, animal dander, pollens, and fungi [20]) can induce and/or aggravate skin lesions in atopic dermatitis patients [8]. Furthermore, IgE sensitization to these allergens is directly correlated with disease severity [11]. Reducing aeroallergen exposure has been shown to relieve atopic dermatitis [8] and thus could be one potential recommendation for reducing atopic flares upon further clinical study [20].

Food allergens may increase the pathogenesis of atopic dermatitis in some patients [8, 11] and may contribute to the severity of disease [8] through inducing pruritus and resulting skin lesions [11]. However, there is current debate in the literature regarding whether food allergies are causal flare factors or whether they merely concur with atopic dermatitis [20]. Nevertheless, food allergen-specific T cells have been cloned from atopic dermatitis skin, suggesting a link between food allergies and allergic skin inflammation [8].

With the impact of environmental agents on precipitating flares of disease becoming increasingly apparent, identifying and reducing patient exposure to environmental triggers may be an effective proactive approach to reducing disease in atopic dermatitis patients.

5.4 Complications that Can Arise from Treatments

Many treatment modalities exist for atopic dermatitis. First-line therapy includes non-pharmacologic interventions to restore skin barrier function, such as emollients, skin hydration, and elimination of environmental flare factors [21]. Other pharmacologic therapies, such as phototherapy, topical corticosteroids, topical calcineurin inhibitors, and antibiotics are secondary therapies given that they are associated with more adverse effects. This section will briefly describe complications that may arise from common treatments.

Phototherapy is a second-line treatment after failure of first-line treatments such as emollient use, topical therapies, and environmental modifications [22]. Though there are relatively few adverse effects directly associated with this therapy, phototherapy can lead to cutaneous sensitivity, pruritus, and erythema and can potentially accelerate skin aging and/or increase the likelihood of more serious cutaneous diseases [8].

More serious complications can arise from antibiotic, steroid, and immunosuppressant therapies. For example, sustained antibiotic therapy can lead to the colonization of antibiotic-resistant strains of *S. aureus* and therefore is not recommended unless topical anti-inflammatory therapies fail to control disease on their own [3]. Topical corticosteroid treatments have extremely well documented efficacy in treating atopic dermatitis [23] and are thus recommended as first-line pharmacological therapy [24]. Though the incidence of side effects is low, the adverse effects associated with topical corticosteroid use are more severe compared to that of phototherapy, for example. Short-term use of topical corticosteroids can result in thinning of the skin, telangiectasia and striae. Furthermore, sustained corticosteroid use can result in skin atrophy and is therefore not recommended [23]. Systemic corticosteroid therapy has transient efficacy with significant systemic adverse effects, and thus should be avoided when possible [22]. Immunosuppressants are an effective treatment option for refractory atopic dermatitis, though their systemic administration can result in nausea, headache, nephrotoxicity, hypersensitivity reactions, leukopenia, and increased risk for skin cancer and lymphoma, among other adverse side effects [22].

There have also been complications reported with use of non-steroidal anti-inflammatory therapies, namely topical calcineurin inhibitors. Topical calcineurin inhibitors are produced by *Streptomyces* bacteria and inhibit T cell activation and thus T cell-induced inflammation [23]. Short-term side effects include itching and burning, though such symptoms usually subside with continued use [23]. Given that topical calcineurin inhibitors are anti-inflammatory, they are not recommended for use during active infection [23].

Given the low risk of adverse effects of non-pharmacologic interventions such as emollients, skin hydration, and elimination of environmental flare factors, such interventions are recommended to support strong skin barrier function [21]. Use of such interventions decreases disease severity and may reduce the necessity for pharmacologic therapies [23]. First-line pharmacologic therapy with topical corticosteroids is recommended for patients who have not responded to non-pharmacologic therapies alone. Using topical steroids for short periods of time balances the effectiveness of the therapy in reducing atopic dermatitis signs and symptoms and avoiding adverse effects [23]. Balancing side effects, effectiveness, and disease burden, second-line pharmacologic therapy with topical calcineurin inhibitors or phototherapy is recommended for patients with moderate to severe and/or refractory atopic dermatitis [23].

5.5 Association of Atopic Dermatitis with Lymphoma

There was previously an association of atopic dermatitis with more serious conditions such as lymphoma, especially with respect to the use of topical calcineurin inhibitors [25]. A black-box warning was formulated based off of theoretical use of high-dose oral therapy in post-transplant patients and extreme exposures animal studies [23]. However, there does not appear to be an increased risk of lymphoma associated with topical calcineurin inhibitor use [26].

5.6 Concluding Remarks

Atopic dermatitis is a complex skin disease marked by abnormal skin barrier function and chronic inflammation of the epidermis. Understanding the dynamic relationship between skin barrier defects and underlying inflammation with respect to infection and environmental flare factors is important for improving disease control and managing comorbidities. Proactive skin care to improve cutaneous barrier function, reduction of environmental triggers, and minimization of adverse treatment effects will aid in preventing and treating outbreaks along with reducing complications in atopic dermatitis patients (Table 5.1).

Table 5.1 Complications of atopic dermatitis

Infectious complications	Complications associated with treatment
Bacterial	Phototherapy
Staphylococcus aureus	Cutaneous sensitivity
Streptococcus pyogenes	Pruritus
Viral	Erythema
Eczema herpeticum	Accelerating of skin aging
Eczema vaccinatum	Increased likelihood for serious skin disease
Molluscum contagiosum	Antibiotics
Fungal	Antibiotic resistance
Malassezia furfur	Topical corticosteroids
Trichophyton rubrum	Skin atrophy
Epidermophyton	Telangiectasia
	Striae
Environmental triggers of flares	Systemic corticosteroids
Allergens	Transient efficacy
House dust mite antigen	Systemic adverse effects
Soaps	Systemic immunosuppressants
Detergents	Systemic adverse effects
Aeroallergens	Topical calcineurin inhibitors
Food antigens	Pruritus
	Burning sensation

References

1. Sun D, Ong PY. Infectious complications in atopic dermatitis. Immunol Allergy Clin North Am. 2017;37(1):75–93. http://www.ncbi.nlm.nih.gov/pubmed/27886912. Accessed 26 Dec 2016.
2. Elias PM, Hatano Y, Williams ML. Basis for the barrier abnormality in atopic dermatitis: outside-inside-outside pathogenic mechanisms. J Allergy Clin Immunol. 2008;121:1337–43.
3. Lin YT, Wang CT, Chiang BL. Role of bacterial pathogens in atopic dermatitis. Clin Rev Allergy Immunol. 2007;33(3):167–77. http://www.ncbi.nlm.nih.gov/pubmed/18163223.
4. Bieber T. Atopic dermatitis. N Engl J Med. 2008;358(14):1483–94.
5. Leung DYM. Our evolving understanding of the functional role of filaggrin in atopic dermatitis. J Allergy Clin Immunol. 2009;124(3):494–5. doi:10.1016/j.jaci.2009.07.041.
6. Ong PY, Leung DYM. Bacterial and viral infections in atopic dermatitis: a comprehensive review. Clin Rev Allergy Immunol. 2016;51(3):329–37. doi:10.1007/s12016-016-8548-5.
7. Higaki S, et al. Comparative study of staphylococci from the skin of atopic dermatitis patients and from healthy subjects. Int J Dermatol. 1999;38(4):265–9.
8. Leung DYM, Bieber T. Atopic dermatitis. Lancet. 2003;361(9352):151–60.
9. Leyden JJ, Marples RR, Kligman AM. Staphylococcus aureus in the lesions of atopic dermatitis. Br J Dermatol. 1974;90(5):525–30.
10. Ong PY, et al. Endogenous antimicrobial peptides and skin infections in atopic dermatitis. N Engl J Med. 2002;347(15):1151–60. doi:10.1056/NEJMoa021481.
11. Novak N, Bieber T, Leung DYM. Immune mechanisms leading to atopic dermatitis. J Allergy Clin Immunol. 2003;112(Suppl 6):128–39.
12. Leung DYM. The role of Staphylococcus aureus in atopic eczema. Acta Derm Venereol. 2008;216:21–7.
13. Lübbe J. Secondary infections in patients with atopic dermatitis. Am J Clin Dermatol. 2003;4(9):641–54. https://www.scopus.com/inward/record.uri?eid=2-s2.0-.
14. Boguniewicz M, Leung DYM. Recent insights into atopic dermatitis and implications for management of infectious complications. J Allergy Clin Immunol. 2010;125(1):4–13. doi:10.1016/j.jaci.2009.11.027.
15. Hung S-H, et al. Staphylococcus colonization in atopic dermatitis treated with fluticasone or tacrolimus with or without antibiotics. Ann Allergy Asthma Immunol. 2007;98(1):51–6. http://www.ncbi.nlm.nih.gov/pubmed/17225720.
16. Gonzalez ME, et al. Cutaneous microbiome effects of fluticasone propionate cream and adjunctive bleach baths in childhood atopic dermatitis. J Am Acad Dermatol. 2016;75(3):481–493.e8. http://linkinghub.elsevier.com/retrieve/pii/S0190962216302067.
17. Leung DYM. Infection in atopic dermatitis. Curr Opin Pediatr. 2003;15(4):399–404.
18. Faergemann J. Atopic dermatitis and fungi. Clin Microbiol Rev. 2002;15(4):545–63.
19. Williams H, et al. Worldwide variations in the prevalence of symptoms of atopic eczema in the international study of asthma and allergies in childhood. J Allergy Clin Immunol. 1999;103(1):125–38.
20. Sidbury R, Tom WL, et al. Guidelines of care for the management of atopic dermatitis: section 4. Prevention of disease flares and use of adjunctive therapies and approaches. J Am Acad Dermatol. 2014;71(6):1218–33. doi:10.1016/j.jaad.2014.08.038.
21. Boguniewicz M, Schmid-Grendelmeier P, Leung DYM. Atopic dermatitis. J Allergy Clin Immunol. 2006;118(1):40–3. http://www.ncbi.nlm.nih.gov/pubmed/16815136.
22. Sidbury R, Davis DM, et al. Guidelines of care for the management of atopic dermatitis: section 3. Management and treatment with phototherapy and systemic agents. J Am Acad Dermatol. 2014;71(2):327–49. doi:10.1016/j.jaad.2014.03.030.
23. Eichenfield LF, et al. Guidelines of care for the management of atopic dermatitis: section 2. Management and treatment of atopic dermatitis with topical therapies. J Am Acad Dermatol. 2014;71(1):116–32. doi:10.1016/j.jaad.2014.03.023.

24. Wasserbauer N, Ballow M. Atopic dermatitis. Am J Med. 2009;122(2):121–5. doi:10.1016/j.amjmed.2008.09.014.
25. Legendre L, et al. Risk of lymphoma in patients with atopic dermatitis and the role of topical treatment: a systematic review and meta-analysis. J Am Acad Dermatol. 2015;72(6):992–1002. doi:10.1016/j.jaad.2015.02.1116.
26. Margolis DJ, et al. Association Between Malignancy and Topical Use of Pimecrolimus. JAMA dermatology. 2015;151(6):594–9. Available at: http://www.pubmedcentral.nih.gov/articlerender.fcgi? artid=4465068&tool=pmcentrez&rendertype=abstract.

Chapter 6
The Psychosocial Impact of Atopic Dermatitis

Heather Gochnauer, Rodrigo Valdes-Rodriguez, Leah Cardwell, and Rachel B. Anolik

Abstract Atopic dermatitis is a chronic skin condition which has significant psychosocial and quality of life impact. The condition causes physical discomfort, emotional distress, embarrassment, social stigma and daily activity limitation. In an effort to assess these aspects of disease burden, quality of life measurement tools were developed. Through use of these tools, we have expanded our knowledge of the psychosocial and quality of life burden of this condition. A variety of quality of life assessment tools exist, yet there is no consensus on which tool is best suited to assess the quality of life impact of atopic dermatitis. Research studies assessing quality of life in atopic dermatitis patients utilize a variety of quality of life measurement tools; this complicates comparisons across research studies. Though comparison across studies is difficult, the data echoes tremendous overall burden of disease, especially pertaining to psychosocial status and life quality.

Keywords Atopic dermatitis • Quality of life index • Psychosocial impact atopic dermatitis

---

H. Gochnauer, B.S. • R. Valdes-Rodriguez, M.D.
Section of Dermatology, Reading Health Physician Network, Wyomissing, PA, USA

Department of Dermatology, Lewis Katz School of Medicine at Temple University, Philadelphia, PA, USA

L. Cardwell, M.D.
Department of Dermatology, Wake Forest University School of Medicine, Winston Salem, NC, USA

R.B. Anolik, M.D. (✉)
Section of Dermatology, Reading Health Physician Network, Wyomissing, PA, USA
e-mail: rchlanolik@gmail.com

E.A. Fortson et al. (eds.), *Management of Atopic Dermatitis*, Advances in Experimental Medicine and Biology 1027, DOI 10.1007/978-3-319-64804-0_6

6.1 Introduction

Atopic dermatitis (AD) is a chronic skin disease that affects both the life of the patient and the lives of the patient's family members. Multiple studies have shown that patients with AD, as well as caregivers and family members, have a low quality of life (QoL). This directly impacts daily activities, sleeping habits, and causes higher levels of fatigue, stress, and depression. The stigma surrounding a chronic skin disease such as AD contributes to decreased interactions between patients, parents of patients, and healthy individuals. In this chapter, we will review the tools currently being used to evaluate quality of life in patients with AD and the impact of AD on quality of life in patients and their families.

6.2 Tools Used to Assess QoL in Atopic Dermatitis Patients

Several tools have been created to evaluate the impact of AD in Quality of Life (Table 6.1). The Quality of Life scale was originally created by John Flanagan in the 1970s and has since been adapted for use in several chronic illness groups [11, 12]. This scale, in addition to the associated Health Related Quality of Life (HRQL), has been used in conjunction with measurements of disease type and severity to better understand the social, emotional, and psychological impacts of disease. Accordingly, the World Health Organization (WHO) has broadened the emphasis from just diagnosis and treatment of disease, to self-management and improved well-being, as these health conditions affect all areas of a patient's life.

There are instruments available to objectively measure the impact of chronic skin diseases on individuals and families. The burden of skin diseases includes physical discomfort, emotional distress, embarrassment, social stigma, and limitations to daily activities. In atopic dermatitis the HRQL scale is useful in understanding how one aspect of the disease, such as itching, may affect other aspects, such as sleeping and mental stress [13].

The Health-Related Quality of Life (HRQL) is a quantitative measure of physical, psychological, and social impact of disease. It can be combined with physical measures of eczema severity to correlate disease severity with other manifestations of the disease [14]. Specific tools have been developed to examine QoL in both adults and children with skin diseases. The Children's Dermatology Quality of Life Index (CDQLI) is a ten-item measure designed as a simple practical questionnaire for children [1]. One potential limitation of this instrument is the low number of questions, which may account for lower scores in diseases with a higher psychological impact but fewer clinical symptoms [14]. Similarly, the Infant's Dermatitis Quality of Life Index (IDQoL) and the Dermatitis Family Index (DFI) are each ten item measures designed primarily to assess symptoms, functioning, and emotional effects. With a limited number of items, it is unknown how comprehensively each questionnaire measures the complex emotional effects of AD [3]. To address this,

Table 6.1 Tools to assess quality of life in patients with atopic dermatitis

Tool name	Target population	Self-reported (Y/N)[a]	Evaluate	References
Children's dermatology quality of life index (CDQLI)	Children with skin disease 4–16 years old	Y	10-item measure	Lewis-Jones and Finlay [1]
Infant's dermatitis quality of life index (IDQoL)	Infants with eczema under 4 years old	N	10-item measure	Lewis-Jones and Finlay [2]
Childhood atopic dermatitis impact scale (CADIS)	Children with eczema 0–6 years old (and parents)	N	45-item; more emphasis on emotional effects	Chamlin et al. [3]
Skindex-teen	Adolescents between 12 and 17 years old	Y	Adolescent-specific	Smidt et al. [4]
Skindex-29	Adults	Y	Changes in QoL in relation to clinical status changes; 29-item measure	Chren et al. [5–7]
Dermatitis family index (DFI)	Families (including caregivers, siblings, and patients)	Y and N[b]	10-item measure	Lawson et al. [8]
Dermatology-specific quality of life (DSQL)	Adults	Y	Varies in item number; e.g., 52-item for contact dermatitis	Anderson and Rajagopalan [9]
Dermatology life quality index (DLQI)	Adults	Y	10-item measure	Finlay and Khan [10]

[a]Self-reported (Y) means that the patient with AD fills in the questionnaire. Otherwise, it is assumed that the primary caregiver of the patients fills in the questionnaire
[b]DFI is completed by caregivers, family members, and patients themselves

Chamlin et al. [3] developed and used the Childhood Atopic Dermatitis Impact Scale (CADIS). This 45-item questionnaire takes approximately 6 min to complete and provides a score (0–180) that emphasizes the emotional effects of AD [3].

The Dermatology Life Quality Index (DLQI) was created by Finlay and Khan in 1994. The DLQI is a ten question survey that was designed to be a simple, practical questionnaire for routine clinical use, only taking about 1–3 min to complete [10]. The DLQI was created to meet the need for a very simple but sensitive method of measuring disability caused by skin diseases [10].

The Skindex-29 is a dermatologic quality of life instrument first developed in 1996 by Chren et al. to measure the impact of skin disease on health-related quality of life in patients with different dermatological conditions and to assess changes in quality of life in relation to clinical status changes [6]. Items were arranged into three areas: physical symptoms, emotions, and functioning. It has been argued that factors influencing adolescents' QoL are fundamentally different from those observed in children and adults, leading to the development of the adolescent-specific Skindex-Teen [4].

The Dermatology-Specific Quality of Life (DSQL) was developed to evaluate treatment effects on well-being. The DSQL is a disease-targeted instrument which has been validated for several disease states in dermatology [9].

There currently exists a plethora of QoL assessment tools used for AD. Unfortunately, the list of QoL scales and measurements prevents consistency among studies and hinders the ability to draw generalized conclusions. A systematic review of QoL instruments for infants, children and adolescents with eczema was recently completed by Heinl et al. [15]. This review examined numerous measurement tools including CADIS, IDQoL, and the CDQLI and found that no QoL instrument for infants, children, or adolescents with eczema could be highly recommended [15]. Nearly all of the existing QoL instruments are lacking significant validation data and many investigate measurement properties in a methodologically poor manner and thus lack interpretability data. Additionally, many of the instruments are reported by the parents of the patient rather than self-reported by the affected child [15].

Hill et al. [16] sought to assess recent trends in the use of disease severity and QoL outcome instruments conducted on patients with AD between July 2010 and July 2015. They limited their assessment to randomized clinical trials and studies published in English. A total of 135 studies were included. Of these 135 studies, only 45 assessed QoL. Sixty two of these studies assessed disease severity measures, and 28 QoL scales were identified. This study aptly demonstrates that the number of tools to measure disease severity and QoL in patients with AD is on the rise. The standardization of these instruments is imperative for comparability among studies and improved quality of evidence. The four most widely used QoL measures included DLQI [10], IDQoL [2], CDLQI [1], and the DFI questionnaire [8]. Approximately 75% of the identified QoL instruments in the above assessment were used only once. If the number of QoL measures continues to rise, it will be increasingly difficult to draw inter-study comparisons [16].

The increasing number of measurements to assess disease severity and QoL in patients with AD hinders their use in studying broader trends and comparisons and limits their translation to clinical practice. To improve the comparability of disease severity and QoL instruments, standardization is needed among studies [16].

6.3 Review of Current Literature on Quality of Life in AD Patients

Multiple studies have shown the devastating impact of this disease in children and adolescents. Atopic dermatitis can either persist into or present in adulthood, manifesting its negative influence on quality of life. Margolis et al. [17] demonstrated that symptoms associated with AD seem to continue well into the second decade of a child's life and likely longer. Considering that the symptoms of AD can persist into adulthood, it follows that the quality of life in adult patients is also negatively affected. Furthermore, several studies have shown that AD not only affects patients' quality of life, but also that of family members and caregivers of patients with AD. In this section, we will review the impact of atopic dermatitis on children and adult patients as well as their family members and caregivers.

6.3.1 Impact on Patients: Children

In a study by Beattie and Lewis-Jones [18], AD caused the greatest impairment in quality of life among children with chronic skin conditions, such as psoriasis and urticaria. Atopic dermatitis also proved to cause a higher impairment when compared with other chronic childhood conditions such as cystic fibrosis and renal disease. Interestingly, AD was second only to cerebral palsy in impact on QoL among children with chronic diseases [18].

Perhaps, this stems from the broad impact of atopic dermatitis. AD affects many physical, social, and emotional aspects of a patient's quality of life. Chamlin et al. [19] interviewed parents of 26 children with AD. At least 20% of participating families listed the following impacts of AD on physical health: itching, scratching, sleep interruptions, pain, bleeding, and dietary limitations. Emotional impacts included behavioral problems, irritability, crying, and treatment related issues such as stress related to application of topical and oral medications. AD interfered with activities such as bathing, playing (especially outside), and swimming. Socially, both adults and children avoided interactions with children with AD, most often for fear the rash was contagious. Chamlin et al. [19] also reported that parents of children with AD avoided other parents to protect themselves and their child from unsolicited advice and fear regarding medications. This study, Chamlin et al. [19], identified important ways that AD affects the life of patients. However, it should be mentioned that this study did not measure disease severity of the children involved and that this study was conducted in a tertiary care setting and the sampled population was likely skewed toward more severe AD.

As stated above, several factors contribute to poor quality of life in patients with AD. Sleep disturbances and itching are consistently named as the greatest causes of discomfort in patients with AD. Itching often presents prior to the onset of the rash and can be quite persistent. Itching is considered the major cause of sleep complications in patients with AD. In a study by Kong et al. [20], 50 pediatric AD patients and 50 adult AD patients were evaluated for severity of disease, sleep habits, and QoL. They found that severity of disease and sleep scores were significantly correlated in children but not in adults. Specifically, children's disease severity, as measured by the SCORing Atopic Dermatitis (SCORAD) index, was significantly associated with five components of the Children's Sleep Habit's Questionnaire (CSHQ): bedtime resistance, sleep onset delay, sleep anxiety, parasomnias, and sleep disordered breathing. Adult patients' SCORAD scores were associated with two components of the Pittsburgh Sleep Quality Index (PSQI): subjective sleep quality and sleep latency. In both children and adults, pruritus scores were associated with sleep disturbances (CSHQ and PSQI scores), which was similar to several other previous studies. Kong et al. [20] also reported that greater disease severity is significantly correlated with poorer QoL and that poorer QoL is significantly correlated with disrupted sleep in both children and adults. One limitation of this study is that they did not account for confounding factors that may also impact sleep, such as obesity. Sleep disturbances, however, remain an important issue for patients with AD. A study by Chamlin et al. [21], reported that of the 270 participating parents, 183 (68%) reported that their child's sleep was disturbed by atopic dermatitis and 166 (61%) reported that their own sleep was disturbed. Additional studies have found that factors impairing QoL in patients with AD include itching and scratching, sleep problems, influence on the child's mood, fears and phobias of treatment, and ability to participate in sports [22–26].

Numerous studies have demonstrated that as disease severity increases, QoL decreases in patients with AD [27] assessed the impact of AD on QoL of Saudi infants and children (n = 630). A positive correlation was observed between the severity of AD and the QoL scores. Three items were identified that negatively impacted the Infant's Dermatitis Quality of Life Index (IDQoL): itching and scratching, the child's mood, and time to get the child to sleep. All of these reached a statistically significantly difference in the severe group as compared with the moderate or mild groups. No significant differences were observed concerning gender or the association with other atopic disorders. Similarly, Maksimovic et al. [28] reported that increasing disease severity was associated with greater impairment on QoL in both children and adults. Patients with AD had inferior social functioning and mental health scores compared with the general population. In a study of Italian children with AD and their families, Monti et al. [29] showed a strong association between severe AD and poor QoL, both in children and mothers. Interestingly, the family's QoL scores were more related to AD severity than the child's QoL, highlighting the strong impact of the disease on the familial unit. Finally, a study by Ho et al. [24] investigated the influence of childhood AD on the health of mothers and its impact on Asian families. This study demonstrated that the severity of childhood AD leads to negative family relationships through reduction of physical and mental health of the mothers, and is independent of patients' Health Related Quality of Life (HRQoL) and socio-demographics.

Mental health of patients is another important aspect of atopic dermatitis. In a large sample (n = 3775) of high school students in Norway, Halvorsen et al. [30] found that mental health problems and suicidal ideation were associated with eczema and that there was an even higher prevalence among students with both eczema and itch.

Atopic dermatitis affects numerous physical, social, emotional, and mental aspects of patients' lives. Each component of a patient's life needs to be considered to provide the best treatment and care possible. Both children and adults with AD face these challenges as this skin disease often persists or presents later in life.

6.3.2 *Impact on Patients: Adults*

It was previously believed that children outgrow AD. However, it is now known that AD can persist into adulthood or the onset of disease can be later in life [17]. A US population based survey by Silverberg et al. [31] demonstrated that adults with eczema and fatigue were more likely to rate their overall health as only fair or poor compared with participants without eczema or fatigue. In addition to the physical limitations seen in children with AD, adults face challenges in the workplace and with intimate relationships [32].

Roosta et al. [33] conducted a survey of college students and found that 25.5% of participants with self-reported eczema believed that it impaired their social life. Halvorsen et al. [30] reported that high school boys with eczema were less likely to have had romantic relationships. Misery et al. [34] report that 57.5% of patients had decreased sexual desire due to AD (n = 266). In the same study, the quality of life of partners did not appear to be particularly impaired, but 36.5% reported that the appearance of eczema had an impact on their sex life. In a community based survey by Anderson and Rajagopalan [13], self-reported patients claimed that social functioning was limited mainly by lack of comfort in groups and not feeling free to do enjoyable things.

Activities of daily living can also be affected in patients with AD. Thirty five per cent of self-reported AD patients faced clothing choice limitations and 32% reported limitations in shaving or wearing makeup [13]. According to this same study, self-perception was another common area of concern, with 20–25% of respondents reporting embarrassment or anger due to their skin disease [13].

Atopic dermatitis also impacts the work life of patients. Nyren et al. [35], analyzed 405 cases of patients with AD as children and found an increased risk for future career changes, sick leave, and medical consultations due to the increased risk of hand eczema. Similarly, Zuberbier et al. [36], found that 32% of participants believed that AD affected their school or work life, and 14% of participating adults believed that their career progression had been hindered. AD is a risk factor for occupational skin disease and patients have reported consequently avoiding specific jobs. Occupations avoided include those in health care, food preparation, cleaning, hairdressing, and automobile repair [35, 37, 38]. These studies highlight the importance of treatment and patient care to address factors outside of the physical symptoms. Adult patients need to be equipped with resources and tools to address challenges faced in the workplace as well as those faced during social interactions.

The correlation between QoL in patients with AD and disease severity seems to be less clear in adults. Chrostowska-Plak et al. [39] examined the relationship between itch and psychological status of adult patients with AD. They reported that patients with symptoms suggesting depression had more intense pruritus compared with other patients. However, the association of QoL with objective disease severity is often modest [28, 39–41]. In a study of 54 patients with severe AD, disease activity correlated better with QoL when disease activity was less severe, and disease extent correlated better with QoL than disease severity [40]. This suggests that factors other than disease activity may influence QoL in patients with AD, such as involvement of certain areas on the body (e.g., face, genitals) [34, 42, 43].

In a survey of 107 adult AD patients (>16 years old), Kiebert et al. [44] examined self-reported disease severity as it relates to Health-Related Quality of Life (HRQL) scores and compared these scores with other chronic conditions. HRQL was measured using the Short Form-36 Health Survey (SF-36) and the Dermatology Life Quality Index (DLQI). Patients with AD had poorer mental health scores compared to those with type 2 diabetes or hypertension, and inferior social functioning scores compared with patients with hypertension. SF-36 mental component scores of patients with AD were significantly worse than patients with psoriasis. Self-reported severity in patients with AD correlated with poorer HRQL scores for both children (n = 132) and adults (n = 107) [44]. Pitfalls of these data include the limitations of recruitment to tertiary care centers and the confounding factors of age and sex when comparing SF-36 scores of the participant population with those of the general population or with those of people with other chronic conditions [45]. Despite these drawbacks, this study does highlight the importance of psychological and social factors in patients with AD.

6.4 QoL in Family Members of Patients with Atopic Dermatitis

Several studies have shown that the family members or caregivers of children with AD also face significant challenges that adversely affect their QoL. This is an important issue to address when caring for patients with AD and for equipping families and caregivers with strategies to overcome these challenges.

In a large, multi-national study of patients with moderate to severe AD, Zuberbier et al. [36] reported that 30% of patients and caregivers believe that AD affects other members of their household (n = 2002). Parents of affected children may experience sleep disturbances, as well as report negative social effects and emotional feelings of guilt, blame, worry, and frustration as a consequence of their child's skin disorder [19]. In a German study using the SF-12 Health Survey, a generic measure of overall health, Warschburger et al. [46] found that maternal mental health scores were significantly impaired on average when compared with mental health scores of parents with healthy children. No association was found between disease severity and parental mental health scores [46]. This study is difficult to generalize to a broader population, however, because it was conducted in a pediatric inpatient AD program [45]. Additionally, a study by Gieler et al. [47] reported that single mothers of children with AD had higher levels of stress than single mothers of healthy children. Though it is unclear as to the exact extent to which family members of patients with AD are affected, it is evident that these family members face additional challenges.

Chamlin et al. [19] reported that the extra time required to care for a child with AD can be a burden for families. However, the amount of extra time that parents spend with their children is variable. Holm and Jemec [48] reported that in patients with relatively severe AD, families spent an average of 63 min per day managing their children's AD. Another study by the same group found only 17 min per day spent on caring for atopic children, despite being conducted in a similar setting [49]. Furthermore, a small study in the United Kingdom showed that mothers spent 78 additional minutes and fathers spent 90 min per night attending to children with AD, compared with no additional time for parents of children with asthma [50]. Regardless of time spent, AD causes disruptions in the daily lives of patients, caregivers, and family members.

6.5 Stigma Associated with Atopic Dermatitis and Tools for Management

Unfortunately, chronic skin diseases often lead to patients' negative self-perceptions and experiencing stigmatization. Atopic dermatitis is no exception to this. According to Schmid-Ott and Steen [51], stigmatization in skin disease is the presence of skin lesions which lead to a person being judged and causes a lack of acceptance, anxiety and dysfunction in social settings. It is important to identify the consequences of stigmatization associated with AD and to provide practical tools to prevent or mitigate this suffering in patients with AD. Commonly encountered stigma include discrimination and bullying. Patient's with AD may be criticized for scratching, bullied/shamed by peers for having skin lesions, or viewed cautiously by people who believe their lesions contagious [52].

As suggested previously, there are social impacts of AD that need to be addressed. In Chamlin et al. [19], over half of parents interviewed stated that adults and other children avoided interacting with their children with AD. Parents also reported that they themselves limited interactions between their children and family and friends so that they would not have to engage in discussion about the child's skin. The International Study on Life with Atopic Eczema found major impacts on the self-esteem of patients with AD. Twenty seven per cent of those surveyed had been teased or bullied because of AD, and 36% said AD affects their self-confidence [36].

LeBocidge et al. [53] list several components of multidisciplinary treatment approaches that should be addressed to effectively manage this condition. These include medical evaluation and management by an AD specialist, education and nursing care, psychological and behavioral support, and nutritional assessment and guidance. They also list components of an education and care plan including important areas such as strategies to break the itch-scratch cycle, stress management, optimal sleep hygiene, and strategies to handle peer questions/teasing [53]. As suggested, patients with AD need both physical treatments and psychological care. As patient's visible symptoms improve, generally so does stigmatization and overall social and psychological well-being of patient and parents.

Table 6.2 Management tools for problems associated with atopic dermatitis

Problem	Tool
Itch-scratch cycle	Cooling, alternative skin stimulation, relaxation, distraction, skin care, habit reversal training
Stress management	Muscle relaxation; meditation; positive outlets such as art or music
Peer questions/teasing	Clearly explain disease without being defensive; explain that it is not contagious
Low self-esteem	Train parents to emphasize positive characteristics of their children; cognitive therapy

Tools are needed to help combat these stigmas and to improve the QoL in patients with AD and their families. Providing education and training to parents and their children regarding these stigmas improves their coping mechanisms [54]. In Table 6.2 we identify several problems encountered by patients with AD and possible tools to help manage these issues such as Habit Reversal Training and alternative skin stimulation [55].

6.6 Conclusion

Atopic dermatitis is a chronic skin disease that has a dramatic impact on the quality of life of both patient and family. Multiple studies have shown that patients with AD, caregivers, and family members suffer from a low quality of life (QoL). Factors such as impaired sleep and itch play a large role in disruption of normal activities of daily living. Furthermore, stigma surrounding chronic skin diseases can create negative social environments and impair intimate relationships. Strategies need to be identified and implemented so those affected can cope with the negative effects of atopic dermatitis and quality of life can be improved for both patients and their families.

References

1. Lewis-Jones MS, Finlay AY. The Children's dermatology life quality index (CDLQI): initial validation and practical use. Br J Dermatol. 1995;132:942–9.
2. Lewis-Jones MS, Finlay AY, Dykes PJ. The infants' dermatitis quality of life index. Br J Dermatol. 2001;144:104–10.
3. Chamlin SL, Cella D, Frieden IJ, Williams ML, Mancini AJ, Lai JS, et al. Development of the childhood atopic dermatitis impact scale: initial validation of a quality-of-life measure for young children with atopic dermatitis and their families. J Invest Dermatol. 2005a;125:1106–11.
4. Smidt AC, Lai JS, Cella D, et al. Development and validation of Skindex-Teen, a quality-of-life instrument for adolescents with skin disease. Arch Dermatol. 2010;146:865–9.
5. Chren MM, Lasek RJ, Quinn LM, et al. Skindex, a quality-of-life measure for patients with skin diseases: reliability, validity and responsiveness. J Invest Dermatol. 1996;107:707–13.

6. Chren MM. The Skindex instruments to measure the effects of skin disease on quality of life. Dermatol Clin. 2012;30(2):231–6. doi:10.1016/j.det.2011.11.003.
7. Chren MM, Lasek RJ, Flocke SA, Zyzanski SJ. Improved discriminative and evaluative capability of a refined version of Skindex, a quality-of-life instrument for patients with skin diseases. Arch Dermatol. 1997;133(11):1433–40.
8. Lawson V, Lewis-Jones MS, Finlay AY, Reid P, Owens RG. The family impact of childhood atopic dermatitis: the dermatitis family impact questionnaire. Br J Dermatol. 1998;138:107–13.
9. Anderson RT, Rajagopalan R. Development and validation of a quality of life instrument for cutaneous diseases. J Am Acad Dermatol. 1997;37:41–50.
10. Finlay AY, Khan GK. Dermatology life quality index (DLQI): a simple practical measure for routine clinical use. Clin Exp Dermatol. 1994;19:210–6.
11. Flanagan JC. A research approach to improving our quality of life. Am Psychol. 1978;33:138–47. doi:10.1037//0003-066X.33.2.138.
12. Flanagan JC. Measurement of the quality of life: current state of the art. Arch Phys Med Rehabil. 1982;63:56–9.
13. Anderson RT, Rajagopalan R. Effects of allergic dermatosis on health-related quality of life. Curr Allergy Asthma Rep. 2001;1:309e15.
14. Lewis-Jones S. Measuring the burden of atopic eczema in young children and the family unit. Soc Invest Dermatol. 2005;125:viii. doi:10.1111/j.0022-202X.2005.23970.x.
15. Heinl D, Prinsen CAC, Sach T, Drucker AM, Ofenloch R, Flohr C, Apfelbacher C. Measurement properties of quality-of-life measurement instruments for infants, children and adolescents with eczema: a systematic review. Br J Dermatol. 2017;176(4):878–89. doi:10.1111/bjd.1496.
16. Hill MK, Pishkenari AK, Braunberger TL, Armstrong AW, Dunnick CA. Recent trends in disease severity and quality of life instruments for patients with atopic dermatitis: a systematic review. J Am Acad Dermatol. 2016;75:906–17.
17. Margolis JS, Abuabara K, Bilker W, Hoffstad O, Margolis DJ. Persistence of mild to moderate atopic dermatitis. JAMA Dermatol. 2014;150:593e600.
18. Beattie PE, Lewis-Jones MS. A comparative study of impairment of quality of life in children with skin disease and children with other chronic childhood diseases. Br J Dermatol. 2006;155:145e5.
19. Chamlin SL, Frieden IJ, Williams ML, Chren MM. Effects of atopic dermatitis on young American children and their families. Pediatrics. 2004;114:607e11.
20. Kong TS, Han TY, Lee JH, Son SJ. Correlation between severity of atopic dermatitis and sleep quality in children and adults. Ann Dermatol. 2016;28(3):321–6. doi:10.5021/ad.2016.28.3.321.
21. Chamlin SL, Mattson CL, Frieden IJ, et al. The price of pruritus: sleep disturbance and cosleeping in atopic dermatitis. Arch Pediatr Adolesc Med. 2005;159:745e50.
22. Ben-Gashir MA, Seed PT, Hay RJ. Quality of life and disease severity are correlated in children with atopic dermatitis. Br J Dermatol. 2004;150:284e90.
23. Ganemo A, Svensson A, Lindberg M, Wahlgren CF. Quality of life in Swedish children with eczema. Acta Derm Venereol. 2007;87:345e9.
24. Ho RC, Giam YC, Ng TP, et al. The influence of childhood atopic dermatitis on health of mothers, and its impact on Asian families. Pediatr Allergy Immunol. 2010;21:501e7.
25. Hon KL, Tsang YC, Pong NH, et al. Correlations among steroid fear, acceptability, usage frequency, quality of life and disease severity in childhood eczema. J Dermatolg Treat. 2015;26:418e25.
26. Ricci G, Bendandi B, Bellini F, Patrizi A, Masi M. Atopic dermatitis: quality of life of young Italian children and their families and correlation with severity score. Pediatr Allergy Immunol. 2007;18:245e9.
27. Alzolibani AA. Impact of atopic dermatitis on the quality of life of Saudi children. Saudi Med J. 2014;35:391e6.
28. Maksimovic N, Jankovic S, Marinkovic J, Sekulovic LK, Zivkovic Z, Spiric VT. Health-related quality of life in patients with atopic dermatitis. J Dermatol. 2012;39:42e7.

29. Monti F, Agostini F, Gobbi F, Neri E, Schianchi S, Arcangeli F. Quality of life measures in Italian children with atopic dermatitis and their families. Ital J Pediatr. 2011;37:59.
30. Halvorsen JA, Lien L, Dalgard F, Bjertness E, Stern RS. Suicidal ideation, mental health problems, and social function in adolescents with eczema: a population-based study. J Invest Dermatol. 2014;134:1847e54.
31. Silverberg JI, Garg NK, Paller AS, Fishbein AB, Zee PC. Sleep disturbances in adults with eczema are associated with impaired overall health: a US population-based study. J Invest Dermatol. 2015a;135:56e66.
32. Holm EA, Wulf HC, Stegmann H, Jemec GB. Life quality assessment among patients with atopic eczema. Br J Dermatol. 2006b;154:719e25.
33. Roosta N, Black DS, Peng D, Riley LW. Skin disease and stigma in emerging adulthood: impact on healthy development. J Cutan Med Surg. 2010;14:285e90.
34. Misery L, Finlay AY, Martin N, et al. Atopic dermatitis: impact on the quality of life of patients and their partners. Dermatology. 2007;215:123e9.
35. Nyren M, Lindberg M, Stenberg B, Svensson M, Svensson A, Meding B. Influence of childhood atopic dermatitis on future worklife. Scand J Work Environ Health. 2005;31:474e8.
36. Zuberbier T, Orlow SJ, Paller AS, et al. Patient perspectives on the management of atopic dermatitis. J Allergy Clin Immunol. 2006;118:226e32.
37. Dickel H, Bruckner TM, Schmidt A, Diepgen TL. Impact of atopic skin diathesis on occupational skin disease incidence in a working population. J Invest Dermatol. 2003;121:37e40.
38. Holm EA, Esmann S, Jemec GB. The handicap caused by atopic dermatitis—sick leave and job avoidance. J Eur Acad Dermatol Venereol. 2006a;20:255e9.
39. Chrostowska-Plak D, Reich A, Szepietowski JC. Relationship between itch and psychological status of patients with atopic dermatitis. J Eur Acad Dermato Venereol. 2013;27:e239e42.
40. Haeck IM, ten Berge O, van Velsen SG, de Bruin-Weller MS, Bruijnzeel-Koomen CA, Knol MJ. Moderate correlation between quality of life and disease activity in adult patients with atopic dermatitis. J Eur Acad Dermatol Venereol. 2012;26:236e41.
41. Wittkowski A, Richards HL, Griffiths CE, Main CJ. The impact of psychological and clinical factors on quality of life in individuals with atopic dermatitis. J Psychomsom Res. 2004;57:195e200.
42. Beikert FC, Langenbruch AK, Radtke MA, Kornek T, Purwins S, Augustin M. Willingness to pay and quality of life in patients with atopic dermatitis. Arch Dermatol Res. 2014;306:279e86.
43. Holm EA, Esmann S, Jemec GB. Does visible atopic dermatitis affect quality of life more in women than in men? Gend Med. 2004;1:125e30.
44. Kiebert G, Sorensen SV, Revicki D, et al. Atopic dermatitis is associated with a decrement in health-related quality of life. Int J Dermatol. 2002;41:151e8.
45. Drucker AM, Wang AR, Li WQ, et al. The burden of atopic dermatitis: summary of a report for the National Eczema Association. J Invest Dermatol. 2017;137(1):26–30. doi:10.1016/j.jid.2016.07.012.
46. Warschburger P, Buchholz HT, Petermann F. Psychological adjustment in parents of young children with atopic dermatitis: which factors predict parental quality of life? Br J Dermatol. 2004;150:304e11.
47. Gieler U, Schoof S, Gieler T, Sibylle S, Schut C, Kupfer J. Atopic eczema and stress among single parents and families: an empirical study of 96 mothers. Acta Derm Venereol. 2017;97(1):42–6. doi:10.2340/00015555-2457.
48. Holm EA, Jemec GB. Time spent on treatment of atopic dermatitis: a new method of measuring pediatric morbidity? Pediatr Dermatol. 2004;21:623e7.
49. Jemec GB, Esmann S, Holm EA, Tycho A, Jorgensen TM. Time spent on treatment (TSOT). An independent assessment of disease severity in atopic dermatitis. Acta Dermatovenerol Alp Pannonica Adriat. 2006;15:119e24.
50. Moore K, David TJ, Murray CS, Child F, Arkwright PD. Effect of childhood eczema and asthma on parental sleep and well-being: a prospective comparative study. Br J Dermatol. 2006;154:514e8.

51. Schmid-Ott G, Steen T. Skin disorders and quality of life. In: Stone JH, Blouin M, editors. International encyclopedia of rehabilitation; 2010. http://cirrie.buffalo.edu/encyclopedia/en/article/152/. Accessed 17 June 2016.
52. Ring J. Atopic dermatitis: eczema. Berlin: Springer; 2016.
53. LeBocidge JS, Elverson RD, Timmons KG, Hawryluk EB, Rea C, Lee M, Schneider LC. Multidisciplinary interventions in the management of atopic dermatitis. J Allergy Clin Immunol. 2016;138:325–34.
54. Kupfer J, Gieler U, Diepgen TL, et al. Structured education program improves the coping with atopic dermatitis in children and their parents-a multicenter, randomized controlled trial. J Psychosom Res. 2010;68:353–8.
55. Schut C, Mollanazar NK, Kupfer J, Gieler U, Yosipovitch G. Psychological interventions in the treatment of chronic itch. Acta Derm Venerol. 2016;96:157–61.

Chapter 7
Stressors in Atopic Dermatitis

Steven Barilla, Kayla Felix, and Joseph L. Jorizzo

Abstract As with other inflammatory skin disorders, atopic dermatitis has a tendency to cause stress and also be exacerbated by it. Patients with atopic dermatitis have several disease-associated stressors, some of which include physical discomfort due to itching and altered appearance due to flare-ups. These stressors have been shown to effect patients psychosocially by altering sleep patterns, decreasing self-esteem and interfering with interpersonal relationships. In combination with its direct effect on patients, atopic dermatitis also causes stress for parents and caregivers. Studies suggest that atopic dermatitis is strongly correlated with co-sleeping habits, which can negatively impact the health and mood of parents or caregivers. It has also been reported to interfere with the formation of a strong mother-child relationship. In order to optimize treatment for patients with atopic dermatitis, it is important to note the impact that it has on quality of life. By implementing patient counseling, sleep-targeted therapies, and the use of quality of life (QoL) indices, atopic dermatitis patients and caregivers have the potential to experience greater satisfaction with treatment.

Keywords Atopic dermatitis • Stress • Quality of life • Sleep impact

7.1 Introduction

Atopic dermatitis is an important clinical disease that not only causes stress and anxiety but also is exacerbated by stress creating a vicious cycle for many of the patients affected by this illness. The key pathomechanism of atopic dermatitis is decreased barrier function of the skin due to filaggrin deficiency in the stratum corneum, but many additional pathogenic factors have been associated with this atopic disease [1]. A complex interconnection between structural, genetic, environmental, social and immunologic factors play a role in the pathogenesis of atopic dermatitis

S. Barilla, B.S., B.A. (✉) • K. Felix, B.S. • J.L. Jorizzo, M.D.
Department of Dermatology, Wake Forest University School of Medicine,
Winston Salem, NC, USA
e-mail: sbarilla@wakehealth.edu

E.A. Fortson et al. (eds.), *Management of Atopic Dermatitis*, Advances in Experimental Medicine and Biology 1027, DOI 10.1007/978-3-319-64804-0_7

as well as in its clinical progression and associated flare ups. One important environmental factor that is thought to play a role is stress, which likely contributes to disease progression through several mechanisms [2]. Atopic dermatitis has been found to have a large impact on the quality of life of affected children and caregivers. It is hypothesized that stress as well as other psychosocial factors alter immune function and neuroendocrine pathways and further alter skin barrier function [2]. The psychobiological model of atopic dermatitis involves psychosocial factors that affect disease progression and severity in a multifactorial manner while atopic dermatitis greatly distresses the affected person [2]. This model is not unique to this disease and has been thought to be involved in other dermatologic conditions, including psoriasis [2, 3].

The importance of preventing excessive stress cannot be underscored enough, as stress has been consistently shown to worsen proinflammatory disorders such as atopic dermatitis [3]. The mechanism of stress induced exacerbation is multifactorial and involves several pathways and inflammatory mediators. Factors that contribute to stress-related change in disease course include but are not limited to a shift to predominantly type 2 T-helper cells (Th2), impaired response to stressful stimuli by the hypothalamic-pituitary axis (HPA axis), cytokine profile alteration and further dysfunction of the barrier function of the skin [2]. The dysregulation of normal immune function causes the body to react to nonspecific environmental allergens that would not typically produce an immune response [2]. Increased predominance of Th2 T-cells as compared to Th1 T-cells can have numerous effects on the immunologic profile of the body, further increasing the likelihood of atopic reactions. Communication between the nervous system and the immune system related to stress further dysregulates the immune system by promoting mast cell degranulation through a number of transmitters released from nerve terminals causing increased release of mediators which promote inflammation and pruritus at the level of the skin [2].

7.2 Chronic Stress and the HPA Axis

This complex immune dysregulation is also seen in other areas of the body's physiologic functioning. Atopic dermatitis leads to numerous disturbances in the life of the patient thus creating an environment of chronic stress and decreased quality of life. Chronic stress has been shown to lead to a blunted response of the HPA axis, thus leaving the body more susceptible to inflammatory conditions including atopic dermatitis [2]. HPA axis hypofunctioning not only creates an environment for worsening disease but also increases the likelihood of stress in the future [2]. Cells in the skin have also been shown to produce corticotropin releasing hormone (CRH), similar to that which is released by the brain in response to stress. This can lead to local inflammatory reactions and mast cell degranulation similar to what is seen with nervous-immune communication [2]. With the added combination of pro-opiomelanocortin peptides, which further suppress proper cell-mediated immune function in the skin as well as the increased stress-related corticosteroid disruption of the stratum corneum, the body and skin become susceptible to chronic inflammatory states perpetuated by stress and in turn create patient distress further exacerbating this vicious cycle [2].

7.3 Stress and the Psychosocial Impact of Atopic Dermatitis

Atopic dermatitis, although not often a condition associated with life threatening complications, still creates a profound impact on the lives of patients with severe psychosocial distress and impairment of normal activities. Not only do patients have to deal with the distress caused by the disease and its treatments, but physical skin lesions can lead to further psychosocial distress, stigmatization and decreased social perception of self [4]. Society has a major focus on physical image and skin disease can generate anxiety, especially in younger patients. Childhood and adolescence are a time when people are trying to establish their place in society and role among peers. Self-image, which is a subjective view of self and one's body, can be altered by atopic dermatitis leading to poor social acceptance and increased social anxiety among children and adolescents [5]. Although psychological impact of atopic dermatitis is studied less often in adults, the disease remains prevalent in the adult population and studies have shown AD to be associated with higher levels of psychological stress and depression [6].

7.4 Sleep Disturbance in Atopic Dermatitis

Atopic dermatitis is a cutaneous disease with health complications reaching far beyond the skin [7]. One major health complication involves sleep disturbance. As many as 50–60% of children with atopic dermatitis experience chronic sleep disturbance, which has a profound impact on quality of life and daily living [8–10]. Sleep disturbances also affect parents, siblings and caretakers living in the home of the affected child [10]. Multiple areas of sleep are affected including difficulty falling asleep (increased sleep latency), difficulty staying asleep (frequent nighttime awakenings) and decreased total sleep time. Poor sleep hygeine can lead to increased irritability, daytime somnolence, aggressive or moody behaviors and discipline problems in school [10, 11]. The reasons behind sleep disturbance may be more complicated than initially thought and may be multifactorial. Classic theories behind sleep disturbance in atopic dermatitis place the blame on the presence of skin inflammation which causes intense and frequent scratching. More severe disease often leads to more severe itching as well as release of a number of inflammatory mediators that further worsen symptoms [12]. Newer theories point to additional causes.

Polysomnography studies in school-aged children with atopic dermatitis have shown frequent episodes of nighttime awakenings due to scratching episodes [13]. In children who reported their happiness was negatively affected by atopic dermatitis, there was an eightfold increase in the prevalence of sleep disturbance [13]. School performance is another aspect of a child's life that is impacted by poor sleep. Dahl et al. demonstrated a significant negative correlation between difficulty falling asleep due to pruritus and ease of waking up in the morning as well as a positive correlation between difficulty falling asleep and major school discipline problems [11].

Co-sleeping is common in patients with atopic dermatitis; whether it is sharing a room with siblings or spending time in the room of parents. One study found 30% of parents of patients with atopic dermatitis reported co-sleeping with their child due to the disease, and this was bothersome for a majority of these parents [13]. Families of patients who suffer from atopic dermatitis also report sleep disturbances due to frequent awakenings of the patient as a result of the disease. There was a significant association between higher SCORAD index scores and parents who reported co-sleeping, as well as in those who reported negative co-sleeping experiences [13]. Parents may use co-sleeping as a way of intervening in the frequent nighttime scratching episodes and awakenings.

Sleep problems secondary to medical conditions such as atopic dermatitis can be difficult to manage as once the medical issues are treated, problems with sleep can often persist. Studies have shown that even when atopic dermatitis is in clinical remission, sleep disturbance may still have an impact as evidenced by polysomnography studies of affected patients [14, 15]. One study found that even in well-controlled atopic dermatitis, objective findings of sleep fragmentation on polysomnographic studies were found that were not associated with the act of scratching, respiratory related arousals or leg movements [15]. This increased sleep fragmentation and frequent arousals in patients without clinically evident atopic disease may cause chronic sleep disturbances leading to daytime sleepiness, difficulty concentrating and ultimately behavior issues [15].

Studies have shown high rates of fatigue and sleep disturbances in adults suffering from atopic dermatitis leading to increased healthcare utilization and negative overall health impact [14]. With almost 10 million AD adults suffering from sleep disturbance, there is potential for significant negative impact on job performance and job satisfaction [14].

New studies point to disruption of the melatonin secretion pathway as contributing to sleep disturbance in AD patients [8, 16]. Melatonin is a small neurohormone secreted by the pineal gland and plays an important role in the body's circadian rhythm and sleep regulation [17]. Melatonin secretion normally increases at night, and peaks in the middle of night before rapidly decreasing towards morning [17]. Studies have demonstrated correlation between decreased melatonin secretion and increased sleep disturbance in AD patients [16]. Conversely, studies have shown correlation between increased levels of melatonin and decreased sleep disturbance in AD patients [8, 16]. Other studies show increased nocturnal melatonin levels in patients with AD, but this may represent compensatory mechanisms by the body to make up for AD induced sleep disturbance [16].

Addressing sleep behaviors is important in this patient population in an effort to minimize other contributing factors to poor sleep hygiene. Inquiring into sleep habits such as bedtime, presence of electronic devices such as computers, televisions, and handheld devices in the bedroom and nighttime routine can help identify additional barriers to quality sleep. The addition of stress-relieving therapies such as massage, hypnosis and cognitive behavioral therapy may also help improve sleep quality [2]. Due to AD often presenting in early childhood, children with atopic dermatitis depend on others for help with disease management. Caregiving usually falls on the shoulders of the parents but in some circumstances can involve siblings, other family remembers, and childcare providers. Dealing with the intricacies of AD including multiple topical medicines, need for specific skin care products, strict avoidance of triggers, chronic sleep deprivation and child irritability can lead to caregiver stress and strain the parent-child relationship [2].

7.5 Atopic Dermatitis and the Mother-Child Relationship

For decades literature has supported a link between presence of childhood AD and a poor mother-child relationship. Theories surrounding this link include maternal hostility towards the child, potential for neglect, and decreased physical bonding [2, 18]. A poor bond between mother and child compounded by presence of chronic disease can lead to abnormal emotional and behavioral development. The theory of object relations is a theory that attempts to qualify the importance of normal emotional development. The theory states that infants are driven by a motivation for closeness and relationship to another mind such as their mother [19]. This relationship with mother helps with healthy behavioral development as the child grows. According to suggestions by Bick in the 1960s, the skin has a unique and important role in early development of the personality [18].

Parents may be hesitant to touch their child due to the presence of cutaneous disease and fear of further exacerbating their child's skin condition [18]. Increased skin sensitivity in AD children may be interpreted as negative stimulation and may be perceived by the parents as causing more distress for the infant [18]. Parents can unintentionally focus on the skin disease to the detriment of the child's emotional needs [18].

7.6 Activities of Daily Living and Atopic Dermatitis

Activities of daily living can become burdensome or associated with negative emotions in families living with AD. Sensitivity to certain foods, personal care products, and fabrics can make daily activities of mealtime, bathing and dressing complicated and difficult. Problems faced by AD patients are often greater than unaffected people fully understand and appreciate. Maintaining a high level of cleanliness in the home to avoid AD triggers or flares can produce large amounts of extra work for caregivers [10]. One study found families who have a child with atopic dermatitis, even in the absence of active disease, describe problems with authority, communication and disruptive conduct within the family unit [20]. Another study reported parents of children with AD spent an average of 3 h a day on disease-related caregiver activities [21].

7.7 Conclusion

This chapter has clearly demonstrated the breadth and depth of stress induced by living with atopic dermatitis. Using quality of life (QoL) indices can help to quantify the impact of a disease on the life of a patient and caregivers [22]. These indices can be used both in the clinical setting and for research purposes. QoL indices can be generic or disease-specific. One benefit to using a generic QoL index is to directly compare QoL between different disease states. One such tool is the health-related quality of life index or HRQoL.

The HRQoL assesses parameters directly related to disease as well as parameters not directly related to disease but affected by disease [22]. A new revised version of the HRQoL includes assessing how life differs from personal expectations due to disease as well as assessing the individual's ability to cope in social situations [22]. This revised HRQoL allows a more nuanced look into a patient's quality of life and to see how the disease has altered the course of their life from their expectations. Using indices such as HRQoL, severe atopic dermatitis demonstrated more QoL impairment than diabetes, asthma, and cystic fibrosis [10]. Childhood AD has shown the highest negative QoL scores compared to all other surveyed chronic childhood illnesses [10]. New questionnaires are now being developed to target emotional, social, financial and occupational aspects of QoL [22].

Although there is less research on the psychological associations of atopic dermatitis as compared to psoriasis, atopic dermatitis has been found to be associated with significant psychological distress [23]. While some patients and families are better able to cope than others, atopic dermatitis is often a burden, causing increased risk of emotional problems in patients and families as well as attention problems in the affected patient [21]. Physicians should counsel families and caretakers on ways to cope with the emotional distress and burden of disease as well as implement targeted interventions to decrease scratching and sleep disturbances, often through a multidisciplinary team approach [21].

Using a multidisciplinary team approach to properly identify and treat the psychosocial stressors associated with atopic dermatitis will likely lead to improved patient and caregiver satisfaction.

References

1. Elias PM, Schmuth M. Abnormal skin barrier in the etiopathogenesis of atopic dermatitis. Curr Opin Allergy Clin Immunol. 2009;9(5):437–46. doi:10.1097/aci.0b013e32832e7d36.
2. Arndt J, Smith N, Tausk F. Stress and atopic dermatitis. Curr Allergy Asthma Rep. 2008;8(4):312–7. doi:10.1007/s11882-008-0050-6.
3. Rapp SR, Exum ML, Reboussin DM, Feldman SR, Fleischer A, Clark A. The physical, psychological and social impact of psoriasis. J Health Psychol. 1997;2(4):525–37. doi:10.1177/135910539700200409.
4. Ograczyk A, Malec J, Miniszewska J, Zalewska-Janowska A. Psychological aspects of atopic dermatitis and contact dermatitis: stress coping strategies and stigmatization. Postepy Dermatologii i Alergologii. 2012;29(1):14.

5. Di Blasi M, Cavani P, Pavia L, Lo Baido R, La Grutta S, Schimmenti A. The relationship between self-image and social anxiety in adolescence. Child Adolesc Ment Health. 2015;20(2):74–80. doi:10.1111/camh.12071.
6. Park H, Kim K. Association of perceived stress with atopic dermatitis in adults: a population-based study in korea. Int J Environ Res Public Health. 2016;13(8):1–7. doi:10.3390/ijerph13080760.
7. Kong TS, Han TY, Lee JH, Son SJ. Correlation between severity of atopic dermatitis and sleep quality in children and adults. Ann Dermatol. 2016;28(3):321–6. doi:10.5021/ad.2016.28.3.321.
8. Chang Y, Lin M, Lee J, et al. Melatonin supplementation for children with atopic dermatitis and sleep disturbance: a randomized clinical trial. JAMA Pediatr. 2016;170(1):35–42. doi:10.1001/jamapediatrics.2015.3092.
9. Camfferman D, Kennedy JD, Gold M, Martin AJ, Lushington K. Eczema and sleep and its relationship to daytime functioning in children. Sleep Med Rev. 2010;14(6):359–69. doi:10.1016/j.smrv.2010.01.004.
10. Lewis-Jones S. Quality of life and childhood atopic dermatitis: the misery of living with childhood eczema. Int J Clin Pract. 2006;60(8):984–92. doi:10.1111/j.1742-1241.2006.01047.x.
11. Dahl RE, Bernhisel-Broadbent J, Scanlon-Holdford S, Sampson HA, Lupo M. Sleep disturbances in children with atopic dermatitis. Arch Pediatr Adolesc Med. 1995;149(8):856–60. doi:10.1001/archpedi.1995.02170210030005.
12. Kelsay K. Management of sleep disturbance associated with atopic dermatitis. J Allergy Clin Immunol. 2006;118(1):198–201. doi:10.1016/j.jaci.2006.04.038.
13. Chamlin SL, Mattson CL, Frieden IJ, et al. The price of pruritus: sleep disturbance and cosleeping in atopic dermatitis. Arch Pediatr Adolesc Med. 2005;159(8):745–50. doi:10.1001/archpedi.159.8.745.
14. Silverberg JI, Garg NK, Paller AS, Fishbein AB, Zee PC. Sleep disturbances in adults with eczema are associated with impaired overall health: a US population-based study. J Invest Dermatol. 2015;135(1):56–66. doi:10.1038/jid.2014.325.
15. Reuveni H, Chapnick G, Tal A, Tarasiuk A. Sleep fragmentation in children with atopic dermatitis. Arch Pediatr Adolesc Med. 1999;153(3):249–53. doi:10.1001/archpedi.153.3.249.
16. Chang Y-S, Chou Y-T, Lee J-H, Lee P-L, Dai Y-S, Sun C, Lin Y-T, Wang L-C, H-H Y, Yang Y-H, Chen C-A, Wan K-S, Chiang B-L. Atopic dermatitis, melatonin, and sleep disturbance. Pediatrics. 2014;134(2):e397. doi:10.1542/peds.2014-0376.
17. Brzezinski A. Melatonin in humans. N Engl J Med. 1997;336(3):186–95.
18. Howlett S. Emotional dysfunction, child–family relationships and childhood atopic dermatitis. Br J Dermatol. 1999;140(3):381–4. doi:10.1046/j.1365-2133.1999.02696.x.
19. Neukrug E. The Sage encyclopedia of theory in counseling and psychotherapy. Thousand Oaks: SAGE; 2015.
20. Rodríguez-Orozco AR, Kanán-Cedeño EG, Martínez EG, MJC G. Family functioning and illness perception of parents of children with atopic dermatitis, living without skin symptoms, but with psychosomatic symptoms. Iran J Allergy Asthma Immunol. 2011;10(1):61–5.
21. Kelsay K, Klinnert M, Bender B. Addressing psychosocial aspects of atopic dermatitis. Immunol Allergy Clin North Am. 2010;30(3):385–96. doi:10.1016/j.iac.2010.05.003.
22. Lifschitz C. The impact of atopic dermatitis on quality of life. Ann Nutr Metab. 2015;66:34–40. doi:10.1159/000370226.
23. Kirby B. The psych and inflammatory skin disease. Br J Dermatol. 2012;166(5):986–93. doi:10.1111/j.1365-2133.2012.10909.x.

Chapter 8
The Economics Burden of Atopic Dermatitis

Adewole S. Adamson

Abstract Atopic dermatitis (AD) is a chronic inflammatory disorder that affects over 30 million people in the United States of America. Given the large and growing prevalence of AD, the associated economic burden is significant. It has been estimated that AD costs over $5 billion dollars annually. These costs include both direct and indirect costs. Direct costs include prescription medicines, visits to health care providers, hospitalizations, and transportation. Indirect costs include missed days or lost productivity at work or school, career modification, and reduced quality of life. Understanding and measuring these costs can be accomplished through rigorous economic evaluation, which is the organized process of considering inputs and outcomes of various activities. Economic evaluation has been used to contextualize the burden of AD in society. It has also been used to inform patients, providers, and other stakeholders on how to deliver the most evidence-based, efficient care possible. Understanding the economic impact of atopic dermatitis is an important aspect of delivering high quality care.

Keywords Economics • Quality of life • Health care costs • Burden of disease

8.1 Introduction

It is estimated that one in three people in the United States is affected by a skin disease at any given time [1]. Studies have attempted to quantify the economic impact of skin disease [2, 3]. It has been estimated that the total annual cost of skin disease in 2004 was $39.3 billion, with $29.1 billion in direct medical costs and $10.2 billion in indirect medical costs [3]. If quality of life factors are added to the economic analysis, it is estimated that the economic cost of skin disease in the United States was $96 billion in 2004 [3].

Atopic dermatitis, one of the most prevalent chronic skin diseases, affects over 30 million Americans, and many of those affected are children. According to the

A.S. Adamson, M.D., M.P.P. (✉)
Department of Dermatology, University of North Carolina School of Medicine, Chapel Hill, NC, USA
e-mail: adewole_adamson@med.unc.edu

E.A. Fortson et al. (eds.), *Management of Atopic Dermatitis*, Advances in Experimental Medicine and Biology 1027, DOI 10.1007/978-3-319-64804-0_8

largest study investigating the burden of skin disease in the United States, it is estimated that total costs for atopic dermatitis in the United States was $4.228 billion in 2004, which would equate to $5.368 billion in 2016 [3].

Measuring the economic impact of disease is an important way to give scope and context to how disease can affect both individuals and society at large. At an individual level, understanding costs can help patients make smarter choices about spending their limited dollars on health care. At a societal level, understanding economic impact can help inform how public health officials and policy makers decide to allocate resources and funding to combat specific health problems. As health care costs continue to rise, the resources available for health care expenditures will become increasingly scarce [4]. As a result, clinicians, patients, and payers will have to become more aware of the economic impact of the management of disease. This is particularly important in atopic dermatitis, a chronic disorder with no cure that can require long-term treatment and, depending upon severity, may involve expensive medication and hospitalizations. Using the tools of economic evaluation, which have been applied in various forms in dermatology, investigators can illuminate the impact of cost at the patient, payer, and societal level.

8.2 Economic Evaluation

Economic evaluation is the ordered consideration of inputs and outcomes associated with alternative actions. The purpose of economic evaluation is to help guide stakeholders in the pursuit of the best course of action based on the best available evidence. In health care, for example, economic evaluation can involve deciding on the most efficient way of treating a disease given two comparable treatment options of differing cost. The goal of economic analysis is not necessarily about finding the cheapest way to deliver care, but about uncovering the most efficient way to deliver care.

Economic evaluations are generally categorized into four groups: cost minimization analysis, cost benefit analysis, cost effectiveness analysis, and cost utility analysis (Table 8.1) [5]. The difference between these groups generally depends upon the health outcome that is measured. In cost minimization, analysis no health outcome is measured; there is simply an accounting of all the inputs (e.g., cost of hospital visits, physician visits, medications) without any assessment of clinical

Table 8.1 Types of economic evaluation

Types	Health outcome measured
Cost minimization analysis	None
Cost benefit analysis	Dollars
Cost effectiveness analysis	Clinical
Cost utility analysis	Quality adjusted life years (QALYs)

Adapted from Hoch et al.

outcome. In cost benefit analysis, many interventions are analyzed, and the health outcome is measured in dollars. This can be ethically fraught given that a health outcome (e.g., disease-free survival) is given a monetary value. In cost-effectiveness, analysis the health outcome is some type of clinical indicator (e.g., itch-free days). Given that the outcomes are often disease specific, comparisons across disease categories are difficult. Cost utility analysis, which is a form of cost-effectiveness analysis, measures patient values, which are reported as utilities, and then combined with a clinical outcome. Cost utility analysis reports its output in Quality Adjusted Life Years (QALYs), which can be compared across disease categories.

Depending on the availability of data any of these types of economic analyses could be used for economic evaluation. In health care, cost effectiveness analyses are the most popular form of economic evaluation performed, likely because of its ease of use and interpretation [6–9]. In the field of dermatology, there are examples of each type of economic evaluation. In the study of atopic dermatitis in particular, economic evaluation spans the breadth of these types of economic evaluation as well [8–12].

8.3 Measuring Economic Impact in Atopic Dermatitis

National health care costs associated with atopic dermatitis are often estimated using large data sets, such as the National Hospital Discharge Survey, the National Ambulatory Medical Care Survey, the Nationwide Inpatient Sample, and the National Hospital Ambulatory Medical Care Survey, which are resources that help estimate use of inpatient and outpatient medical services. Other databases such as Truven Health Analytics MarketScan™ data or publically available Medicare data can be used to assess the costs for products (e.g., medications) and services rendered to patients.

Understanding and measuring the financial impact of atopic dermatitis is an important consideration and involves quantification beyond the direct expenses associated with the disorder. In particular, there are certain non-financial opportunity costs associated with atopic dermatitis that must also be taken into account. These non-financial costs can indirectly exact an economic toll on patients and society. Some of these costs have a profound effect on the lived experiences of patients and their caregivers. Atopic dermatitis may not be a life-threatening disorder, but the symptoms of itching, emotional distress, disfigurement, and discomfort can take a toll on patients' quality of life. In health care, these non-financial economic consequences can be measured in utility, which is determined by state of health, consumption of health-related goods and services, and the opportunity costs associated with other activities in their daily lives. Importantly, patients with atopic dermatitis report decrements in quality of life greater than patients with asthma, hypertension, and angina [13].

Quantifying the economic impact of disease involves carefully measuring inputs at many different levels, including individual, family, insurance payer, government,

Table 8.2 Direct and indirect cost in atopic dermatitis

Direct cost	Indirect cost
Medication	Missed school/work (absenteeism)
Provider office visits (co-pays)	Reduce productivity (presenteeism)
Over-the-counter medication/supplies	Reduced quality of life
Hospitalization	Career modification
Transportation	
Home environment modifications	

Adapted from Mancini et al.

societal, or at some other aggregation of these units. Depending upon the level of the analysis, economic evaluation can be microeconomic or macroeconomic in scope. Both these approaches of assessing economic impact are different but complementary and have been used in the economic evaluation of atopic dermatitis [12, 14–16].

The economic impact of atopic dermatitis is directly related to the severity of disease, which has been shown in many studies [17–19]. However, calculating the total cost associated with atopic dermatitis can be difficult because there are so many factors that must be considered. Both direct and indirect financial costs are associated with atopic dermatitis. Direct costs can include medications, over-the-counter treatments, provider appointments, and hospitalizations. Indirect costs can include financial losses associated with missed work or decreased work productivity. Missed school, also known as absenteeism, can affect scholastic performance and overall achievement. There are also intangible costs related to decrements in quality of life related to disease, which can have an economic effect on patients and society as a whole (Table 8.2) [20].

Indirect costs can represent a significant amount of the burden associated with atopic dermatitis. According to the ISOLATE (International Study on Life with Atopic Eczema) study, atopic dermatitis is associated with over € 2 billion ($2.44 billion in 2004) in annual indirect costs [21]. The sources of these indirect costs are mostly related to missed workdays during flares. Nearly one third of patients indicated that atopic dermatitis affected their school-work life. The average number of absent days from school or work because of a flare was 2.5 days in mild-moderate patients, and for patients with severe atopic dermatitis it was 5.3 days. Fourteen percent of adult patients believed that their career progression was encumbered and 11% believe they have been discriminated against because of their disorder. This represents a significant potential burden to both children and adults affected by atopic dermatitis. Given that atopic dermatitis can persist into adulthood, the economic burden of disease may continue for a long time in patients' lives.

A Danish survey study found that 38% of survey respondents refrained from participating or seeking certain educational or job opportunities because of atopic dermatitis [22]. The mean number of workdays missed for patient with eczema was 148% higher than the national average. This could adversely affect the incomes of patients with atopic dermatitis.

An important consideration is that studies which measure indirect costs are potentially biased or misestimate given bias when reporting on survey data. National surveys in particular rely on patients being able to correctly identify their skin disorder. It is possible that survey participants could confuse their inflammatory skin disease as eczema, when their actual diagnosis is psoriasis or some other similar disorder. Despite these shortcomings, measuring indirect costs are an important window into the economic impact of the disease.

Several studies have examined economic impact through large insurance data. In an analysis of a population-based claims database covering over 5 million beneficiaries on an employer-based health plan, it was found that 38% of the cost burden resulted from employee disability and increased sick days [23]. In another retrospective study of a large managed care organization, researchers found that atopic dermatitis imposed a financial burden on both the health care system and patients. The mean annual cost per patient was $609 with only 27% of the total burden borne by third-party payers. The rest of the financial burden came from missed work and out-of-pocket expenses from medications and household items [19].

There is increasing evidence to suggest that atopic dermatitis is more than just a skin disease with a few extra-cutaneous manifestations; rather, atopic dermatitis is a systemic disorder with many associated co-morbidities, including asthma, allergic conjunctivitis, allergic rhinitis, and eosinophilic esophagitis. Atopic dermatitis has also been associated with malignancies, cardiovascular disease, and neuropsychiatric disorders [24]. These co-morbidities are not easily economically quantifiable but certainly influence the cost of treatment and quality of life of patients with atopic dermatitis.

8.4 Societal Economic Impact of Atopic Dermatitis

According to the 2010 National Health Interview Survey, a questionnaire collected by the National Center for Health Statistics (NCHS) of the Centers for Disease Control (CDC), 10.2% of 27,157 respondents had eczema [12]. Extrapolated to the rest of society means that well over 30 million people are affected by the disorder in the United States. The prevalence of AD is increasing worldwide, especially in developing countries [25]. The cost of treating atopic dermatitis could increase significantly in the future given novel therapeutic agents for the disorder. According to the Global Burden of Disease Study 2013, dermatitis, of which atopic dermatitis is a significant proportion, is responsible for the biggest global burden of disability-adjusted life years and years lived with disability [26].

There have been several efforts undertaken to characterize the economic burden of atopic dermatitis on a societal level. The most far-reaching economic evaluation of societal burden of atopic dermatitis in the United States found that in 2004 the total annual economic burden of atopic dermatitis was $4.223 billion, much greater than the cost of psoriasis [3]. These estimates were based on data that include direct, indirect, and quality of life costs. A significant burden of the associated cost was from indirect costs. However, this study did not consider costs of over-the-counter products or missed workdays not related to clinic visits. In addition, with new biologic medications and possible changes in prescribing patterns, the previous estimation of costs associated with atopic dermatitis is likely an under-estimation of the true burden of disease [27].

Atopic dermatitis has a greater impact on patient quality of life than those with asthma or hypertension [13]. Of note, patients with atopic dermatitis have an associated increase in health care use. In a study of the effect of atopic dermatitis on total burden of illness in a large managed care organization, patients who had eczema had an increased likelihood of emergency department visits, hospitalizations, receiving home care, and outpatient physician visits compared with patients without eczema. However, this study was limited in that it could not assess whether these visits were associated with atopic dermatitis [19].

8.5 Cost of Atopic Dermatitis in Children

Atopic dermatitis is one of the most common chronic inflammatory skin diseases worldwide, especially among children. It is estimated that 10–20% of children in the United States have atopic dermatitis [28, 29]. In children the impact of the disease is felt not only among patients with the disorder, but also their family members and caretakers. The direct financial impact of atopic dermatitis on children and their caretakers is similar to those with juvenile type I diabetes [17]. The financial burden of childhood atopic dermatitis involves both direct and indirect costs. Direct costs include provider visits, prescription medication, over-the-counter medication, moisturizers, soaps, and other environmental modifications required to reduce atopic dermatitis flares. Indirect costs are more challenging to quantify and include missed work, cost of transportation to physician appointments, caretaker career choices, and reduced productivity. There have been numerous studies attempting to quantify the economic costs associated with atopic dermatitis. These studies have varying methods of measuring costs. Some studies take a societal perspective, while others take an individual perspective or third-party payer perspective.

Understanding how atopic dermatitis financially impacts patients, families, and society is important in order to demonstrate the broad scope and effect of the disorder [15, 30]. However, the burden of disease in children is difficult to measure in economic terms because a significant proportion of the cost is indirect—missed school, reduced school performance, psychosocial stress, and other opportunity costs. Most studies have focused on direct costs of atopic dermatitis given that the analysis is easier to define and the results simpler to interpret. The definition of what qualifies as an indirect cost is not entirely consistent across the literature, and its effects may depend on context.

One of the first U.S.-based studies to measure health care costs associated with atopic dermatitis measured only direct cost based on emergency room use by children with atopic dermatitis at one institution, which was then extrapolated to a national cost using national data sets [31]. The study was published in 1993 and it estimated that the total cost of atopic dermatitis in the United States was $364 million. This was likely an underestimate, particularly considering that indirect costs, including those related to quality of life were not calculated.

Use of the dermatology-specific Children's Dermatology Quality of Life Index (CDLQI) has demonstrated that eczema in children can have greater impact on quality of life than other chronic skin disorders such as psoriasis [32]. Patient quality of life correlates with disease activity and severity in both children and adults [33, 34]. Parents often agree with children in terms of quality of life measures for atopic dermatitis [35]. As a result, reliable quality of life measures can be elicited either from children or their parents.

Cost of care for atopic dermatitis is a real worry for families that take care of children with the disorder [36]. A significant amount of this cost is manifested in indirect losses. An estimated 40% of total indirect annual cost associated with atopic dermatitis is related to workdays lost by caregivers [3]. Several studies have shown that indirect costs related to caregivers constitute a significant amount of costs associated with atopic dermatitis [16, 17]. One study that examined the time spent on the treatment of atopic dermatitis showed that families of children with atopic dermatitis spend an average of 63 min/day on the disorder [37]. Sleep disturbance is a problem in patients with atopic dermatitis. Poor sleep has been associated with reduced performance at school and work. Poor sleep has been associated with significant economic implications [38]. Atopic dermatitis in children can potentially affect future job choices, and ultimately economic productivity. A history of childhood atopic dermatitis has been associated with an increased likelihood of job change, sick leave, and physician visits, mostly because of the disease [39].

There is a direct relationship between severity of atopic disease and associated health care use. Health care use among children with atopic dermatitis is higher than those of the same age without eczema. This is likely because of the increase in comorbid disease associated with having atopic dermatitis [40]. A study of administrative claims showed that atopic dermatitis patients were more likely to be diagnosed with asthma, allergic rhinitis, and allergic conjunctivitis than those without the diagnosis. Those patients with atopic dermatitis that developed these associated clinical disorders had a doubling of their associated total medical costs in the subsequent 12 months [41]. The majority of admissions in one large hospital dermatology consult service were for management of atopic dermatitis, representing over 86% of total admissions [42].

The direct and indirect costs of atopic dermatitis care is of concern in many countries. In one Italian study measuring the impact of atopic dermatitis on family, 44% of respondents indicated that economic cost as a high concern [43]. In a 2001 study of preschool children in the United Kingdom, direct and indirect costs associated with atopic dermatitis, regardless of severity, was £80 ($125) per child over a 12-month period. Most of the costs were associated with physician visits and prescription medication. However, 36% of the total cost of disease was associated with family care, which included transportation, workdays missed, over-the-counter medications, and visits to alternative medicine practitioners [44]. In a 1999 Australian study of costs of atopic dermatitis, researchers found that annual costs were $A1142 ($894) per child for mild atopic dermatitis and $A6099 ($4774) per child for severe atopic dermatitis. These figures include direct costs such as hospitalization, drug costs, visits to the doctors, and the indirect costs of missed work.

As the prevalence of atopic dermatitis continues to increase over time, particularly in children, there will be increasing urgency to address costs associated with the disorder. Further research is ongoing to figure out the most cost effective way to prevent and treat atopic dermatitis.

8.6 Access to Care

Access to care for patients with atopic dermatitis can be challenging given the chronic nature of the disorder, which can require high levels of health care use. This is particularly challenging for children—many patients do not have access to a pediatric dermatologist or pediatric allergist. As a result, general pediatricians treat most children with atopic dermatitis [45].

Adult patients with eczema also have problems with access to care. When compared with patients without eczema, adults with eczema report more trouble reaching their provider, getting a timely appointment, having reliable transportation, and being able to afford their medications [12]. Patient with eczema more frequently report delaying their care because of health-related costs. When patients with eczema are hospitalized, they have higher odds of a prolonged hospitalization. With the advent of more costly biologic medications to treat atopic dermatitis, access issues may become more problematic over time.

Teledermatology is a potential innovative technology that could improve access to care for patients with chronic skin disorders such as atopic dermatitis. Routine follow-up care is a significant part of the atopic dermatitis process of care and could be streamlined with the use of teledermatology. Armstrong et al. demonstrated that the use of a teledermatology model for atopic dermatitis follow-up resulted in equivalent outcomes when compared with in-person clinic visits [46]. Teledermatology represents a promising strategy for delivering health care services to patients with atopic dermatitis.

8.7 Out-of-Pocket Cost of Atopic Dermatitis

Out-of-pocket costs include co-pays, transportation, prescription medications, over-the-counter medications, home environment adjustments and other costs associated with managing atopic dermatitis. Out-of-pocket costs can have a significant effect on household budgets depending on patient insurance status and severity of disease. It is estimated that more than 75% of total out-of-pocket spending is for household items and medications [19].

The estimated out-of-pocket cost for the treatment of atopic dermatitis in the United States was $37.8 million in 2010 [12]. On an average per patient basis, eczema patients incurred higher out-of-pocket costs when compared with patients with hypertension and diabetes. Eczema is associated with more than 68 million days of lost work; nearly 6 million of those days were directly caused by eczema [12]. When compared with adults without eczema, adults with eczema had an increased likelihood of missing more than six workdays for any cause.

Despite the significant cost of treatment, atopic dermatitis ranks in the top five among major skin disorders by willingness to pay for symptom relief [3]. Willingness to pay for relief of skin disease has been calculated as $125–260/month, which is comparable to many other serious chronic medical conditions [13]. Willingness to pay is a way to measure the perceived value that patients have for any choice. Having a sense of this figure is important to prioritize what patients' value in terms of outcomes for medical decisions. This is particularly important when evaluating trade-offs between treatments with differing cost [47]. Using willingness to pay as a way to reliably measure preferences is controversial; however, it could be an important measure to inform treatment decisions that affect patient out-of-pocket costs [48].

Given its high prevalence worldwide, atopic dermatitis can be an economic burden in many countries. In a 2002 study of the cost of atopic dermatitis, health care costs resulting from atopic dermatitis varied between $71 in the Netherlands to $2559 in Germany. This variance was due to differences of study population and cost variability across countries [49].

8.8 Ways to Reduce Costs

Health care costs continue to rise in the United States and around the world. Finding ways to reduce cost by more efficiently managing atopic dermatitis will continue to be important for physicians, patients, and society. Given its high prevalence there has been a renewed focus on finding ways to prevent the disorder from developing in young children [50]. A majority of childhood atopic dermatitis develops before 5 years of age. Studies suggest that application of daily moisturizer beginning in the first few weeks of life reduced that risk of developing atopic dermatitis in infants at high risk of developing the disorder [51, 52]. These studies reduced the incidence by 32–50%. In a subsequent cost-effectiveness study, it was shown that prophylactic moisturization of high-risk newborns was cost-effective. Overall, the study demonstrated that the use of moisturizers was cost-effective across a range of moisturizers with Vaseline petroleum jelly being the most cost-effective at $353 per quality adjusted life year. Therefore, this type of low-cost intervention could reduce future societal economic burden of atopic dermatitis. By reducing the incidence of atopic dermatitis, it is possible that fewer patients will require more expensive interventions, which is of particular concern as emerging biologics become available for this disorder.

There is some evidence to suggest that exclusive breastfeeding is associated with a lower incidence of atopic dermatitis in infants [53]. Prebiotics and probiotics, together known as synbiotics, have been advocated for the use in prevention of atopic dermatitis. While a meta-analysis showed some evidence to support this view, current studies are heterogeneous and of limited quality [54]. More rigorous prospective trials are needed to confirm the effects of synbiotics on the risk of atopic dermatitis development in children. If a beneficial effect is found, synbiotics could be a low-cost population-based strategy to reduce atopic dermatitis incidence and thus lower its associated costs.

Cost utility and cost-effectiveness analyses can also be used to figure out which treatments are more cost-effective for atopic dermatitis patients. In a study of clinical efficacy and economic impact, twice-weekly treatment with topical tacrolimus 0.03% ointment in children between 2 and 15 years old was shown to be cost-effective over a 12-month period [55]. This study was conducted in 267 European children across 10 countries. Tacrolimus use prolonged the time to first flare to 146 days as compared with 17 days for children using vehicle. Despite tacrolimus being more expensive, the reduction in flares made it cost-neutral for children with moderate atopic dermatitis and possibly cost-saving for children with severe atopic dermatitis. These findings may not necessarily be generalizable to other countries, particularly in the United States, where patients often pay more for prescription medication [56]. However, decreasing flares can have a significant economic impact if it leads to reduced physician visits and costly hospitalizations.

In a modeling study of cost-effectiveness analysis of pimecrolimus 1% cream for management of mild-to-moderate atopic dermatitis in children, it was shown that pimecrolimus was $38,231 per QALY gained compared with standard therapy [57]. By convention, a QALY under $50,000 is seen as reasonable. However, in a cost utility analysis by Pitt et al. comparing pimecrolimus as a treatment for mild and moderate atopic eczema with conventional treatments (i.e., topical corticosteroids), investigators found few situations where pimecrolimus was cost effective. QALYs were negative, meaning that compared with topical steroids pimecrolimus was not as cost effective. However, when compared with emollient only, pimecrolimus was cost effective.

Corticosteroids, pimecrolimus, and tacrolimus are potential topical treatments for atopic dermatitis; however, corticosteroids are usually less expensive. Few comparative effectiveness trials have been conducted comparing these medications head to head. A systematic review and cost effectiveness analysis analyzed randomized controlled trials of pimecrolimus and tacrolimus before 2005. The review concluded that pimecrolimus was not cost-effective for the treatment of mild-to-moderate eczema in adults or children compared with topical corticosteroids. While pimecrolimus offered fewer quality adjusted life years compared with topical corticosteroids, there was a certain degree of uncertainty around those results given the small absolute differences in QALY. At a QALY of £30,000 (~$55,000), tacrolimus was found to be cost-effective in moderate-to-severe facial atopic dermatitis in adults and non-facial eczema in children. However, authors suggested that these results should be interpreted with caution given the high level of uncertainty of their analysis [9]. Since these cost effectiveness studies were conducted, tacrolimus is now generic and the patent on pimecrolimus will expire in 2018, therefore cost-effectiveness may differ [58].

Substitution of high-cost providers (physicians) for low-cost providers (nurses) for the treatment and management of atopic dermatitis could potentially be cost-saving. In a study from the Netherlands, investigators randomized children to nurse practitioner-led care versus dermatologist-led care and found that it was cost-effective without a difference in quality of life [8]. These findings are not necessarily generalizable to other countries; however, they offer another possible strategy to reduce cost associated with the management of atopic dermatitis.

8.9 Conclusion

All resources in health care are finite, including money, time, technology and space. Understanding the economic impact of skin disease, particularly chronic skin disease such as atopic dermatitis, can help physicians, patients, payers, and other stakeholders improve their decision making related to disease management. Economic evaluation is an important tool to provide context to disease and clarify the consequences of choices we make. Using the best available evidence economic evaluation can help in making wise choices with our limited resources.

References

1. Thorpe KE, Florence CS, Joski P. Which medical conditions account for the rise in health care spending?. Health Aff (Millwood). 2004; Suppl Web Exclusives:W4-437445.
2. Dehkharghani S, Bible J, Chen JG, Feldman SR, Fleischer AB Jr. The economic burden of skin disease in the United States. J Am Acad Dermatol. 2003;48(4):592–9.
3. Bickers DR, Lim HW, Margolis D, et al. The burden of skin diseases: 2004 a joint project of the American Academy of Dermatology Association and the Society for Investigative Dermatology. J Am Acad Dermatol. 2006;55(3):490–500.
4. Martin AB, Hartman M, Washington B, Catlin A, National Health Expenditure Accounts T. National health spending: faster growth in 2015 as coverage expands and utilization increases. Health Aff (Millwood). 2017;36(1):166–76.
5. Hoch JS, Dewa CS. A clinician's guide to correct cost-effectiveness analysis: think incremental not average. Can J Psychiatry. 2008;53(4):267–74.
6. Pak HS, Datta SK, Triplett CA, Lindquist JH, Grambow SC, Whited JD. Cost minimization analysis of a store-and-forward teledermatology consult system. Telemed J E Health. 2009;15(2):160–5.
7. Chen S, Shaheen A, Garber A. Cost-effectiveness and cost-benefit analysis of using methotrexate vs Goeckerman therapy for psoriasis. A pilot study. Arch Dermatol. 1998;134(12):1602–8.
8. Schuttelaar ML, Vermeulen KM, Coenraads PJ. Costs and cost-effectiveness analysis of treatment in children with eczema by nurse practitioner vs. dermatologist: results of a randomized, controlled trial and a review of international costs. Br J Dermatol. 2011;165(3):600–11.

9. Pitt M, Garside R, Stein K. A cost-utility analysis of pimecrolimus vs. topical corticosteroids and emollients for the treatment of mild and moderate atopic eczema. Br J Dermatol. 2006;154(6):1137–46.
10. Ellis CN, Drake LA, Prendergast MM, et al. Cost-effectiveness analysis of tacrolimus ointment versus high-potency topical corticosteroids in adults with moderate to severe atopic dermatitis. J Am Acad Dermatol. 2003;48(4):553–63.
11. Xu S, Immaneni S, Hazen GB, Silverberg JI, Paller AS, Lio PA. Cost-effectiveness of prophylactic moisturization for atopic dermatitis. JAMA Pediatr. 2017;171(2):e163909.
12. Silverberg JI. Health care utilization, patient costs, and access to care in US adults with eczema: a population-based study. JAMA Dermatol. 2015;151(7):743–52.
13. Parks L, Balkrishnan R, Hamel-Gariepy L, Feldman SR. The importance of skin disease as assessed by “willingness-to-pay”. J Cutan Med Surg. 2003;7(5):369–71.
14. Ellis CN, Drake LA, Prendergast MM, et al. Cost of atopic dermatitis and eczema in the United States. J Am Acad Dermatol. 2002;46(3):361–70.
15. Carroll CL, Balkrishnan R, Feldman SR, Fleischer AB Jr, Manuel JC. The burden of atopic dermatitis: impact on the patient, family, and society. Pediatr Dermatol. 2005;22(3):192–9.
16. Filanovsky MG, Pootongkam S, Tamburro JE, Smith MC, Ganocy SJ, Nedorost ST. The financial and emotional impact of atopic dermatitis on children and their families. J Pediatr. 2016;169:284–290.e5. e285
17. JC S, Kemp AS, Varigos GA, Nolan TM. Atopic eczema: its impact on the family and financial cost. Arch Dis Child. 1997;76(2):159–62.
18. Handa S, Jain N, Narang T. Cost of care of atopic dermatitis in India. Indian J Dermatol. 2015;60(2):213.
19. Fivenson D, Arnold RJ, Kaniecki DJ, Cohen JL, Frech F, Finlay AY. The effect of atopic dermatitis on total burden of illness and quality of life on adults and children in a large managed care organization. J Manag Care Pharm. 2002;8(5):333–42.
20. Mancini AJ, Kaulback K, Chamlin SL. The socioeconomic impact of atopic dermatitis in the United States: a systematic review. Pediatr Dermatol. 2008;25(1):1–6.
21. Zuberbier T, Orlow SJ, Paller AS, et al. Patient perspectives on the management of atopic dermatitis. J Allergy Clin Immunol. 2006;118(1):226–32.
22. Holm EA, Esmann S, Jemec GB. The handicap caused by atopic dermatitis—sick leave and job avoidance. J Eur Acad Dermatol Venereol. 2006;20(3):255–9.
23. Fowler JF, Duh MS, Rovba L, et al. The direct and indirect cost burden of atopic dermatitis: an employer-payer perspective. Manag Care Interface. 2007;20(10):26–32.
24. Brunner PM, Silverberg JI, Guttman-Yassky E, et al. Increasing comorbidities suggest that atopic dermatitis is a systemic disorder. J Invest Dermatol. 2017;137(1):18–25.
25. Asher MI, Montefort S, Bjorksten B, et al. Worldwide time trends in the prevalence of symptoms of asthma, allergic rhinoconjunctivitis, and eczema in childhood: ISAAC phases one and three repeat multicountry cross-sectional surveys. Lancet. 2006;368(9537):733–43.
26. Karimkhani C, Dellavalle RP, Coffeng LE, et al. Global skin disease morbidity and mortality: an update from the global burden of disease study 2013. JAMA Dermatol. 2017;153:406–12.
27. Simpson EL, Bieber T, Guttman-Yassky E, et al. Two phase 3 trials of dupilumab versus placebo in atopic dermatitis. N Engl J Med. 2016;375(24):2335–48.
28. Laughter D, Istvan JA, Tofte SJ, Hanifin JM. The prevalence of atopic dermatitis in Oregon schoolchildren. J Am Acad Dermatol. 2000;43(4):649–55.
29. Shaw TE, Currie GP, Koudelka CW, Simpson EL. Eczema prevalence in the United States: data from the 2003 National Survey of Children’s health. J Invest Dermatol. 2011;131(1):67–73.
30. Balkrishnan R, Housman TS, Grummer S, et al. The family impact of atopic dermatitis in children: the role of the parent caregiver. Pediatr Dermatol. 2003;20(1):5–10.
31. Lapidus CS, Schwarz DF, Honig PJ. Atopic dermatitis in children: who cares? Who pays? J Am Acad Dermatol. 1993;28(5):699–703.
32. Lewis-Jones MS, Finlay AY. The Children’s dermatology life quality index (CDLQI): initial validation and practical use. Br J Dermatol. 1995;132(6):942–9.

33. Holm EA, Wulf HC, Stegmann H, Jemec GB. Life quality assessment among patients with atopic eczema. Br J Dermatol. 2006;154(4):719–25.
34. Ben-Gashir MA, Seed PT, Hay RJ. Quality of life and disease severity are correlated in children with atopic dermatitis. Br J Dermatol. 2004;150(2):284–90.
35. Beattie PE, Lewis-Jones MS. A comparative study of impairment of quality of life in children with skin disease and children with other chronic childhood diseases. Br J Dermatol. 2006;155(1):145–51.
36. Chren MM, Weinstock MA. Conceptual issues in measuring the burden of skin diseases. J Investig Dermatol Symp Proc. 2004;9(2):97–100.
37. Holm EA, Jemec GB. Time spent on treatment of atopic dermatitis: a new method of measuring pediatric morbidity? Pediatr Dermatol. 2004;21(6):623–7.
38. Colten HR, Altevogt BM, Institute of Medicine (U.S.). Committee on Sleep Medicine and Research. Sleep disorders and sleep deprivation : an unmet public health problem. Washington, DC: Institute of Medicine: National Academies Press; 2006.
39. Nyren M, Lindberg M, Stenberg B, Svensson M, Svensson A, Meding B. Influence of childhood atopic dermatitis on future worklife. Scand J Work Environ Health. 2005;31(6):474–8.
40. Silverberg JI, Simpson EL. Association between severe eczema in children and multiple comorbid conditions and increased healthcare utilization. Pediatr Allergy Immunol. 2013;24(5):476–86.
41. Suh DC, Sung J, Gause D, Raut M, Huang J, Choi IS. Economic burden of atopic manifestations in patients with atopic dermatitis—analysis of administrative claims. J Manag Care Pharm. 2007;13(9):778–89.
42. Storan ER, McEvoy MT, Wetter DA, et al. Pediatric hospital dermatology: experience with inpatient and consult services at the Mayo Clinic. Pediatr Dermatol. 2013;30(4):433–7.
43. Neri E, Agostini F, Gremigni P, et al. Italian validation of the childhood atopic dermatitis impact scale: a contribution to its clinical application. J Invest Dermatol. 2012;132(11):2534–43.
44. Emerson RM, Williams HC, Allen BR. What is the cost of atopic dermatitis in preschool children? Br J Dermatol. 2001;144(3):514–22.
45. Tollefson MM, Bruckner AL, Section On Dermatology. Atopic dermatitis: skin-directed management. Pediatrics. 2014;134(6):e1735–44.
46. Armstrong AW, Johnson MA, Lin S, Maverakis E, Fazel N, Liu FT. Patient-centered, direct-access online care for management of atopic dermatitis: a randomized clinical trial. JAMA Dermatol. 2015;151(2):154–60.
47. Olsen JA, Smith RD. Theory versus practice: a review of 'willingness-to-pay' in health and health care. Health Econ. 2001;10(1):39–52.
48. Cookson R. Willingness to pay methods in health care: a sceptical view. Health Econ. 2003;12(11):891–4.
49. Verboom P, Hakkaart-Van L, Sturkenboom M, De Zeeuw R, Menke H, Rutten F. The cost of atopic dermatitis in the Netherlands: an international comparison. Br J Dermatol. 2002;147(4):716–24.
50. Foisy M, Boyle RJ, Chalmers JR, Simpson EL, Williams HC. Overview of reviews the prevention of eczema in infants and children: an overview of cochrane and non-cochrane reviews. Evid Based Child Health. 2011;6(5):1322–39.
51. Horimukai K, Morita K, Narita M, et al. Application of moisturizer to neonates prevents development of atopic dermatitis. J Allergy Clin Immunol. 2014;134(4):824–830.e6. e826
52. Simpson EL, Chalmers JR, Hanifin JM, et al. Emollient enhancement of the skin barrier from birth offers effective atopic dermatitis prevention. J Allergy Clin Immunol. 2014;134(4):818–23.
53. Gdalevich M, Mimouni D, David M, Mimouni M. Breast-feeding and the onset of atopic dermatitis in childhood: a systematic review and meta-analysis of prospective studies. J Am Acad Dermatol. 2001;45(4):520–7.
54. Chang YS, Trivedi MK, Jha A, Lin YF, Dimaano L, Garcia-Romero MT. Synbiotics for prevention and treatment of atopic dermatitis: a meta-analysis of randomized clinical trials. JAMA Pediatr. 2016;170(3):236–42.

55. Thaci D, Chambers C, Sidhu M, Dorsch B, Ehlken B, Fuchs S. Twice-weekly treatment with tacrolimus 0.03% ointment in children with atopic dermatitis: clinical efficacy and economic impact over 12 months. J Eur Acad Dermatol Venereol. 2010;24(9):1040–6.
56. Kesselheim AS, Avorn J, Sarpatwari A. The high cost of prescription drugs in the united states: origins and prospects for reform. JAMA. 2016;316(8):858–71.
57. Ellis CN, Kahler KH, Grueger J, Chang J. Cost effectiveness of management of mild-to-moderate atopic dermatitis with 1% pimecrolimus cream in children and adolescents 2–17 years of age. Am J Clin Dermatol. 2006;7(2):133–9.
58. Garside R, Stein K, Castelnuovo E, et al. The effectiveness and cost-effectiveness of pimecrolimus and tacrolimus for atopic eczema: a systematic review and economic evaluation. Health Technol Assess. 2005;9(29):iii. xi–xiii,1–230

Chapter 9
Defining and Measuring the Scope of Atopic Dermatitis

Mary Laird and Kristen Lo Sicco

Abstract Atopic dermatitis (AD) has no definitive diagnostic test and has a large range of phenotypes, making it a difficult disease to assess and define. However, an agreed-upon definition of AD is important for clinical trials, population-based studies, and clinical practice. Several diagnostic criteria systems have been proposed to fill these needs, with none considered the gold standard. To further aid in standardized assessment of AD patients, numerous disease severity and quality of life measurement tools have been proposed. There is similarly no gold standard and efforts are ongoing to develop a single consensus scale. Finally, assessment of AD-associated comorbidities, including allergic/immunologic conditions, psychiatric disorders, and metabolic/cardiac conditions, is important when evaluating this patient population.

Keywords Comorbidities • Diagnosis • Diagnostic criteria • Disease severity • Quality of life

9.1 Introduction

Atopic dermatitis (AD) remains a clinical diagnosis, with no definitive diagnostic test. Its wide range of phenotypes, which depend on factors including the patient's age, disease severity, and disease chronicity, make it a particularly difficult entity to define. An agreed-upon definition of AD is of particular value in clinical trials, in order to properly define the study populations; however, it is also beneficial for population-based studies and clinical practice, especially for the non-dermatologist. As such, there has been great effort to develop diagnostic criteria over the last several decades (Table 9.1).

M. Laird, B.A. • K. Lo Sicco, M.D. (✉)
The Ronald O. Perelman Department of Dermatology, New York University Langone Health, New York, NY, USA
e-mail: Kristen.LoSicco@nyumc.org

E.A. Fortson et al. (eds.), *Management of Atopic Dermatitis*, Advances in Experimental Medicine and Biology 1027, DOI 10.1007/978-3-319-64804-0_9

Table 9.1 List of significant criteria developed for the definition or diagnosis of atopic dermatitis

Criteria	Year
Hanifin and Rajka [1]	1980
Kang and Tian [2]	1989
Diepgen [3]	1989
Schultz-Larsen [4]	1992
Lillehammer [5]	1994
UK Working Party [6–8]	1994
JDA [9]	1994
ISAAC Questionnaire [10]	1995
Diepgen [11]	1996
Millenium [12]	1996
DARC [13]	2005
KDA [14]	2006
AAD Consensus [15, 16]	2003, 2014
REACH [17]	2016

ISAAC International Study of Asthma and Allergies in Childhood; *JDA* Japanese Dermatological Association; *DARC* Danish Allergy Research Centre; *KDA* Korean Dermatological Association; *AAD* American Academy of Dermatology; *REACH* Reliable Estimation of Atopic Dermtitis in ChildHood

9.2 Defining Atopic Dermatitis: Diagnostic Criteria in Clinical Practice Versus Research Studies

Widely recognized as the earliest diagnostic criteria, the 1980 Hanifin and Rajka criteria were primarily developed to clearly define the AD population for research studies [1]. They proposed a system in which the diagnosis is made if 3 of 4 major criteria and 3 of 23 minor criteria are met (Table 9.2). These criteria have had widespread use in research studies and have also been used as the reference standard against which newer criteria were measured [18]. However, several studies have found some minor criteria to be nonspecific, uncommon, overly subjective or poorly defined, or variable depending on factors such as age or ethnicity of the study population [3, 19–24]. These factors, in addition to the length of the criteria, made it an unrealistic diagnostic tool for many settings, including population-based studies or clinical practice [6, 16, 18].

In response to these limitations, numerous other groups have proposed their own diagnostic criteria for AD, many of which were based on the original Hanifin and Rajka criteria (Table 9.1). Some of these were targeted toward specific populations (e.g., the Kang and Tian criteria for the Chinese population [2]), while others attempted to perform better in the population-based community setting (e.g., International Study of Asthma and Allergies in Childhood (ISAAC) questionnaire [10]). In 1994, the U.K. Working Party's Diagnostic Criteria for Atopic Dermatitis attempted to condense the Hanifin and Rajka criteria and develop a simpler definition

Table 9.2 Comparison of the Hanifin and Rajka, UK Working Party and AAD consensus criteria for AD

1980 Hanifin and Rajka [1]	1994 UK Working Party Diagnostic Criteria for Atopic Dermatitis [6–8]	2003/2014 American Academy of Dermatology Consensus [15, 16]
Major criteria (3/4) 1. Pruritus 2. Typical morphology and distribution (a) Flexural in adults (b) Facial/extensor in infants/children 3. Chronic or chronically relapsing course 4. Personal or family history of atopy *Minor criteria* (3/23) 1. Xerosis 2. Ichthyosis/palmar hyperlinearity/keratosis pilaris 3. Immediate type 1 skin test reactivity 4. Elevated serum IgE 5. Early age of onset 6. Tendency toward cutaneous infections 7. Tendency toward non-specific hand/foot dermatitis 8. Nipple eczema 9. Cheilitis 10. Recurrent conjunctivitis 11. Dennie-Morgan infraorbital fold 12. Keratoconus 13. Anterior subcapsular cataracts 14. Orbital darkening 15. Facial pallor/facial erythema 16. Pityriasis alba 17. Anterior neck folds 18. Itch when sweating 19. Intolerance to wool and lipid solvents 20. Perifollicular accentuation 21. Food intolerance 22. Course influenced by environmental/emotional factors 23. White dermographism/delayed blanch	*Mandatory* 1. Pruritus • For children: Parental report of scratching/rubbing *Major criteria* (3/5) 1. History of flexural involvement 2. Personal history of atopy • For children <4: history of atopic disease in first degree relative 3. History of dry skin in the last year 4. Onset <2 years old • For children <4: criteria not used 5. Visible flexural eczema • For children <4: visible flexural eczema or eczema involving cheeks, forehead or outer limbs	*Essential features* (must be present) 1. Pruritus 2. Eczema (acute, subacute or chronic) • Typical morphology and age-specific patterns • Chronic or relapsing history *Important features* (add diagnostic support) 1. Early age at onset 2. Atopy (a) Personal and/or family history (b) IgE reactivity 3. Xerosis *Associated features* (helpful but nonspecific) 1. Atypical vascular responses (e.g., facial pallor, white dermatographism, delayed blanch response) 2. Keratosis pilaris/hyperlinear palms/ichthyosis 3. Ocular/periorbital changes 4. Other regional findings (e.g., perioral changes, periauricular lesions) 5. Perifollicular accentuation/lichenification/prurigo nodules *Exclusionary conditions* (must exclude to diagnose) 1. Scabies 2. Seborrheic dermatitis 3. Allergic contact dermatitis 4. Ichthyoses 5. Cutaneous lymphoma 6. Psoriasis 7. Immune deficiency diseases 8. Photosensitivity dermatoses 9. Erythroderma of other causes

of AD that could be used in both population-based and clinical trials [6–8]. Their criteria defined AD based on one mandatory criterion (pruritus) in addition to 3 of 5 major criteria, with some modifications based on age. Although one major criterion requires an observer to note visible dermatitis, it can be adapted to a purely question-based format for greater ease in population-based studies [7, 18]. Validation studies showed highly variable sensitivity depending on the study population, and the authors were less confident in their criteria for infants less than 1 year [7, 18]. However, this set of criteria is the most validated overall, and is the only set to be tested for repeatability, in both hospital and community settings [18].

More recently, a 2003 consensus from the American Academy of Dermatology (AAD) proposed a new refinement to the Hanifin and Rajka criteria [15]. This outlined two essential features of AD that must be present for diagnosis—pruritus and chronic or relapsing eczema in an age-specific pattern—as well as important and associated features that can help support the diagnosis. This definition also featured the importance of excluding other conditions including scabies and allergic contact dermatitis. This definition was recommended by the 2014 AAD clinical guidelines on AD, which stressed its applicability to a broad age range and the practicality of its use in a clinical setting [16]. Although elevated IgE levels are included as an "important" criterion, the AAD clinical guidelines recommend against their routine use in clinical practice, as IgE elevations are not specific or sensitive [16]. While the lack of validation of this definition may make it less attractive for clinical studies, it may be most useful in clinical practice, particularly to non-dermatologists.

Of the numerous proposed criteria, none emerge as ideal. Some criteria have not been validated at all, and even those that have face issues including lack of independent validation and wide variations in results based on factors including study population, use of point versus 1-year prevalence, non-English translation discrepancies, and methodological differences [18]. Furthermore, with no definitive diagnostic test, the reference or "gold standard" against which criteria are validated is frequently clinical diagnosis by a dermatologist or an earlier set of criteria, which can introduce bias [18]. In addition to these issues, the ideal criteria for a clinical trial will necessarily differ from ideal criteria for population-based studies or clinical practice, making it challenging to create a unifying definition.

9.3 Disease Severity and Quality of Life Measurement Tools

Effective, valid, and reliable outcome measurements are critical to rigorously assess new and existing therapeutics for AD. Both disease severity, which refers to condition-specific parameters of disease activity, and quality of life, which looks at the global impact of a disease on a patient's life and function, are important outcome measures that researchers have attempted to capture using numerous instruments. At least 28 disease severity scales have been described or used for measuring disease severity in AD, which widely vary in the clinical signs assessed, extent of subjective symptom inclusion, and degree and result of rigorous testing on measures including validity, reliability, responsiveness to change, and minimal clinically important difference [16, 25, 26]. At least 22 quality of life instruments have been used to measure outcomes in AD, which are similarly highly variable [16, 25].

The most commonly used disease severity scores in clinical trials in AD are the Severity Scoring of Atopic Dermatitis (SCORAD) and the Eczema Area and Severity Index (EASI) (Table 9.3) [25]. These instruments are also the most rigorously validated and currently have the highest quality measurement properties [26]. The SCORAD was developed by the European Task Force on Atopic Dermatitis [27]. This severity instrument assesses three major categories: extent of disease, clinical signs and subjective symptoms. Extent of disease is a body surface area estimate made using the "rule of nines." A "representative" or "average intensity" area is chosen to evaluate six key signs of disease: erythema, edema/papulation, oozing/crusts, excoriation, lichenification, and dryness (evaluated on an uninvolved area). Subjective symptoms are incorporated by asking the patient to rank their pruritus and sleep loss on a scale from 1 to 10 (Table 9.3).

The EASI was developed using the template of the Psoriasis Area Severity Index (PASI), a well-established disease severity score for psoriasis [28]. This tool uses measurements of involved body surface area of four body sites (head, upper limbs, trunk, and lower limbs) and evaluates four key signs of disease: erythema, induration/papulation/edema, excoriations, and lichenification (Table 9.3) One advantage of the EASI over the SCORAD is evaluating clinical signs in many areas of the body, as opposed to choosing only one representative area [26]. While some believe that the subjective symptoms of the SCORAD capture key information, others believe that the lack of that subjectivity is a key strength of the EASI [25, 26].

As no single disease severity instrument has become the gold standard, the Harmonising Outcome Measures for Eczema (HOME) group was established aimed at achieving international consensus on a single, valid and reliable tool to be used in all clinical trials [29, 30]. This would allow for greater comparison between various clinical trials and AD therapies, creating the opportunity for stronger evidence-based medicine.

As AD is known to significantly impact the lives of patients and their families, measurements of quality of life are also used as important outcome measurements in AD research. Similar to disease severity scales, numerous quality of life instruments have been developed or used in AD, with no gold standard [16, 25]. The most frequently used quality of life instrument in clinical trials is the Children's Dermatology Life Quality Index (CDLQI), followed by the Dermatitis Family Impact (DFI), the Dermatology Life Quality Index (DLQI), and the Infant's Dermatology Quality of Life (IDQOL) [25].

Although outcome measurements would be helpful in guiding individual treatment in routine clinical practice, the existing severity and quality of life scales were generally not designed for this purpose, and are usually too cumbersome to be used in that setting. Efforts at addressing this, including the simplified Three Item Severity (TIS) score [31], show promise but currently need further validation [26]. Ultimately, current evidence does not support the routine clinical use of the available disease severity and quality of life scales; however, providers should ask patients about key aspects of AD's effect on overall wellbeing, including itch, sleep, disease persistence and impact on daily activity [16].

Table 9.3 Comparison of SCORAD and EASI scores for disease severity in atopic dermatitis

	SCORAD [27]	EASI [28]
Score components	*Extent (A)* • Use rule of nine's to estimate area involved *Clinical signs/intensity (B)*—each scored from 0 to 3 (none, mild, moderate, severe)[a] • Erythema • Edema/papulation • Oozing/crust • Excoriation • Lichenification • Dryness *Subjective symptoms (C)*—each scored from 0 to 10 • Pruritus • Sleep loss	*Body regions* (proportionate body surface areas[b]) • Head (10%) • Upper limbs (20%) • Trunk (30%) • Lower limbs (40%) *Clinical signs*—each scored from 0 to 3 (none, mild, moderate, severe) • E = Erythema • I = Induration/papulation/edema • Ex = Excoriations • L = Lichenification *Area score*—each site scored on 7-point scale based on area involved • 0 = none • 1 = <10% • 2 = <10–29% • 3 = <30–49% • 4 = <50–69% • 5 = <70–89% • 6 = >90–100%
Score calculation	A/5 + 7B/2 + C	Head: (E+I+Ex+L) × Area × 0.1 Upper limbs: (E+I+Ex+L) × Area × 0.2 Trunk: (E+I+Ex+L) × Area × 0.3 Lower limbs: (E+I+Ex+L) × Area × 0.4 EASI = sum of above body region scores[b]

SCORAD severity scoring of atopic dermatitis; *EASI* eczema area and severity index

[a]These are calculated based on a representative or average intensity area, with the exception of dryness which is calculated based on an uninvolved area

[b]For patients >8 years old. For patients 0–7 years old, modifications are made to the proportionate body surface area assigned to each body region: head/neck, 20%; upper limbs, 20%; trunk, 30%; lower limbs, 30%

9.4 Assessment of Comorbidities (Table 9.4)

9.4.1 Atopic Diseases: Asthma and Allergic Rhinitis

The association between AD and other atopic diseases has been well established, with children with AD having an increased risk of asthma and allergic rhinitis [32–35]. AD is often described as the beginning of the "atopic march," with individuals first developing AD in early childhood or infancy, and then progressing to allergic rhinitis and asthma as older children. In this theory, it is thought that skin barrier disruption in AD allows for sensitization, which ultimately leads to asthma and allergic rhinitis. However, these diseases are complex and multifactorial and a

Table 9.4 Atopic dermatitis associated comorbidities

Allergy/immunology/dermatologic
Food allergy
Asthma
Allergic rhinitis
Allergic contact dermatitis
Psychiatric
Depression
Anxiety
ADHD
Metabolic/cardiac
Obesity
Pre-diabetes
Hypertension

ADHD attention-deficit hyperactivity disorder

precise causal relationship has not been established; additionally, AD patients may not go on to develop other atopic diseases or may develop them in a different order [32–34, 36].

Nonetheless, treating physicians should be aware of these associations and counsel patients and their parents accordingly [16, 33]. Work-up for a true allergy to an aeroallergen, including specific IgE antibodies and skin prick testing, should be performed based on a relevant clinical history [37]. For those AD patients sensitized to house dust mites, one study found that house dust mite covers (for the mattress, pillows, etc.) may lead to improvement, particularly in children [38]; however, others have shown no impact on overall disease activity [39].

9.4.2 Food Allergy

AD is also strongly associated with food allergies, with up to a third of AD patients also having an IgE-mediated food allergy [40–42]. An even larger proportion of AD patients may demonstrate sensitization to a food (with positive skin prick testing or allergen-specific IgE levels). However, sensitization on testing often does not have clinical relevance, and a true food allergy requires a reproducible, specific immune response on food exposure [40, 42, 43].

The treating physician should be aware of the association with food allergies, with testing guided by a relevant clinical history. The National Institute of Allergy and Infectious Diseases (NIAID) Food Allergy Expert Panel recommends testing for food allergy to milk, egg, peanut and soy in moderate-to-severe AD patients less than 5 years old with at least one of the following: [1] a history of persistent AD despite optimized management and/or [2] a reliable history of immediate reaction after ingestion of a specific food. Skin prick testing and allergen-specific IgE levels, followed by confirmatory oral food challenges, are recommended to diagnose food allergy [40].

Despite the strong association, it is controversial whether a proven food allergy plays a role in the exacerbation of AD symptoms, and it is therefore not fully clear if elimination diets are useful in disease management [40, 44]. There is some limited evidence that egg-free diets in infants with suspected egg allergy and a positive egg-specific IgE decreased AD severity. Regardless of the impact on AD, patients with a true food allergy should already be practicing specific food avoidance. It is important to note that many children with food allergy "outgrow" or become tolerant to foods over time, and that these foods can be reintroduced into diets without worsening of AD symptoms [45].

In patients without proven food allergy, elimination diets or avoidance of potentially allergenic foods is not recommended. This strategy has not been shown to have benefit on AD severity, and overly restrictive diets may place patients at risk of nutritional or growth deficiencies [40, 44].

9.4.3 Allergic Contact Dermatitis

Allergic contact dermatitis (ACD) is in the differential diagnosis for AD, and can be hard to clinically distinguish. However, it is important to recognize that AD and ACD may be concomitant. Studies have shown that ACD is at least as common in patients with AD as in the general population, if not more common [37, 46]. Some believe that AD patients are more susceptible to ACD because of skin barrier defects [47]. On patch testing, nickel is the most common positive result; emollients, antiseptics and topical corticosteroids used for treatment of AD are positive in a small but non-trivial proportion of patients [46, 48]. However, much of this data reflects sensitization, and it is important to recognize that not all positive patch test results are clinically relevant [37, 47]. Patch testing should be considered in patients with a history or exam suggestive of ACD (i.e., marked facial/eyelid involvement, worsening after topical medication), atypical distribution of disease, later onset of disease, and new significant worsening or recalcitrant disease [37, 47].

9.4.4 Obesity, Hypertension, Pre-diabetes

A recent study using two US population cohorts demonstrated that adults with AD are more likely to have lower rates of vigorous activity and higher rates of cigarette smoking and alcohol consumption [49]. Although these are modifiable risk factors, multivariable models controlling for these behaviors still demonstrated a statistically significant association of AD with obesity, hypertension, and pre-diabetes [49]. This suggests that AD confers an additional risk of developing these comorbidities. However, discussion of lifestyle modifications such as smoking and alcohol cessation, and increasing physical activity remains an important part of patient counseling.

It remains unclear if obesity increases the risk of developing AD. A meta-analysis of 30 studies suggests that patients who are overweight or obese have higher odds of AD than normal weight patients [50]. However, the effect sizes were modest and causality cannot be determined from this analysis. Additionally, there may be regional variation, as this association did not hold when looking at European populations specifically. While underlying mechanisms have been postulated, including obesity's association with impaired skin barrier function and chronic inflammation, the mechanism of this association is still unclear [50].

9.4.5 Psychiatric Disorders

AD is known to take a psychiatric toll, particularly due to sleep loss that may result in impaired work or school performance and mood disturbances. Children are also vulnerable to embarrassment and social difficulties [51]. AD has also been associated with increased odds of several psychiatric disorders in adults and children including depression, anxiety and attention-deficit hyperactivity disorder (ADHD) [52–58]. In several cases, studies have shown that severity of AD may further increase the risk of a given psychiatric disorder and sleep disturbance has been associated with increased risk of ADHD specifically [56, 58–60].

In all associations with psychiatric disorders, the mechanisms underlying these associations are not yet understood. It is possible that AD and psychiatric disorders share a common etiological basis, that AD triggers or exacerbates the psychiatric condition, that the psychiatric condition triggers or exacerbates AD, or a that a more complex interaction exists [56, 59, 61]. While awareness of these associations is important, recommendations on specific interventions cannot be made until the causal relationships are further elucidated.

References

1. Hanifin JM, Rajka G. Diagnostic features of atopic dermatitis. Acta Derm Venereol Suppl (Stockh). 1980;92:44–7.
2. Kang KF, Tian RM. Criteria for atopic dermatitis in a Chinese population. Acta Derm Venereol Suppl (Stockh). 1989;144:26–7.
3. Diepgen TL, Fartasch M, Hornstein OP. Evaluation and relevance of atopic basic and minor features in patients with atopic dermatitis and in the general population. Acta Derm Venereol Suppl (Stockh). 1989;144:50–4.
4. Schultz Larsen F, Hanifin JM. Secular change in the occurrence of atopic dermatitis. Acta Derm Venereol Suppl (Stockh). 1992;176:7–12.
5. Schultz Larsen F, Diepgen T, Svensson A. Clinical criteria in diagnosing atopic dermatitis: the Lillehammer criteria 1994. Acta Derm Venereol Suppl (Stockh). 1996;96:115–9.
6. Williams HC, Burney PG, Hay RJ, Archer CB, Shipley MJ, Hunter JJ, et al. The U.K. Working Party's Diagnostic Criteria for Atopic Dermatitis. I. Derivation of a minimum set of discriminators for atopic dermatitis. Br J Dermatol. 1994;131:383–96.

7. Williams HC, Burney PG, Pembroke AC, Hay RJ. The U.K. Working Party's Diagnostic Criteria for Atopic Dermatitis. III. Independent hospital validation. Br J Dermatol. 1994;131:406–16.
8. Williams HC, Burney PG, Strachan D, Hay RJ. The U.K. Working Party's Diagnostic Criteria for Atopic Dermatitis. II. Observer variation of clinical diagnosis and signs of atopic dermatitis. Br J Dermatol. 1994;131:397–405.
9. Association TJD. Definition and diagnostic criteria for atopic dermatitis. Jpn J Dermatol. 1994;104:1210.
10. Asher MI, Keil U, Anderson HR, Beasley R, Crane J, Martinez F, et al. International Study of Asthma and Allergies in Childhood (ISAAC): rationale and methods. Eur Respir J. 1995;8:483–91.
11. Diepgen TL, Sauerbrei W, Fartasch M. Development and validation of diagnostic scores for atopic dermatitis incorporating criteria of data quality and practical usefulness. J Clin Epidemiol. 1996;49:1031–8.
12. Bos JD, Van Leent EJ, Sillevis Smitt JH. The millennium criteria for the diagnosis of atopic dermatitis. Exp Dermatol. 1998;7:132–8.
13. Johnke H, Vach W, Norberg LA, Bindslev-Jensen C, Host A, Andersen KE. A comparison between criteria for diagnosing atopic eczema in infants. Br J Dermatol. 2005;153:352–8.
14. Park Y, Kim H, Kim K, Kim M, Kim J, Ro Y, et al. Report from ADRD: a study on the diagnostic criteria of Korean atopic dermatitis. Korean. J Dermatol. 2006;44:659–63.
15. Eichenfield LF, Hanifin JM, Luger TA, Stevens SR, Pride HB. Consensus conference on pediatric atopic dermatitis. J Am Acad Dermatol. 2003;49:1088–95.
16. Eichenfield LF, Tom WL, Chamlin SL, Feldman SR, Hanifin JM, Simpson EL, et al. Guidelines of care for the management of atopic dermatitis: section 1. Diagnosis and assessment of atopic dermatitis. J Am Acad Dermatol. 2014;70:338–51.
17. Lee S-C, Bae JM, Lee H-J, Kim HJ, Kim B-S, Li K, et al. Introduction of the reliable estimation of atopic dermatitis in ChildHood: novel, diagnostic criteria for childhood atopic dermatitis. Allergy Asthma Immunol Res. 2016;8:230–8.
18. Brenninkmeijer EE, Schram ME, Leeflang MM, Bos JD, Spuls PI. Diagnostic criteria for atopic dermatitis: a systematic review. Br J Dermatol. 2008;158:754–65.
19. Kang KF, Tian RM. Atopic dermatitis. An evaluation of clinical and laboratory findings. Int J Dermatol. 1987;26:27–32.
20. Kanwar AJ, Dhar S, Kaur S. Evaluation of minor clinical features of atopic dermatitis. Pediatr Dermatol. 1991;8:114–6.
21. Kim KH, Chung JH, Park KC. Clinical evaluation of minor clinical features of atopic dermatitis. Ann Dermatol. 1993;5:9–12.
22. Mevorah B, Frenk E, Wietlisbach V, Carrel CF. Minor clinical features of atopic dermatitis. Evaluation of their diagnostic significance. Dermatologica. 1988;177:360–4.
23. Mevorah B, Marazzi A, Frenk E. The prevalence of accentuated palmoplantar markings and keratosis pilaris in atopic dermatitis, autosomal dominant ichthyosis and control dermatological patients. Br J Dermatol. 1985;112:679–85.
24. Rudzki E, Samochocki Z, Rebandel P, Saciuk E, Galecki W, Raczka A, et al. Frequency and significance of the major and minor features of Hanifin and Rajka among patients with atopic dermatitis. Dermatology. 1994;189:41–6.
25. Rehal B, Armstrong AW. Health outcome measures in atopic dermatitis: a systematic review of trends in disease severity and quality-of-life instruments 1985-2010. PLoS One. 2011;6:e17520.
26. Schmitt J, Langan S, Deckert S, Svensson A, von Kobyletzki L, Thomas K, et al. Assessment of clinical signs of atopic dermatitis: a systematic review and recommendation. J Allergy Clin Immunol. 2013;132:1337–47.
27. Severity scoring of atopic dermatitis: the SCORAD index. Consensus Report of the European Task Force on Atopic Dermatitis. Dermatology. 1993;186:23–31.
28. Hanifin JM, Thurston M, Omoto M, Cherill R, Tofte SJ, Graeber M. The eczema area and severity index (EASI): assessment of reliability in atopic dermatitis. EASI evaluator group. Exp Dermatol. 2001;10:11–8.

29. Schmitt J, Spuls P, Boers M, Thomas K, Chalmers J, Roekevisch E, et al. Towards global consensus on outcome measures for atopic eczema research: results of the HOME II meeting. Allergy. 2012;67:1111–7.
30. Schmitt J, Williams H. Harmonising outcome measures for eczema (HOME). Report from the first International Consensus Meeting (HOME 1), 24 July 2010, Munich, Germany. Br J Dermatol. 2010;163:1166–8.
31. Wolkerstorfer A, de Waard van der Spek FB, Glazenburg EJ, Mulder PG, Oranje AP. Scoring the severity of atopic dermatitis: three item severity score as a rough system for daily practice and as a pre-screening tool for studies. Acta Derm Venereol. 1999;79:356–9.
32. Bantz SK, Zhu Z, Zheng T. The atopic march: progression from atopic dermatitis to allergic rhinitis and asthma. J Clin Cell Immunol. 2014;5 doi:10.4172/2155-9899.1000202.
33. Dharmage SC, Lowe AJ, Matheson MC, Burgess JA, Allen KJ, Abramson MJ. Atopic dermatitis and the atopic march revisited. Allergy. 2014;69:17–27.
34. van der Hulst AE, Klip H, Brand PL. Risk of developing asthma in young children with atopic eczema: a systematic review. J Allergy Clin Immunol. 2007;120:565–9.
35. von Kobyletzki LB, Bornehag CG, Hasselgren M, Larsson M, Lindstrom CB, Svensson A. Eczema in early childhood is strongly associated with the development of asthma and rhinitis in a prospective cohort. BMC Dermatol. 2012;12:11.
36. Spergel JM. From atopic dermatitis to asthma: the atopic march. Ann Allergy Asthma Immunol. 2010;105:99–106. quiz 7-9, 17
37. Sidbury R, Tom WL, Bergman JN, Cooper KD, Silverman RA, Berger TG, et al. Guidelines of care for the management of atopic dermatitis: section 4. Prevention of disease flares and use of adjunctive therapies and approaches. J Am Acad Dermatol. 2014;71:1218–33.
38. Friedmann PS, Tan BB. Mite elimination—clinical effect on eczema. Allergy. 1998;53:97–100.
39. Gutgesell C, Heise S, Seubert S, Seubert A, Domhof S, Brunner E, et al. Double-blind placebo-controlled house dust mite control measures in adult patients with atopic dermatitis. Br J Dermatol. 2001;145:70–4.
40. Boyce JA, Assa'ad A, Burks AW, Jones SM, Sampson HA, Wood RA, et al. Guidelines for the diagnosis and management of food allergy in the United States: report of the NIAID-sponsored expert panel. J Allergy Clin Immunol. 2010;126:S1–58.
41. Eigenmann PA, Calza AM. Diagnosis of IgE-mediated food allergy among Swiss children with atopic dermatitis. Pediatr Allergy Immunol. 2000;11:95–100.
42. Eller E, Kjaer HF, Host A, Andersen KE, Bindslev-Jensen C. Food allergy and food sensitization in early childhood: results from the DARC cohort. Allergy. 2009;64:1023–9.
43. Garcia C, El-Qutob D, Martorell A, Febrer I, Rodriguez M, Cerda JC, et al. Sensitization in early age to food allergens in children with atopic dermatitis. Allergol Immunopathol. 2007;35:15–20.
44. Bath-Hextall F, Delamere FM, Williams HC. Dietary exclusions for established atopic eczema. Cochrane Database Syst Rev. 2008;1:Cd005203.
45. Sampson HA. The evaluation and management of food allergy in atopic dermatitis. Clin Dermatol. 2003;21:183–92.
46. Fonacier LS, Aquino MR. The role of contact allergy in atopic dermatitis. Immunol Allergy Clin North Am. 2010;30:337–50.
47. Kwan JM, Jacob SE. Contact dermatitis in the atopic child. Pediatr Ann. 2012;41:422–8.
48. Mailhol C, Lauwers-Cances V, Rance F, Paul C, Giordano-Labadie F. Prevalence and risk factors for allergic contact dermatitis to topical treatment in atopic dermatitis: a study in 641 children. Allergy. 2009;64:801–6.
49. Silverberg JI, Greenland P. Eczema and cardiovascular risk factors in 2 US adult population studies. J Allergy Clin Immunol. 2015;135:721–8.e6.
50. Zhang A, Silverberg JI. Association of atopic dermatitis with being overweight and obese: a systematic review and metaanalysis. J Am Acad Dermatol. 2015;72:606–16.e4.
51. Lewis-Jones S. Quality of life and childhood atopic dermatitis: the misery of living with childhood eczema. Int J Clin Pract. 2006;60:984–92.

52. Bashir K, Dar NR, Rao SU. Depression in adult dermatology outpatients. J Coll Physicians Surg Pak. 2010;20:811–3.
53. Chen MH, TP S, Chen YS, Hsu JW, Huang KL, Chang WH, et al. Is atopy in early childhood a risk factor for ADHD and ASD? A longitudinal study. J Psychosom Res. 2014;77:316–21.
54. Cheng CM, Hsu JW, Huang KL, Bai YM, TP S, Li CT, et al. Risk of developing major depressive disorder and anxiety disorders among adolescents and adults with atopic dermatitis: a nationwide longitudinal study. J Affect Disord. 2015;178:60–5.
55. Schmitt J, Buske-Kirschbaum A, Roessner V. Is atopic disease a risk factor for attention-deficit/hyperactivity disorder? A systematic review. Allergy. 2010;65:1506–24.
56. Schmitt J, Romanos M, Pfennig A, Leopold K, Meurer M. Psychiatric comorbidity in adult eczema. Br J Dermatol. 2009;161:878–83.
57. Slattery MJ, Essex MJ, Paletz EM, Vanness ER, Infante M, Rogers GM, et al. Depression, anxiety, and dermatologic quality of life in adolescents with atopic dermatitis. J Allergy Clin Immunol. 2011;128:668–671.e3.
58. Yaghmaie P, Koudelka CW, Simpson EL. Mental health comorbidity in patients with atopic dermatitis. J Allergy Clin Immunol. 2013;131:428–33.
59. Romanos M, Gerlach M, Warnke A, Schmitt J. Association of attention-deficit/hyperactivity disorder and atopic eczema modified by sleep disturbance in a large population-based sample. J Epidemiol Community Health. 2010;64:269–73.
60. Strom MA, Fishbein AB, Paller AS, Silverberg JI. Association between atopic dermatitis and attention deficit hyperactivity disorder in U.S. children and adults. Br J Dermatol. 2016;175:920–9.
61. Buske-Kirschbaum A, Schmitt J, Plessow F, Romanos M, Weidinger S, Roessner V. Psychoendocrine and psychoneuroimmunological mechanisms in the comorbidity of atopic eczema and attention deficit/hyperactivity disorder. Psychoneuroendocrinology. 2013;38:12–23.

Chapter 10
Prescription Treatment Options

Brad Ackerson, Ryan Thorpe, and Matilda W. Nicholas

Abstract Atopic dermatitis frequently requires the use of over-the-counter and prescription medications for effective management. Emollients and topical corticosteroids are effective for most patients and are the most commonly utilized agents by experienced dermatologists. Antihistamines, antibiotics, and calcineurin inhibitors may also prove helpful in the correct clinical scenarios. Severe atopic dermatitis, however, can be difficult to manage and not infrequently require substantial immunomodulatory medications. Targeted molecular therapies, such as dupilumab, are promising, emerging atopic dermatitis therapies. The medication pearls reviewed in this chapter will assist providers in managing atopic dermatitis patients.

Keywords Topical steroids • Atopic dermatitis • Systemic immunosuppressents • Non-steroid topical treatments

10.1 Introduction

Atopic dermatitis frequently requires the use of over-the-counter and prescription medications for effective management. Emollients and topical corticosteroids are effective for most patients and are the most commonly utilized agents by experienced dermatologists. Antihistamines, antibiotics, and calcineurin inhibitors may also prove helpful in the correct clinical scenarios. Severe atopic dermatitis, however, can be difficult to manage and not infrequently require substantial immunomodulatory medications. Targeted molecular therapies, such as dupilumab, are promising, emerging atopic dermatitis therapies. The medication pearls reviewed in this chapter will assist providers in managing atopic dermatitis patients.

B. Ackerson, B.S. • R. Thorpe, M.D. • M.W. Nicholas, M.D., Ph.D. (✉)
Department of Dermatology, Duke University Hospital, Durham, NC, USA
e-mail: matilda.nicholas@duke.edu

E.A. Fortson et al. (eds.), *Management of Atopic Dermatitis*, Advances in Experimental Medicine and Biology 1027, DOI 10.1007/978-3-319-64804-0_10

10.2 Topical Prescription Agents

10.2.1 Topical Corticosteroids

Topical corticosteroids (TCSs) are the first-line prescription treatment for atopic dermatitis and are used in the management of both adults and children. They exert their effect by acting on T lymphocytes, monocytes, dendritic cells, macrophages, and other immune cells to suppress the actions of proinflammatory cytokines. Given their side effect profile, they are considered after proper skin care and moisturizers alone have failed to provide adequate control of lesions [1]. Their use is well-validated by over 100 randomized controlled trials (RCT) performed to date [2], and they are typically the standard against which other therapies are compared [1]. These trials show the ability of TCSs to reduce acute and chronic signs of AD, as well as reduce associated pruritus [3].

Great variability exists in institution-specific TCS preference in terms of duration, strength, and quantity of application, and no current universal standard exists. Trials evaluating the efficacy of one TCS compared to another are limited resulting in insufficient data to recommend any specific formulation; [1] however, practitioners should contemplate several meaningful components when selecting the appropriate TCS, including potency, patient vehicle preference, cost, and availability [1]. Potency is a crucial consideration, and TCSs are broken into seven classes from very low/lowest potency (class VII) to very high/super potency (class I) [1]. Some prefer a short duration of a high-potency class I or II TCS to quickly control active flares, followed by a taper. Others prefer to use the lowest-potency TCS that adequately controls the disease, gradually increasing the dose until the optimal result is achieved [1].

TCS choice, including vehicle selection, is dependent on the anatomic area to be treated, and therapeutic response and potential side effects must both be considered. Ointments increase hydration of the stratum corneum via an occlusive effect and are preferred for thicker plaques or more severe disease [4]. In the authors' experiences, however, patients often prefer creams that are less greasy. Creams are also preferred when used on moist skin or intertriginous areas [4]. Fluocinolone oil is useful for the scalp areas in patients with coarse hair types, but be sure to counsel patients that the shower cap that comes packaged with the scalp oil may be discarded and that the directions to apply in the evening and wash out in the morning may be ignored. It can be applied once daily as needed for scalp involvement. Some patients also prefer the oil for application to the body. Some patients may prefer other options including sprays, foams, lotions and solutions. It should be noted that the use of alcohol containing vehicles (solutions or foams), creams or lotions often leads to burning and stinging upon application to inflamed or excoriated skin. In these cases, ointments are much better tolerated.

Areas of particular concern for atrophy include the face, skin folds, and the groin, and low potency steroids, such as desonide 0.05% ointment, are recommended for these areas. For example, the absorption of applied drug on the forearm, scalp, and scrotum has been reported to be 1%, 4%, and 35%, respectively [4, 5]. Furthermore, the skin of patients with acute dermatitis demonstrates a defective barrier function resulting in increased intraindividual absorption rates by a factor of 2–10 times baseline during times of acute flares [6]. If low potency TCSs are ineffective, however, short courses of a more potent TCS may be appropriate, but their use may require management by a dermatologist, particularly in high-risk areas. In general, the authors recommend the use of the lowest potency topical steroid which is able to control disease rapidly (ideally within 3 days of twice daily use) and provides a reasonable period before relapse (3–5 days). Often, a class I or II TCS is required to achieve this. It is our belief that use of a higher potency steroid which is able to completely clear disease leads to less overall topical steroid use over the long term and has better patient adherence.

No agreed-upon standard exists for the quantity of TCS application, but many providers use the adult fingertip unit which provides approximately 0.5 g applied over an area the size of two adult palms. It is especially important to consider that children have a greater body surface area - to - weight ratio, about 2.5 to 3 fold higher than adults, leading to higher overall absorption for given amounts applied compared to adults [4]. Regardless of the amount used, studies have shown that mid- and even higher-potency TCSs for short courses are safe and are indicated if rapid control of symptoms is needed, even in children.

Most trials and providers recommend twice daily application of TCSs. That said, a systematic review identified 10 RCTs that found no clear evidence that TCS application more than once daily produced significantly better clinical outcomes [7]. Some new TCS formulations like fluocinonide 0.1% cream specifically recommend once-daily applications [8]. TCS use is recommended daily until control of lesions is achieved, which is best indicated by the inability to appreciate the lesions on palpation when the eyes are closed. It is crucial to recognize that pigment changes, however, may last far longer and will not improve with topical steroid use; in fact, TCSs may exacerbate color change. This should be emphasized through patient education.

There is a role for TCSs in maintenance for patients plagued by repeated outbreaks at the same body sites. A recent meta-analysis of eight vehicle-controlled trials suggests that twice weekly application of fluticasone propionate is efficacious for preventing flares [9].

A detrimental mistake committed by many patients and some providers is not continuing emollient use alongside topical steroids. Unequivocally, atopic dermatitis patients should always use emollients, particularly when being treated with TCSs. They may be applied before or after the use of corticosteroids [10]. However, application of emollients directly after TCS application may lead to spreading of medication beyond the intended area of treatment (see Chap. 11).

While side effects of TCSs are rarely reported, they are very relevant and of particular concern to patients receiving high potency or long courses of TCSs. The risk of skin atrophy increases with higher-potency agents, age, and use on areas of thinner skin, such as the face, groin, and skin folds [4]. Specifically, the use of mid or high potency TCS use should be minimized at periocular sites or corticosteroid-induced glaucoma can develop, which can be resistant to therapy even after discontinuing the TCS [11]. Other side effects include atrophy, striae (stretch marks), focal hypertrichosis, telangiectasias, purpura, and acneiform or rosacea-like eruptions. These typically resolve after discontinuation of TCS use, but patients should be informed that it may take weeks to months [4]. If persistent erythema is noted in treated areas, it is important to differentiate between the erythema from inflammation and the erythema that can result when atrophy allows significant visualization of the superficial vascular plexus, lest the effect be made worse by continued TCS application.

Long-term potent TCS use is also associated with perioral dermatitis, which manifests as erythematous papules and pustules in a perioral distribution sparing the skin immediately adjacent to the vermillion border [4, 12, 13]. While typically associated with TCS us on the face, the authors have seen this side effect with TCS used elsewhere on the body and it has even been reported with inhaled corticosteroids [14]. Notably, maintenance therapy of once to twice weekly application of fluticasone propionate in clinical trials does not appear to cause these side effects, and this likely applies to other TCS formulations [9].

Systemic side effects are rare, but enough absorption can occur with higher potency TCSs applied over a large body surface area to lead to these events. Hyperglycemia, hypertension, and suppression of the hypothalamic-pituitary-adrenal axis are potential risks with long courses of continuous use [4]. These risks increase with concurrent use of inhaled, intranasal, or oral corticosteroids [1]. Nevertheless, the relative safety of TCSs and the benefits afforded to patients with their judicious use almost always outweigh the risks of these infrequent systemic side effects. Furthermore, the rarity of these side effects supports no specific monitoring and none is recommended routinely. When suspicion arises, a cortisol stimulation test can assess adrenal response. If high potency TCSs over a large surface area are required for extended periods of time, referral to a dermatologist is warranted.

10.2.2 Topical Calcineurin Inhibitors

Topical calcineurin inhibitors (TCIs) are anti-inflammatory therapies produced by *Streptomyces* bacteria, which work by inhibiting calcineurin-dependent T-cell activation, thus blocking cytokines involved in the inflammatory reaction [15]. Topical tacrolimus ointment (0.03% and 0.1%) and pimecrolimus cream (1%) are two TCIs have been effective in both short-term (3–12 weeks) and long-term (up to 12 months) control of disease in both children and adults [16]. Tacrolimus is indicated for more severe disease and is often used in combination with TCSs, and pimecrolimus is indicated for mild to moderate presentations of AD. They have a similar efficacy to TCSs, depending on TCS potency. RCTs have found that both topical pimecrolimus and topical tacrolimus are effective in the treatment of atopic dermatitis. In a meta-analysis of 25 RCTs, tacrolimus fared similar to potent topical corticosteroids [17].

Current recommendations encourage TCI use for the treatment of acute and chronic disease. They are recommended for use in mild to severe disease as well as a steroid-sparing agent for long-term use. TCIs can also be used concurrently with TCSs and is in fact recommended by some experts when there is a flare in moderate disease or prior to initiating systemic agents in severe disease. Other providers start with a TCS to control the flare, then switch to a TCI. These medicines are also used for maintenance therapy and can be applied 2–3 times per week on sites of recurrent flares to prevent relapse. This may also reduce the need for TCSs and provides better control than emollients alone. TCIs can be preferable to TCSs in steroid-recalcitrant cases or when TCS side effects, such as steroid-induced atrophy, become an issue. Accordingly, they are particularly useful on the face and skin folds where the risks of TCSs use are increased. TCIs may also be preferred when TCS use is long-term and uninterrupted [1, 17].

The application of tacrolimus ointments twice daily has been shown to be more effective at disease control than either vehicle or once-daily use [18]. A RCT evaluating 3-times-weekly use of tacrolimus for maintenance therapy showed significantly more flare-free days and a longer time until first disease relapse [19]. For maintenance therapy, studies have shown that application of TCIs 2–3 times/week over 40–52 weeks is similarly efficacious compared to TCSs for maintenance therapy [9]. Local reactions (stinging and burning) are the most common side effects seen with TCI use and are reported more often than with TCS use [17]. It is important to inform patients that they may experience this initially, but these effects generally decrease after several applications. More serious, rare side-effects include allergic contact dermatitis and a rosacea-like granulomatous reaction [1]. Continued TCI use during acute infection is not recommended, mostly due to the lack of appropriate studies and the theoretical risk of immunosuppression. The authors have found that pimecrolimus cream can cause significant ocular stinging with accidental contact, so we prefer tacrolimus ointment for the periocular area.

There is a controversial block box warning on the use of TCI stating that long-term safety has not been established, and that although no causal relationship has been confirmed, rare cases of malignancy (skin and lymphoma) have been reported in patients treated with TCI. Importantly, follow-up of 8000 patients treated with TCIs has shown no evidence of increased malignancy risk relative to the general population [20]. Furthermore, a large case-control study of nearly 300,000 patients noted that severity of AD correlated with an increased risk of lymphoma, but not with the use of TCIs [21]. It is important to inform patients and particularly parents of pediatric patients of this warning balanced with the follow-up data that fails to support the black box warning.

10.2.3 Topical Antibiotics

AD predisposes patients to skin infections, and *Staphylococcus aureus* is frequently involved. This is due to both a breakdown of the physical skin barrier and an impaired immune response to various microbes. The use of topical antibiotics is controversial, but the current guidelines derived from a 2010 Cochrane review do not recommend their use, reporting that no benefit for topical antibiotics/antiseptics, antibacterial soaps, or antibacterial bath additives has been found, regardless of the presence of clinical infection [22]. This conclusion is contradicted in part by at least one RCT that reported that the severity of AD in patients with clinical signs of secondary bacterial infections improved with regular dilute bleach baths combined with intermittent intranasal mupirocin [23].

10.3 Oral Antibiotics and Oral Antihistamines

10.3.1 Oral Antibiotics

Evaluating AD patients for infection is difficult. The most common bacterial infection is due to *Staphylococcus aureus,* a microbe isolated in skin culture from greater than 90% of adult patients with AD [24]. While substantially higher than the estimated 5% of the general population colonized with *Staphylococcus aureus*, the majority of the AD patients are not symptomatic, and therefore systemic antibiotics should be reserved for cases of high clinical suspicion of infection. Routine skin swabs are not recommended and, in the authors' opinion, lead to overprescribing of antibiotics.

Weeping purulence, pustules, honey-colored crusting, and other signs of clinical infection validate culture and antibiotic use [25]. Oral antibiotic use can safely be used concurrently with other treatments for AD. Other clinical signs that are important to note include the presence of vesicles and punched-out erosions, which are characteristic of eczema herpeticum, necessitating the prompt use of systemic antivirals. Prior to the use of acyclovir, mortality for untreated eczema herpeticum was 10–50%; whereas, a contemporary retrospective chart review of 1331 patients found no deaths with systemic antiviral therapy [26]. More recently, an entity akin to eczema herpeticum involving the coxsackie virus has been noted in some children.

10.3.2 Oral Antihistamines

In AD, histamine is secreted by mast cells and causes vasodilation and pruritus by stimulating local blood vessels and nerves [25]. Scratching caused by histamine worsens the perceived pruritus in what is described as the itch-scratch cycle. This contributes to breakdown of the physical skin barrier, increasing the risk for infection. Additionally, pruritus is one of the most common complaints of patients with AD, and significantly affects quality of life [27]. Both sedating oral antihistamines such as diphenhydramine, hydroxyzine, and cyproheptadine, as well as non-sedating preparations such as cetirizine, fexofenadine, and loratidine are often prescribed to alleviate pruritus.

A meta-analysis of 16 RCTs comparing sedating and non-sedating oral antihistamines for the treatment of AD concluded that sedating antihistamines may be indicated in cases where symptom severity affects sleep quality; however, there is no evidence to advocate the use of non-sedating antihistamines in the treatment of AD [28]. Furthermore, no evidence has suggested that oral antihistamines have any significant effect on the underlying disease process. The latest guidelines state that there is insufficient evidence to recommend their use for anything other than sleep-loss associated itch [25].

Common side effects of systemic antihistamines include sedation and anticholinergic symptoms such as tachycardia, dry mouth, and blurred vision. It is not necessary to perform any monitoring, unless toxicity is suspected, in which case an electrocardiogram might be indicated. It is important to appreciate that, in the pediatric setting, the use of sedating antihistamines can negatively affect school performance [29]. Paradoxically, however, significant sleep interruption from pruritus can also detrimentally effect academic performance and must be balanced against side effects. In adults, particularly those with poor response or intolerance to antihistamines and/or a component of anxiety, oral doxepin can be considered as a sedating anti-pruritic and is generally very well-tolerated and effective at low doses.

10.4 Systemic Immunomodulators

In the majority of cases, patients with AD see satisfactory clinical improvement with non-pharmacologic interventions, environmental modifications, and the aforementioned conventional topical therapies. However, failure in both disease and symptomatic control necessitates the use of systemic agents [25]. Specifically, patients suffering frequent flares, requiring unsafe levels of topical therapies, or experiencing a persistently negative effect on quality of life inspire the utilization of a systemic immunomodulator.

10.4.1 Cyclosporine

The use of Cyclosporin A (CSA) for the treatment of refractory AD was first reported in 1991 [30]. CSA binds to cyclophilin of lymphocytes, inhibiting calcineurin. This decreases T-cell activity and the transcription of interleukin-2, which causes its immunosuppressant effects. Various RCTs have proven CSA's efficacy in the treatment of AD. Schmitt et al. performed a double-blind, placebo-controlled trial comparing prednisolone vs. CSA, reporting a much higher rate of stable remission for patients treated with CSA [31]. A meta-analysis of 272 RCTs found evidence to support the use of oral cyclosporine in AD [2], and there have also been studies showing that long-term, low-dose use of CSA is safe and effective [32].

There have been studies comparing high- and low-starting doses of CSA for AD treatment. Czech et al. found that a higher starting dose of 300 mg/day in adult patients is more effective than 150 mg/day in controlling AD; however, they recommended 150 mg/day due to greater renal tolerability [33]. The actual starting dose depends on many factors such as patient age, disease severity, medical comorbidities, and tolerability. All formulations of CSA have proven efficacious in the treatment of AD, however one study showed that the microemulsion formulation had greater efficacy and a faster onset of action [34].

The side effect profile includes nephrotoxicity, hypertension, infection, tremor, hypertrichosis, gingival hyperplasia, headache, and increased risk of lymphoma and skin cancer [25]. Monitoring includes bimonthly blood pressure and serum creatinine checks for the first 3 months of treatment followed by monthly monitoring of the same. Significant increases in blood pressure or evidence of renal toxicity are indications to either lower the dose or stop treatment. It is important to remember that many common medications increase cyclosporine levels, including the azole antifungals, furosemide, thiazides, carbonic anhydrase inhibitors, calcium channel blockers, high-dose methylprednisolone, metoclopramide, fluoroquinolones, amiodarone, antimalarials, antiretrovirals, and the SSRI's, fluoxetine and sertraline. Other medications decrease CSA levels, including antibiotics such as nafcillin, rifabutin rifampin, and rifapentine, antiepileptics such as carbamazepine, phenytoin, phenobarbital, and valproic acid, octreotide, rifampicin, and bexarotene.

CSA is also effective in children, and both continuous long-term and intermittent short-term dosing schemes can be appropriate options. It is typically given at a dose of 2.5–5 mg/kg/day in two divided doses for 6 weeks. After 6 weeks, adjustment is made to the lowest effective dose.

It is recommended that with the clearance of acute disease, CSA be tapered, discontinued, and/or replaced by an alternative maintenance therapy with a preferable side effect profile. Overall, most dermatologists favor CSA as a short-term agent for immediate control given its rapid onset of action, but more extensive side effect profile. Maintenance therapies include emollients, topical agents, methotrexate or other systemic agent, or phototherapy [25].

10.4.2 Methotrexate

MTX is an immunosuppressant which exerts its effects by multiple pathways. As an antifolate, it inhibits the synthesis of DNA and RNA. It is also believed to inhibit enzymes involved in purine metabolism, which leads to the accumulation of adenosine. Accumulated adenosine inhibits T-cell activation and deactivates other enzymes related to immune system function [35]. MTX is often used for oncologic, inflammatory, and autoimmune disorders. Along with its FDA approved use for the treatment of mycosis fungoides and psoriasis, MTX has off-label use in treating AD.

Schram et al. conducted a single-blind trial of 42 patients, assigning them to either MTX (dosage, 10–22.5 mg/week) or azathioprine (dosage, 1.5–2.5 mg/kg/day). Both groups had significant mean reduction in severity scoring of AD index, with the MTX group seeing a 42% reduction [36]. A prospective trial of 12 patients showed a 45–60% improvement in disease activity, with significant reduction in the body surface area affected while showing improvements in quality of life, sleep, and itch scores [37]. Lyakhovitsky et al. also concluded that MTX is safe and efficacious in a 20 patient trial [38]. MTX is also safe for use in children. El-Khalawany et al. compared MTX to CSA use in children and found a mean absolute reduction in severity scoring for atopic dermatitis (SCORAD) to be 25.25 in the MTX arm and no statistical difference between MTX and CSA [39].

MTX is available in both an injectable solution and oral tablet forms. Although patients tend to avoid injections, MTX's once weekly dosing makes either feasible and injections may be preferred in the event of gastrointestinal upset from the oral form. Dosing is grounded on its use for psoriasis and is generally 7.5–25 mg weekly (pediatric dosing is 0.2–0.7 mg/kg/week) in the oral form [25, 40]. The lowest possible dose to achieve disease remission is recommended. It takes an average of 10 weeks to achieve maximum effect, and further dose escalation after 12–16 weeks appears to provide no increased efficacy [37]. After clearance of active disease, tapering off of MTX in favor of maintenance therapies is desired, if tolerated. If patients fail to respond to a sufficient dose after a 12- to 16-week trial, physicians should consider discontinuing MTX [25]. Folate supplementation should be given while treating with MTX and is recommended to be taken daily (1–5 mg) except for the 1 day each week on which MTX is taken. Authors generally recommend starting with 1 mg on non-MTX days, but this should be increased by 1 mg/day up to 5 mg/day as needed to ameliorate side effects.

The side effect profile is well-known to frequent prescribers, although limited studies have addressed its safety specifically in cases of AD. One of the more serious side effects is hepatotoxicity, and traditionally some experts advise that a liver biopsy be done once patients reach a cumulative dose of 3.5–4 g; however, patients without risk factors for hepatic fibrosis may not need biopsies. The Fibroscan in conjunction with blood testing has been replacing this approach [41, 42]. In general, liver evaluation by a gastroenterologist is recommended for persistent elevation of LFTs or at cumulative doses of methotrexate of 3.5–4 g.

Common side effects include nausea, GI symptoms, and fatigue. Rare, yet more serious, side effects include bone marrow suppression and pulmonary fibrosis. Caution should be taken when prescribing MTX to patients with asthma, chronic cough, or other pulmonary disease, and a complete pulmonary evaluation is suggested prior to initiating therapy in these patients. Recently, MTX was associated with an increased risk of nonmelanoma skin cancer formation in rheumatoid arthritis and inflammatory bowel disease patients, but the authors are unaware of similar data specific to AD patients [43].

Notably, most side effects are reversible by increasing the folic acid dose, reducing the methotrexate dose, or altering dosing schedule [25]. MTX interacts with other hepatotoxic drugs such as barbiturates to increase the risk of liver damage. Sulfamethoxazole, NSAIDs, and penicillins interfere with the renal clearance of MTX, and it is important not to use MTX with other folic acid antagonists such as trimethoprim. Prior to beginning therapy, baseline hepatic and renal function should be assessed. After initiation, providers should check traditional liver function tests weekly for 2–4 weeks, then every 2 weeks for 1 month. Once patients are on stable doses, labs should be re-evaluated every 2–3 months [25]. The authors have found that higher doses may be needed in atopic dermatitis and suggest a starting dose of 15 mg/week for adults, increasing the dose, if tolerated, to 20 mg/week which can be tapered once control is achieved.

10.4.3 Mycophenolate Mofetil

Mycophenolate mofetil (MMF) is an immunosuppressant that inhibits inosine monophosphate dehydrogenase thereby blocking purine synthesis selectively in T cells and B cells. While it is currently only FDA approved in cases of solid organ transplantation, its off-label use in patients with AD is a viable option in refractory cases.

There is very limited data proving efficacy of MMF in the treatment of refractory AD. A trial performed by Haeck et al. treated 55 patients with CSA for 6 weeks. Twenty-four of these patients were then switched from CSA to MMF for 30 weeks. In the first 10 weeks after the switch, the patients who remained on CSA did better. However, after week 10 both CSA- and MMF-treated patients showed equal efficacy and comparable side effect severity [44]. No studies have attempted to study relapse rates or establish dosing recommendations. Retrospective studies report dose ranges from 0.5 to 3 g/day [45]. It is administered twice daily and is available in oral suspension, tablets, and capsules. The most common side effects include nausea, vomiting, and abdominal cramping. These do not seem to be dose dependent. There are rare reports of hematologic side effects such as anemia, leukopenia, and thrombocytopenia, as well as genitourinary symptoms such as urgency, frequency, and dysuria. As with other immunosuppressant medications, increased rates of infections, skin cancer, and lymphoma are potential risks. MMF interacts with calcium, iron, cholestyramine, high-dose salicylates, phenytoin, xanthine bronchodilators, probenecid, antacids containing aluminum and magnesium, and the -cyclovirs. Antibiotics such as cephalosporins, fluoroquinolones, macrolides, -penems, penicillins, and sulfonamides all decrease MMF levels.

MMF can be considered safe and efficacious in children. A retrospective analysis of 14 pediatric patients with severe AD who were treated with MMF as systemic monotherapy showed encouraging results. Only one child had no response, while four (29%) enjoyed a complete clearance, four (29%) experienced >90% improvement, and five (35%) showed 60–90% improvement [46]. The pediatric dosing of 600–1200 mg/m^2 is based on body surface area due to increased hepatic metabolism [25].

10.4.4 Azathioprine

Azathioprine (AZA) is an immunosuppressant that exerts its effect by inhibiting DNA production. It is a prodrug of mercaptopurine whose metabolites are incorporated into replicating DNA; therefore, its effects are greatest on rapidly proliferating cells such as T cells and B cells. It is FDA approved for the treatment of renal transplant rejection prophylaxis and rheumatoid arthritis, but it is used off-label for the treatment of inflammatory disorders such as AD. It is recommended only for AD cases refractory to more conservative options.

There have been several RCTs evaluating AZA's effectiveness for the treatment of AD. Berth-Jones et al. conducted a double-blind, randomized, placebo-controlled, crossover trial of AZA. Thirty-seven adult patients with severe AD were assigned to either AZA 2.5 mg/kg/day or placebo. Disease activity and severity of symptoms were monitored. They concluded that there was a significant reduction in disease activity for patients treated with AZA. There was a significant mean improvement for disruption of work/daytime activity, but not for pruritus or sleep disturbance [47]. Meggitt et al. conducted a placebo-controlled trial which assigned 63 patients to treatment with AZA or placebo for 12 weeks. They found a 17% mean improvement in disease activity with AZA (95% CI 4.3–29%). They also found significant improvements in pruritus, area of involvement, and quality of life [48]. Schram et al. conducted an RCT comparing MTX to AZA, finding clinically significant improvement in both, but no significant difference between the two treatments [36].

Most studies have chosen a dose rate between 1–3 mg/kg/day. The metabolism of AZA depends on individual activity levels of thiopurine methyltransferase (TPMT), and some patients have genetic polymorphisms that predispose them to AZA toxicity. Meggitt et al. controlled for TPMT activity, finding equal efficacy, but a reduction in side effects compared to traditional dosing [48]. It is strongly recommended to obtain baseline TPMT levels prior to AZA initiation and to adjust dosing accordingly.

Side effects include nausea, vomiting, bloating, anorexia, and cramping. These are common reasons for patient non-compliance. Less common side-effects include headache, hypersensitivity reactions, leukopenia, and elevated liver enzymes. Infection, skin cancer, and lymphoma are potential risks. AZA interacts with allopurinol, increasing the risk of pancytopenia. Its use with captopril increases the risk of anemia and leukemia. The warfarin effect and pancuronium effect are reduced. When used with cotrimoxazole there is an increased risk of hematologic toxicity.

Monitoring consists of a complete blood count, liver function panel, and evaluation of renal function twice per month for 2 months, then monthly for 4 months. Providers should continue with labs every other month and with any dose increases.

A retrospective study of AZA use in children with severe AD concluded that it was both safe and effective in children with normal TPMT activity [49]. A dose range of 2.5–3.5 mg/kg/day in children with normal TPMT levels is recommended. Again, assessment of TPMT level should be done prior to therapy initiation. Prescribing physicians must appreciate that TPMT-deficient patients are at risk for myelosuppression; whereas, those with supraphysiologic TMPT activity, which is less common, may not demonstrate a therapeutic response to standard dosage [49].

10.4.5 Omalizumab

Heil et al. conducted a randomized, placebo-controlled study of omalizumab, an injectable monoclonal antibody against IgE. Twenty patients were given omalizumab or placebo subcutaneously and assessed. They found that omalizumab lowered free serum IgE, but did not significantly improve control of disease [50]. In general this treatment is reserved for patients with extremely high IgE levels as an adjuvant therapy.

10.4.6 Emerging Therapies

Emerging therapies for the treatment of AD focus on the blockade of inflammatory cytokines. Of particular interest are the cytokines derived from type 2 T helper cells (Th2) which participate in the sensitization of immunoglobulin E (IgE). The most promising therapeutic targets include the chemoattractant receptor-homologous molecule expressed on Th2 cells (CRTH2), IgE, thymic stromal lymphopoietin (TSLP), the JAK/STAT pathway, phosphodiesterase-4 (PDE-4), and the interleukin-4/interleukin-13 receptor alpha chain.

For details on novel therapeutics which are currently being developed and tested in clinical trials, please see Chap. 15.

10.4.7 The Pediatric Patient

As with any disease, it is important to consider the differences in treating children versus adults with AD, including both the pathophysiological and social differences. Furthermore, it is important to be more cautious regarding long-term side effects, particularly when using systemic medications. This means following the patient's weight to monitor for needed dose changes and tracking the cumulative dose reached. As referenced above, children have a higher body surface area - to - weight ratio resulting in increased absorption than in the adult patient [4]. Though the risks of systemic side effects of TCSs remain rare, they are greater in children, and include suppression of the hypothalamic-pituitary-adrenal axis and can affect growth [4]. However, high-potency TCSs often controls flaring disease much more quickly and may be preferable to long-term use of a lower potency TCS. Prevention of disease flares is also important in order to limit exposure to these medications. Topical tacrolimus 0.03% used 2–3 times/weekly has been shown to decrease the number of flares requiring further medication [9].

Lack of understanding by families often leads to non-compliance. Steroid phobia is well documented. A questionnaire-based study of 200 patients with AD showed that 72.5% of patients worried about using TCSs on their own or their child's skin. Thirty-one percent of patients using hydrocortisone either did not know its potency or incorrectly classified it as strong or very strong [51]. While it is always important to inform parents regarding the side effects of TCSs, it is also imperative to inform them of the benefit and importance of treatment in order to improve patient compliance. The authors have heard first-hand parents of pediatric patients preferring systemic immunomodulators such as CSA over TCSs due to misappropriating risks.

The social and developmental impact of AD is much more pronounced in children. Severe pruritus causes significant distress, both for children and caregivers, and AD in a child can be disabling for whole families by affecting sleep, school performance, and quality of life. Studies have attempted to evaluate the effectiveness of psychological and educational approaches to manage itching, scratching, and sleep disturbances with generally positive results. These approaches include relaxation techniques, behavioral interventions, cognitive behavioral therapy, and educational interventions. A study of 185 parent-child pairs compared a group receiving a training program on the aforementioned approaches to a waiting control group. At 1-year follow-up, they found improvements—not only in AD severity—but also in both the children's and parents' coping behavior [52]. Recognition and treatment of psychosocial stresses leads to better outcomes.

Some research suggests that emollient therapy from birth may help prevent AD. Simpson et al. conducted a study with 22 neonates at high risk for AD. They were instructed to begin emollient therapy at birth. Results were compared to historical controls and suggested a protective effect against developing atopic dermatitis [53].

Recently, introducing peanuts early to infants at high risk for peanut allergy modulated the immune response resulting in a decreased likelihood of acquiring a peanut allergy [54]. While the correlation of this finding to developing AD is not clear, the American Academy of Pediatrics (AAP) has stated that nutritional decisions during the first year of life may affect the development of atopic disease, including food allergies, asthma, as well as AD [55]. Congruently, in 2008 the AAP guidelines recommended against delaying the introduction of complementary foods beyond 4–6 months and encouraged breastfeeding or hydrolyzed formulas for the first 4 months of life to delay or prevent the development of AD [55].

For children who do develop AD, research suggests that only one third of children affected with refractory, moderate-severe AD have an IgE-mediated reactivity to food proteins. (Eigenmann) Evaluating and treating a food allergy can prove helpful in this subset patients; however, in the authors' experience, these types of evaluations and interventions often lead to needless disruptions in the lives of AD patients through diet restrictions and allergy testing that do not result in any benefit. For this reason, physicians should be judicious with food and allergy testing in AD patients.

References

1. Eichenfield LF, Tom WL, Berger TG, et al. Guidelines of care for the management of atopic dermatitis: section 2. Management and treatment of atopic dermatitis with topical therapies. J Am Acad Dermatol. 2014;71:116–32.
2. Hoare C, Li Wan Po A, Williams H. Systematic review of treatments for atopic eczema. Health Technol Assess. 2000;4:1–191.
3. Stein SL, Cifu AS. Management of atopic dermatitis. JAMA. 2016;315:1510–1.
4. Hengge UR, Ruzicka T, Schwartz RA, Cork MJ. Adverse effects of topical glucocorticosteroids. J Am Acad Dermatol. 2006;54:1–15. quiz 6-8
5. Feldmann RJ, Maibach HI. Regional variation in percutaneous penetration of 14C cortisol in man. J Invest Dermatol. 1967;48:181–3.
6. Turpeinen M, Lehtokoski-Lehtiniemi E, Leisti S, Salo OP. Percutaneous absorption of hydrocortisone during and after the acute phase of dermatitis in children. Pediatr Dermatol. 1988;5:276–9.
7. Williams HC. Established corticosteroid creams should be applied only once daily in patients with atopic eczema. BMJ. 2007;334:1272.
8. Woods MT, Brown PA, Baig-Lewis SF, Simpson EL. Effects of a novel formulation of fluocinonide 0.1% cream on skin barrier function in atopic dermatitis. J Drugs Dermatol. 2011;10:171–6.
9. Schmitt J, von Kobyletzki L, Svensson A, Apfelbacher C. Efficacy and tolerability of proactive treatment with topical corticosteroids and calcineurin inhibitors for atopic eczema: systematic review and meta-analysis of randomized controlled trials. Br J Dermatol. 2011;164:415–28.
10. Ng SY, Begum S, Chong SY. Does order of application of emollient and topical corticosteroids make a difference in the severity of atopic eczema in children? Pediatr Dermatol. 2016;33:160–4.
11. Kersey JP, Broadway DC. Corticosteroid-induced glaucoma: a review of the literature. Eye (London, England). 2006;20:407–16.
12. Sneddon I. Perioral dermatitis. Br J Dermatol. 1972;87:430–4.
13. Mihan R, Ayres S Jr. Perioral dermatitis. Arch Dermatol. 1964;89:803–5.
14. Poulos GA, Brodell RT. Perioral dermatitis associated with an inhaled corticosteroid. Arch Dermatol. 2007;143:1460.
15. Breuer K, Werfel T, Kapp A. Safety and efficacy of topical calcineurin inhibitors in the treatment of childhood atopic dermatitis. Am J Clin Dermatol. 2005;6:65–77.
16. El-Batawy MM, Bosseila MA, Mashaly HM, Hafez VS. Topical calcineurin inhibitors in atopic dermatitis: a systematic review and meta-analysis. J Dermatol Sci. 2009;54:76–87.
17. Ashcroft DM, Dimmock P, Garside R, Stein K, Williams HC. Efficacy and tolerability of topical pimecrolimus and tacrolimus in the treatment of atopic dermatitis: meta-analysis of randomised controlled trials. BMJ. 2005;330:516.

18. Reitamo S, Harper J, Bos JD, et al. 0.03% Tacrolimus ointment applied once or twice daily is more efficacious than 1% hydrocortisone acetate in children with moderate to severe atopic dermatitis: results of a randomized double-blind controlled trial. Br J Dermatol. 2004;150:554–62.
19. Breneman D, Fleischer AB Jr, Abramovits W, et al. Intermittent therapy for flare prevention and long-term disease control in stabilized atopic dermatitis: a randomized comparison of 3-times-weekly applications of tacrolimus ointment versus vehicle. J Am Acad Dermatol. 2008;58:990–9.
20. Koo JY, Fleischer AB Jr, Abramovits W, et al. Tacrolimus ointment is safe and effective in the treatment of atopic dermatitis: results in 8000 patients. J Am Acad Dermatol. 2005;53:S195–205.
21. Arellano FM, Wentworth CE, Arana A, Fernandez C, Paul CF. Risk of lymphoma following exposure to calcineurin inhibitors and topical steroids in patients with atopic dermatitis. J Invest Dermatol. 2007;127:808–16.
22. Bath-Hextall FJ, Birnie AJ, Ravenscroft JC, Williams HC. Interventions to reduce Staphylococcus aureus in the management of atopic eczema: an updated Cochrane review. Br J Dermatol. 2010;163:12–26.
23. Huang JT, Abrams M, Tlougan B, Rademaker A, Paller AS. Treatment of Staphylococcus aureus colonization in atopic dermatitis decreases disease severity. Pediatrics. 2009;123:e808–14.
24. Boguniewicz M, Sampson H, Leung SB, Harbeck R, Leung DY. Effects of cefuroxime axetil on Staphylococcus aureus colonization and superantigen production in atopic dermatitis. J Allergy Clin Immunol. 2001;108:651–2.
25. Sidbury R, Davis DM, Cohen DE, et al. Guidelines of care for the management of atopic dermatitis: section 3. Management and treatment with phototherapy and systemic agents. J Am Acad Dermatol. 2014;71:327–49.
26. Aronson PL, Yan AC, Mittal MK, Mohamad Z, Shah SS. Delayed acyclovir and outcomes of children hospitalized with eczema herpeticum. Pediatrics. 2011;128:1161–7.
27. Sher LG, Chang J, Patel IB, Balkrishnan R, Fleischer AB Jr. Relieving the pruritus of atopic dermatitis: a meta-analysis. Acta Derm Venereol. 2012;92:455–61.
28. Klein PA, Clark RA. An evidence-based review of the efficacy of antihistamines in relieving pruritus in atopic dermatitis. Arch Dermatol. 1999;135:1522–5.
29. Schad CA, Skoner DP. Antihistamines in the pediatric population: achieving optimal outcomes when treating seasonal allergic rhinitis and chronic urticaria. Allergy Asthma Proc. 2008;29:7–13.
30. Sowden JM, Berth-Jones J, Ross JS, et al. Double-blind, controlled, crossover study of cyclosporin in adults with severe refractory atopic dermatitis. Lancet. 1991;338:137–40.
31. Schmitt J, Schakel K, Folster-Holst R, et al. Prednisolone vs. ciclosporin for severe adult eczema. An investigator-initiated double-blind placebo-controlled multicentre trial. Br J Dermatol. 2010;162:661–8.
32. Haw S, Shin MK, Haw CR. The efficacy and safety of long-term oral cyclosporine treatment for patients with atopic dermatitis. Ann Dermatol. 2010;22:9–15.
33. Czech W, Brautigam M, Weidinger G, Schopf E. A body-weight-independent dosing regimen of cyclosporine microemulsion is effective in severe atopic dermatitis and improves the quality of life. J Am Acad Dermatol. 2000;42:653–9.
34. Zurbriggen B, Wuthrich B, Cachelin AB, Wili PB, Kagi MK. Comparison of two formulations of cyclosporin A in the treatment of severe atopic dermatitis. Aa double-blind, single-centre, cross-over pilot study. Dermatology. 1999;198:56–60.
35. Wessels JA, Huizinga TW, Guchelaar HJ. Recent insights in the pharmacological actions of methotrexate in the treatment of rheumatoid arthritis. Rheumatology (Oxford). 2008;47:249–55.
36. Schram ME, Roekevisch E, Leeflang MM, Bos JD, Schmitt J, Spuls PI. A randomized trial of methotrexate versus azathioprine for severe atopic eczema. J Allergy Clin Immunol. 2011;128:353–9.

37. Weatherhead SC, Wahie S, Reynolds NJ, Meggitt SJ. An open-label, dose-ranging study of methotrexate for moderate-to-severe adult atopic eczema. Br J Dermatol. 2007;156:346–51.
38. Lyakhovitsky A, Barzilai A, Heyman R, et al. Low-dose methotrexate treatment for moderate-to-severe atopic dermatitis in adults. J Eur Acad Dermatol Venereol. 2010;24:43–9.
39. El-Khalawany MA, Hassan H, Shaaban D, Ghonaim N, Eassa B. Methotrexate versus cyclosporine in the treatment of severe atopic dermatitis in children: a multicenter experience from Egypt. Eur J Pediatr. 2013;172:351–6.
40. Menter A, Korman NJ, Elmets CA, et al. Guidelines of care for the management of psoriasis and psoriatic arthritis: section 4. Guidelines of care for the management and treatment of psoriasis with traditional systemic agents. J Am Acad Dermatol. 2009;61:451–85.
41. Strober BE. Practice gaps. Methotrexate-induced liver toxicity: replacing the liver biopsy. JAMA Dermatol. 2014;150:862–3.
42. Afdhal NH. Fibroscan (transient elastography) for the measurement of liver fibrosis. Gastroenterol Hepatol. 2012;8:605–7.
43. Scott FI, Mamtani R, Brensinger CM, et al. Risk of nonmelanoma skin cancer associated with the use of immunosuppressant and biologic agents in patients with a history of autoimmune disease and nonmelanoma skin cancer. JAMA Dermatol. 2016;152:164–72.
44. Haeck IM, Knol MJ, Ten Berge O, van Velsen SG, de Bruin-Weller MS, Bruijnzeel-Koomen CA. Enteric-coated mycophenolate sodium versus cyclosporin A as long-term treatment in adult patients with severe atopic dermatitis: a randomized controlled trial. J Am Acad Dermatol. 2011;64:1074–84.
45. Murray ML, Cohen JB. Mycophenolate mofetil therapy for moderate to severe atopic dermatitis. Clin Exp Dermatol. 2007;32:23–7.
46. Heller M, Shin HT, Orlow SJ, Schaffer JV. Mycophenolate mofetil for severe childhood atopic dermatitis: experience in 14 patients. Br J Dermatol. 2007;157:127–32.
47. Berth-Jones J, Takwale A, Tan E, et al. Azathioprine in severe adult atopic dermatitis: a double-blind, placebo-controlled, crossover trial. Br J Dermatol. 2002;147:324–30.
48. Meggitt SJ, Gray JC, Reynolds NJ. Azathioprine dosed by thiopurine methyltransferase activity for moderate-to-severe atopic eczema: a double-blind, randomised controlled trial. Lancet. 2006;367:839–46.
49. Murphy LA, Atherton D. A retrospective evaluation of azathioprine in severe childhood atopic eczema, using thiopurine methyltransferase levels to exclude patients at high risk of myelosuppression. Br J Dermatol. 2002;147:308–15.
50. Heil PM, Maurer D, Klein B, Hultsch T, Stingl G. Omalizumab therapy in atopic dermatitis: depletion of IgE does not improve the clinical course—a randomized, placebo-controlled and double blind pilot study. J Dtsch Dermatol Ges. 2010;8:990–8.
51. Charman CR, Morris AD, Williams HC. Topical corticosteroid phobia in patients with atopic eczema. Br J Dermatol. 2000;142:931–6.
52. Kupfer J, Gieler U, Diepgen TL, et al. Structured education program improves the coping with atopic dermatitis in children and their parents-a multicenter, randomized controlled trial. J Psychosom Res. 2010;68:353–8.
53. Simpson EL, Berry TM, Brown PA, Hanifin JM. A pilot study of emollient therapy for the primary prevention of atopic dermatitis. J Am Acad Dermatol. 2010;63:587–93.
54. Du Toit G, Roberts G, Sayre PH, et al. Randomized trial of peanut consumption in infants at risk for peanut allergy. N Engl J Med. 2015;372:803–13.
55. Greer FR, Sicherer SH, Burks AW. Effects of early nutritional interventions on the development of atopic disease in infants and children: the role of maternal dietary restriction, breastfeeding, timing of introduction of complementary foods, and hydrolyzed formulas. Pediatrics. 2008;121:183–91.

Chapter 11
Non-Prescription Treatment Options

Sandy François, Kayla Felix, Leah Cardwell, Taylor Edwards, and Zakiya Rice

Abstract The pathogenesis of atopic dermatitis (AD) is complex and multifactorial. However, recent advancements in the genetics and pathophysiology of AD suggest that epidermal barrier dysfunction is paramount in the development and progression of the condition (Boguniewicz and Leung, Immunol Rev 242(1):233–246, 2011). In addition to standard therapy for AD, there are a plethora of non-prescription treatment modalities which may be employed. Over-the-counter treatments for atopic dermatitis can come in the form of topical corticosteroids, moisturizers/emollients, and oral anti-histamines. Though these treatments are beneficial, prescription treatments may be quicker acting and more efficacious in patients with moderate to severe disease or during flares. OTC agents are best used for maintenance between flares and to prevent progression of mild disease. Alternative and complementary treatments lack strong efficacy evidence. However, wet wraps, bleach baths, and other treatments appear to be promising when used in conjunction with conventional treatments. With the financial burden of atopic dermatitis ranging from 364 million to 3.8 billion dollars each year in the United States, we suspect this topic will gain further research attention.

Keywords Alternative treatment • Natural oils • Emollients • Textile

---

S. François, B.S., M.Sc. • Z. Rice, M.D. (✉)
Department of Dermatology, Emory School of Medicine, Atlanta, GA, USA
e-mail: zpressl@emory.edu

K. Felix, B.S. • L. Cardwell, M.D.
Department of Dermatology, Wake Forest University School of Medicine, Winston Salem, NC, USA

T. Edwards, B.S.
Ohio University Heritage College of Osteopathic Medicine, Athens, OH, USA

E.A. Fortson et al. (eds.), *Management of Atopic Dermatitis*, Advances in Experimental Medicine and Biology 1027, DOI 10.1007/978-3-319-64804-0_11

11.1 Introduction

The pathogenesis of atopic dermatitis (AD) is complex and multifactorial. However, recent advancements in the genetics and pathophysiology of AD suggest that epidermal barrier dysfunction is paramount in the development and progression of the condition [1]. In addition to standard therapy for AD, there are a plethora of non-prescription treatment modalities which may be employed. In this chapter, we will discuss non-prescription options for treating atopic dermatitis. These items include over-the-counter (OTC) topical and systemic medications, emollients, and skin care regimens. These alternative treatment modalities may improve the symptoms associated with this burdensome condition.

11.2 Non-Prescription Treatments in Atopic Dermatitis

11.2.1 Topical Corticosteroids

Low potency topical corticosteroids such as hydrocortisone are a commonly used OTC treatment for atopic dermatitis. Typically, topical hydrocortisone is available in concentrations of 1% or less, with 1% concentrations being the maximum strength available without a prescription.

Hydrocortisone efficacy was observed prior to the 1970s, however several trials were done to evaluate its efficacy in different vehicle types. In 1973, a double-blind study evaluated a preparation of 1% hydrocortisone in a 10% urea cream compared to 0.1% betamethasone 17-valerate [2]. During this time, highly-potent fluorinated steroids were widely in use and the introduction of hydrocortisone cream was a movement toward less potent topical preparations. Urea cream was used to aid in drug penetration and to improve ichthyosis of the skin [3]. In the study (n = 50), each patient was supplied with both medications and instructed to use one treatment per side of the body for 2–3 weeks. Progress was measured by physician exam and disease progress was labelled as excellent, good, none, or deterioration. Twelve patients showed greater improvement due to the hydrocortisone in urea, 15 showed greater improvement using betamethasone 17-valerate, while the remaining 23 patients had equal improvement by both treatments. There was no significant difference in treatment which, at the time, confirmed the ability of implementing hydrocortisone as a safer treatment option for atopic dermatitis [2]. Soon after, another double-blind study was done evaluating the efficacy of 1% hydrocortisone in a novel carbamide delivery system (n = 36) [4]. The study had an identical design as explained above, and treatment was applied 3 times daily for 2 weeks. Participants who were not responsive to either treatment after 42 weeks continued in the study for 4 weeks. Eleven patients had greatest improvement with the hydrocortisone in carbamide, 5 had greatest improvement using betamethasone 17-valerate, and 17 had equal responses to both. Hydrocortisone was shown to be, at the least, equally efficacious to betamethasone 17-valerate—an already widely-used treatment for atopic dermatitis.

Additional vehicle formulations have also been evaluated. In 1980, a comparison of two hydrocortisone formulations was done. Both were efficacious, and no side effects were reported [5]. In a 2004 study (n = 624), 0.03% Tacrolimus ointment was more efficacious for the treatment of moderate to severe atopic dermatitis in children than 1% hydrocortisone [6]. Subjects using tacrolimus once or twice daily for 3 weeks had decreases in mEASI (66.7% and 76.7%, respectively) that were significantly greater than the decrease due to 1% hydrocortisone acetate (47.6%, $p < 0.001$). A 6 week comparison to 0.1% mometasone furoate cream yielded a comparable result, with 1% hydrocortisone cream again being less efficacious in treating pediatric patients with moderate to severe atopic dermatitis (n = 48) [7].

11.2.2 Oral Anti-Histamines

Oral anti-histamines have also been evaluated for efficacy in treating dermatitis, though there is not much conclusive data on their efficacy [8]. Pruritus in atopic dermatology is not completely understood, but a proposed mechanism is the release of histamine from IgE sensitized mast cells and basophils [9, 10]. Anti-histamines work to reduce the amount of histamine present and, theoretically, to reduce itch as a result. One of the anti-histamines that appear to be beneficial in relieving pruritus is cetirizine, though only in extremely high amounts (4×–8× OTC dosage) and with a high amount of adverse events [8, 11]. Fexofenadine has also been effective in reducing pruritus in one trial when used with a 0.1% hydrocortisone butyrate [12]. Patients (n = 400) were randomized to either receive topical steroid and placebo, or topical steroid with fexofenadine HCl 60 mg twice per day. Pruritus was evaluated twice daily using a five point scale. Compared to placebo, the treatment group had significant improvement in pruritus both day ($p = 0.0001$) and night ($p= 0.013$). The treatment group also experienced a significant reduction in pruritic area to body surface area (BSA) compared to placebo. Additional studies should be done, as this is one of the only confirming efficacy of an OTC histamine in the treatment of pruritus in atopic dermatitis patients.

11.2.3 Role of Emollients

When given the choice of emollient type, creams are selected most frequently by patients [13]. Moisturizing creams and other emollients are believed to enhance the skin barrier by providing a source of exogenous lipids to the skin [14]. Although the mechanism of topical creams is not well understood their effectiveness and tolerability have been well documented. The natural moisturizing factor (NMF), is a naturally occurring compound in the skin containing amino acids, lactates, urea and electrolytes. Many companies have attempted to emulate NMF in the innovation of moisturizing creams containing these agents.

Two of the most commonly used ointments in the United States are Aquaphor healing ointment and Vaseline petroleum jelly and both have been used safely for many years. Vaseline petroleum jelly accelerates skin barrier recovery [15]. Despite their effectiveness and affordability, ointments are often not preferred by patients presumably due to the greasiness factor [13, 15, 16]. Therefore, their presumed effectiveness needs to be weighed against the likelihood of patient compliance (Table 11.1).

In a study on infants deemed high risk for AD, regular emollient application from birth was an effective approach for atopic dermatitis prevention [13]. Infants were considered high risk if they had a first degree relative diagnosed with AD, asthma, or allergic rhinitis. Subjects in the intervention arm received sunflower seed oil, Cetaphil cream, or Aquaphor Healing Ointment [13]. Daily emollient use reduced the incidence of atopic dermatitis at 6 months (43% in the control group vs. 22% in the emollient group) [13]. This corresponds to a relative risk reduction of 50% (relative risk, 0.50; 95% CI, 0.28–0.90; $P = .017$). If confirmed in larger trials, emollient therapy in infants may be a simple intervention to decrease the worldwide prevalence of atopic dermatitis.

11.2.4 Natural Oils

Sunflower seed oil is one of the oldest oilseeds in America and has three variants of fatty acid composition: high linoleic, mid-oleic and high oleic [19]. Sunflower seed oil has been reported to have anti-inflammatory, moisturizing, and skin barrier restoring effects [20]. The use of sunflower seed oil preserves the stratum corneum integrity and improves hydration [21]. This option may appeal to patients who seek a natural and affordable treatment for AD, however additional studies are needed to determine clinical efficacy.

Virgin coconut oil is defined by the method in which it is processed which allows it to retain its natural antioxidant and antimicrobial properties [22]. In contrast to coconut oil, virgin coconut oil is obtained by wet-milled, cold-press with the absence of chemical use, which allows it to maintain its antioxidant status [22, 23]. In mild to moderate atopic dermatitis, topical application of virgin coconut oil improved skin capacitance, reduced SCORing of Atopic Dermatitis (SCORAD) score, and decreased transepidermal water loss [24]. Extensive studies are warranted in order to firmly establish this as a recommendation [21].

Evening primrose oil (EPO) is obtained by cold expression of the seed of the evening primrose plant [23, 25]. It is best known for its anti-inflammatory properties and use in dermatitis, eczema and rheumatoid arthritis [25]. EPO seeds are high in omega-6 essential fatty acid, which includes linoleic and gamma-linolenic acid (GLA), which may play a role in eczema, as GLA seems to reduce inflammation [26]. Ingested EPO increased gamma-linoleic acid levels and decreased the

Table 11.1 Efficacy of various emollient preparations

Emollient	References	Study design	Number of subjects	Regimen	Outcome measure	Results
Choice of: sunflower seed oil, Cetaphil Cream, Aquaphor Healing Ointment (US)	Simpson et al. [13]	Multicenter, multinational 2 arm parallel group, assessor blinded, randomized (1:1) control pilot study	124	Daily emollient application from birth (maximum age of 3 weeks) to entire body surface area except scalp	Rate of development of AD in intervention arm versus control arm	Relative Risk Reduction of 50%; 95% CI (.2–.9); $p = .017$
Choice of: sunflower seed oil, Doublebase Gel, liquid paraffin 50% in white paraffin						
Water in oil emollient cream	Lane and Drost [17]	Prospective analysis	34	Twice daily cream application for 16 days	1.Clinical skin condition	1. significantly decreased rates of dermatitis
					2. fungal cultures and quantitative bacterial cultures	2. no change in cutaneous flora

(continued)

Table 11.1 (continued)

Emollient	References	Study design	Number of subjects	Regimen	Outcome measure	Results
8% synthetic pseudo-ceramide cream	Imokawa and Ishida [18]	Prospective clinical comparison	24	Daily application of 8% synthetic pseudo-ceramide cream to nonlesional forearm skin	1. Clinical condition of skin treated with 8% synthetic pseudo-ceramide cream versus 0.3% mucopolysaccaride cream	1. pseudo-ceramide cream = 50% of subjects marked improvement, 36% had moderate improvement,15% had slight improvement mucopolysaccaride cream arm = 80% subjects slight improvement, 20% moderate improvement
					2. TEWL values for skin treated with 8% synthetic pseudo-ceramide cream versus 0.3% mucopolysaccaride cream	2. pseudo-ceramide cream = greater reduction in TEWL ($p < .0001$)

SCORAD 4–12 weeks after initiation of treatment. There was improvement of AD symptoms in both pediatric and adult groups. However, this was a small, non-randomized study without a placebo or control group [27]. There is insufficient evidence to establish the efficacy of this agent in the treatment of AD.

11.2.5 Role of Ceramides

For several years, researchers have been hypothesizing that decreased ceramides in the skin may be a factor in the development of atopic dermatitis. Ceramides form lamellar structures in combination with other lipids between cells in the stratum corneum [28]. Ceramides, along with other structures, allow the skin to retain moisture [29]. There is a deficiency of ceramides even in the non-lesional skin of adults with AD [30]. Decreased ceramides in the stratum corneum is hypothesized to lead to decreased functionality of the skin barrier, allowing irritants and allergens to permeate the skin, initiating the inflammatory process of AD.

In a study assessing the utility of ceramides in the treatment of AD, subjects were treated for 4 weeks with 8% synthetic pseudo-ceramide cream or 0.3% mucopolysaccharide cream. In the synthetic pseudo-ceramide cream treatment arm, 50% of subjects had marked improvement in AD symptoms, 36% had moderate improvement in AD symptoms, and 15% of subjects had slight improvement in AD symptoms. In the mucopolysaccharide cream arm, 80% of AD subjects had slight improvement while 20% had moderate improvement [18]. There was a greater reduction in transepidermal water loss at 4 weeks in the pseudo-ceramide cream group compared to the mucopolysaccharide cream group [18]. House dust mite antigen applied under occlusive conditions easily penetrated the dermis of non-lesional skin in AD patients, but with pre-application of synthetic ceramide there was a reduction in mite antigen cutaneous allergic reaction [31]. Patients with AD should incorporate the use of a daily moisturizer with ceramide technology in to their daily skin care regimen.

11.2.6 Cost of Emollients

With a world-wide prevalence of up to 18.1% for individuals under the age of 18 and US annual costs ranging from 364 million to 3.8 billion each year, finding a cost effective way to decrease the burden of atopic dermatitis is a noble venture [32, 33]. Recent research has shown that regular emollient use from birth can decrease the incidence of atopic dermatitis in infants at 6 months by 50% [13, 34]. With this knowledge, along with the realization that almost half of the cases of atopic dermatitis develop before the first year of life, researchers set out to compare the cost of some of the most popular moisturizers on the market in order to evaluate the

Table 11.2 Cost-effectiveness analysis of seven moisturizers for 1 year of use

Moisturizer	Cost per ounce	Cost per application	Cost of daily application for 1 year
Vaseline petroleum jelly	$0.13	$0.04	$14.60
Sunflower seed oil	$0.25	$0.10	$36.50
CeraVe moisturizing cream	$0.79	$0.25	$91.26
Aquaphor baby healing ointment	$0.94	$0.31	$113.16
Cetaphil moisturizing cream	$1.00	$0.32	$116.82
Aveeno eczema therapy moisturizing cream	$1.40	$0.45	$164.26
Vaniply ointment	$2.96	$0.95	$346.78

*Xu et al.

The cost per ounce was determined by averaging the listed price of the product across four major retailers by Xu et al. in July of 2016. Cost per application was determined by averaging BSA of average sex-neutral child from 0 to 6 months of age

cost-effectiveness of using a daily moisturizer as a prevention strategy against atopic dermatitis [16].

In this section we look at the results of a cost-effectiveness analysis of seven common moisturizers as a prophylactic measure against atopic dermatitis (Table 11.2). In the aforementioned study, the ratio of moisturizer per meters squared was determined to be 17 g/m^2 based on the fact that 30 g of topical moisturizer covers an adult with average body surface area of 1.73 m^2 [16]. Age specific body surface area was calculated with the Mosteller formula and the World Health Organization 50th percentile growth chart for boys and girls at ages 0 and 6 months. This led to a calculated amount of .12 oz. g needed for full body moisturization per application at birth and .22 oz. at 6 months of age [16]. Investigators averaged the cost of each product using prices listed for online retailers Walmart, Amazon, Target, and Walgreens [16]. Six moisturizers were included: petroleum jelly, Vaniply Ointment, Aveeno Eczema Therapy Moisturizing Cream, Cetaphil Moisturizing Cream, CeraVe Moisturizing Cream as well as sun-flower seed oil. Researchers assumed that from 0 to 6 months, children would have linear growth enabling them to determine average body surface area requiring moisturization to calculate the cost per application [16]. Quality-adjusted life-years (QALYs) for AD were determined via the prevalence of pediatric atopic dermatitis for mild, moderate, and severe disease as previously reported with health utility values of .86 for mild disease, .69 for moderate disease, and .59 in severe disease [35, 36]. The cost effectiveness of prophylactic moisturization was calculated assuming a relative risk reduction of 50% [16]. They calculated the $/QALY value by dividing the cost of moisturization with standard care ($0) with a window of health utility set at 6 months [16]. Of the seven products evaluated in this study the average price was $1.07/oz. Petroleum jelly was the most economical option totaling $7.30 for 6 months of use and Vaniply Ointment was the most expensive option at $173.39 for 6 months of use. QALY gain of moisturizers was .030, .021, and .0041 for a relative risk of .28, .5, and .9 respectively using a 6-month time window. Assuming equal efficacy among the moisturizers compared in this study petroleum jelly was the most cost-effective option at \$353/QALY [16].

11.2.7 *Bleach Baths*

Sodium hypochlorite (bleach) baths have been recommended as a complimentary treatment in patients with atopic dermatitis and secondary bacterial infections. The mechanism of action is believed to be related to the antiseptic effects of bleach and its possibility of reducing skin colonization by *S. aureus* [37]. A 2009 study ($n = 31$) revealed a significant reduction in body surface area affected and EASI score following treatment by bleach baths twice per week and intranasal mupirocin. In a study assessing the utility of bleach baths as a complement to topical medications, patients were randomized into a treatment arm or a placebo arm. For 2 months, patients in the treatment arm were on a stable regimen of topical medications and using bleach baths (0.005% concentration) 2 times per week. At 1 month, subjects in the treatment group had a statistically significant reduction in EASI score ($p < 0.001$). Body surface area affected by atopic dermatitis was significantly reduced in the treatment group after 2 months. Skin cultures following treatment revealed a 53.3% reduction in density of *S. aureus* compared to baseline measures [38].

11.2.8 *Wet Wraps*

Wet wrap therapy is a technique, used to treat several pruritic conditions, that involves wrapping a wet bandage, or "wet wrap", over a topical treatment to theoretically increase moisturization and steroid absorption [39]. It has been used for the treatment of atopic dermatitis; however, few studies have been completed evaluating its efficacy.

A study of 50 pediatric patients was completed in 2006 to evaluate the efficacy of wet wraps compared to traditional treatment [40]. The conventional treatment ($n = 22$) used in the study involved as-needed emollient use, as-needed 1% hydrocortisone ointment use, and access to more potent steroids, if necessary. Wet wrap therapy ($n = 28$) involved once per week use of wet wraps for a 24-h period over 1% hydrocortisone, or more potent steroids if necessary. Additional wet wraps could be used for 12–24 h per day if recommended by a clinician. The SCORAD index was used to assess efficacy. At the end of the study period, both groups showed improvement in SCORAD, and there was no statistically significant difference in SCORAD reduction between the traditional and wet wrap groups (59% vs. 55%). A larger ($n = 72$), and more recent, also indicated improvement in symptoms with use of wet wrap therapy (Nicol 2014). All 72 participants were part of an atopic dermatitis treatment program. Patients were treated using a wet wrap therapy for varying durations depending on the length of stay in the program that was necessary to improve atopic dermatitis flare. No other treatments for AD were used. SCORAD was used to measure improvements. There was a significant decrease in SCORAD from admission to discharge ($p < 0.001$). Of the 33 participants with severe atopic dermatitis, 25 improved to mild and 8 improved to moderate [40].

11.2.9 Textiles

Functional textiles are being developed as an option for the management of atopic dermatitis. Fabrics impregnated with antimicrobial material such as silver, zinc, anion and coated silks have been explored [22].

The innovation of textile has a promising future in treatment and maintenance of AD. A 2013 ($n = 12$) study showed significant improvement in atopic dermatitis severity and sleep quality with the use of ZnO textile overnight with pants and a long-sleeved shirt. Clinical symptoms such as erythema, edema and papules, and excoriations all decreased in severity. The textile was comprised of zinc-coated fibers with a significant antibacterial activity and antioxidant capacity against reactive oxygen species and reactive nitrogen species. The results should be interpreted cautiously, since this was a small sample size with short-term use, (3 nights) and it was non-controlled [41]. Other types of material, such as wool, are also being revisited. Wool was previously seen as an irritant and was avoided, but the size of the fiber could possibly have beneficial effects. In a 2017 study ($n = 39$), superfine merino wool clothing decreased the severity of mild and moderate pediatric atopic dermatitis in infants [42]. Participants were assigned to wear either wool or cotton for a 6 week period, and those wearing superfine wool had a reduction in mean SCORAD and ADSI at the conclusion of the study. These were preliminary results; environmental influences may have played a role in results and should be further explored [42].

Textiles are a great approach to care since they are in contact with the skin for extended periods of time. The long-term use and the cost of the specialized garments is a concern. The current studies are limited in data and warrant further exploration.

11.3 Conclusion

Over-the-counter treatments for atopic dermatitis can come in the form of topical corticosteroids, moisturizers/emollients, and oral anti-histamines (Table 11.3). Though these treatments are beneficial, prescription treatments may be quicker acting and more efficacious in patients with moderate to severe disease or during flares. OTC agents are best used for maintenance between flares and to prevent progression of mild disease.

Table 11.3 Efficacy of non-prescription treatment options

Drug/Tx	References	n=	Regimen	Outcome measure	Results
Hydrocortisone	Almeyda [2]	50	1% HC in 10% urea vs. betamethasone 17-valerate over 2–3 weeks	Improvement on physical exam compared to baseline. Progress labelled as excellent, good, no improvement, or deterioration	HC equally efficacious to betamethasome 17-valerate when used in urea
	Almeyda [2]	36	1% HC in carbamide vs. betamethasone 17-valerate over 2–4 weeks	Improvement on physical exam compared to baseline. Progress labelled as excellent, good, no improvement, or deterioration	HC equally efficacious to betamethasome 17-valerate when used in carbamide
	Jorizzo 1995	113	0.05% desonide vs. 1% hydrocortisone over 5 weeks (6 months extension)	Changes in IGA, occurrence of adverse events compared to baseline	Desonide use resulted in 35% improvement in IGA vs. 20% by HC
	Reitamo [6]	624	0.03% Tacrolimus vs. 1% HC over 3 weeks	Change in EASI, BSA compared to baseline	Tacrolimus resulted in greater decrease in mEASI than HC
	Vernon [7]	48	mometasone furoate vs. 1% hydrocortisone for 6 weeks	Change in BSA from baseline	Momentasone furoate use resulted in greater improvements than HC use

(continued)

Table 11.3 (continued)

Drug/Tx	References	n=	Regimen	Outcome measure	Results
Emollients/Moisturizers	Lucky 1997	25	2.5% HC with Eucerin® Moisturizer as steroid-sparing treatment	Decrease in mean lesion sizes and skin condition scores	No difference in progress with moisturizer use
	Loden 1999	15	Canoderm emollient as treatment for 20 days	TEWL, skin capacitance, reaction to sodium lauryl sulfate	TEWL improved and irritation improved with use of emollient alone, compared to control
	Angelova-Fischer 2014	18	emollient use only vs. 1% hydrocortisone with emollient for 4 weeks	Improvement in VAS, TEWL, severity score, decrease in density of bacterial culture	Emollient as stand-alone treatment resulted in significant improvement in severity and VAS for pruritis
	Weber [43]	45	body cleanser with moisturizer vs. cleanser alone. Moisturizing flare treatment on active sites as needed for 4 weeks	Reduction in risk of flare, incidence of flare, and greater time to flare compared to baseline	Lower incidence of flare with moisturizer use, longer time to flare with moisturizer use. OTC flare treatment effective in clearing flares within 4 weeks
Oral anti-histamines	Kawashima [12]	400	Treatment with 0.1% hydrocortisone butyrate (HCB) with fexofenadine HCl 60 mg twice daily vs. 0.1% HCB with placebo for 1 week	Change in pruritis based on a five-point scale, change in pruritis to BSA	Treatment group had significantly lower pruritis each day of treatment compared to placebo and lower pruritis to BSA

Drug/Tx	References	n=	Regimen	Outcome measure	Results
	Grundmann-Kollmann 1999	5	phototherapy with NB_UVB once daily, 5 times per week, for 3 weeks	Improvement in SCORAD from baseline	NB-UVB use resulted in significant reduction in SCORAD at 3 weeks and complete clearance at 4.5 weeks in all patients
	Reynolds 2001	73	NB-UVB treatment vs. UVA, administered twice per week for 12 weeks	Improvement in SASSAS compared to visible light therapy	Mean reduction in SASSAD with NB-UVB was greater than reduction using UVA.
Bleach baths	Huang [37]	31	bleach baths twice per week with intranasal mupirocin	Reduction in BSA, EASI compared to baseline	significant reduction in both BSA and EASI at end of study due to bleach bath
	Wong [38]	36	stable topical regimen with bleach baths as a compliment, twice per week for 2 months	Reduced EASI, BSA compared to control. Decreased density in bacterial culture.	Significant decrease in EASI of treatment group after 1 and 2 months, decreased BSA, 53.3% reduction in bacterial density in skin cultures
Wet wraps	Hindley [40]	50	conventional treat ment with emollients and 1%HC vs. wet wraps over 1% HC for 24 h	Improvement in SCORAD compared to control	Both treatment groups showed improvement in SCORAD, there ws no significant difference between treatments.
	Nicol 2014	72	use of wet wraps for varying duration	Decrease in SCORAD from admission to discharge	Significant improvement in SCORAD at discharge, 25/33 severe cases progressed to mild, 8/33 to moderate

(continued)

Table 11.3 (continued)

Drug/Tx	References	n=	Regimen	Outcome measure	Results
Textiles	Wiegand 2013	12	treatment by conventional methods, followed by overnight treatment with ZnO textiles for three nights	Decreased impairment of sleep and decreased severity of clinical symptoms	Distinct reductions of clinical symptoms, such as erythema and excoriations. Reduction in pruritis and impairment of sleep.
	Su [42]	39	infants randomized to wear superfine wool clothing vs. cotton clothing for 6 weeks	Reduction in SCORAD and ADSI, improvement in IDQOL from baseline	Infants wearing superfine wool experienced decreases in severity and improvement in mean SCORAD
Evening primrose oil	Simon [27]	21	Patients were administered 4–6 g EPO daily for 12 weeks	Increase in GLA and DGLA with treatment, decrease in SCORAD compared to baseline	Mean reduction in SCORAD that was inversely correlated with GLA/DGLA levels

Alternative and complementary treatments lack strong efficacy evidence. However, wet wraps, bleach baths, and other treatments appear to be promising when used in conjunction with conventional treatments.

Promising data suggests that emollients may be an effective way to prevent the development of atopic dermatitis if used consistently in high risk infants. Regular moisturize use decreases trans-epidermal water loss of the skin. Emollients containing ceramide technology reduced transepidermal water loss to a greater degree than emollients without ceramides. While moisturizers containing ceramide technology are a promising development, experienced physicians agree that the most effective emollient is the one that the patient can commit to using regularly.

With the financial burden of atopic dermatitis ranging from 364 million to 3.8 billion dollars each year in the United States, we suspect this topic will gain further research attention.

References

1. Boguniewicz M, Leung DYM. Atopic dermatitis: a disease of altered skin barrier and immune dysregulation. Immunol Rev. 2011;242(1):233–46. doi:10.1111/j.1600-065X.2011.01027.x.
2. Almeyda J, Fry L. Controlled trial of the treatment of atopic eczema with a urea-hydrocortisone preparation versus betamethasone 17-valerate. Br J Dermatol. 1973;88(5):493–5. doi:10.1111/j.1365-2133.1973.tb15456.x.
3. Swanbeck GA. new treatment of ichthyosis and other hyperkeratotic conditions. Acta Derm Venereol. 1968;48(2):123–7. http://www.ncbi.nlm.nih.gov/pubmed/4171281. Accessed 16 June 2017.
4. Almeyda J, Burt BW. Double blind controlled study of treatment of atopic eczema with a preparation of hydrocortisone in a new drug delivery system versus betamethasone 17-valerate. Br J Dermatol. 1974;91(5):579–83. http://www.ncbi.nlm.nih.gov/pubmed/4611469. Accessed 16 June 2017.
5. Pilgaard CE, Norholm A. Hydrocortisone in an improved vehicle. J Int Med Res. 1980;8(1):81–5. doi:10.1177/030006058000800114.
6. Reitamo S, Harper J, Bos JD, et al. 0.03% tacrolimus ointment applied once or twice daily is more efficacious than 1% hydrocortisone acetate in children with moderate to severe atopic dermatitis: results of a randomized double-blind controlled trial. Br J Dermatol. 2004;150(3):554–62. doi:10.1046/j.1365-2133.2004.05782.x.
7. Vernon HJ, Lane AT, Weston W. Comparison of mometasone furoate 0.1% cream and hydrocortisone 1.0% cream in the treatment of childhood atopic dermatitis. J Am Acad Dermatol. 1991;24(4):603–7. http://www.ncbi.nlm.nih.gov/pubmed/2033138. Accessed 16 June 2017.
8. Herman SM, Vender RB. Antihistamines in the treatment of dermatitis. J Cutan Med Surg. 2003;7(6):467–73. doi:10.1177/120347540300700608.
9. Klein GL, Galant SPA. comparison of the antipruritic efficacy of hydroxyzine and cyproheptadine in children with atopic dermatitis. Ann Allergy. 1980;44(3):142–5. http://www.ncbi.nlm.nih.gov/pubmed/7362092. Accessed 16 June 2017.
10. Reitamo S, Ansel JC, Luger TA. Itch in atopic dermatitis. J Am Acad Dermatol. 2001;45(1 Suppl):S55–6. http://www.ncbi.nlm.nih.gov/pubmed/11423876. Accessed 16 June 2017.
11. La Rosa M, Ranno C, Musarra I, Guglielmo F, Corrias A, Bellanti JA. Double-blind study of cetirizine in atopic eczema in children. Ann Allergy. 1994;73(2):117–22. http://www.ncbi.nlm.nih.gov/pubmed/8067594. Accessed 16 June 2017.

12. Kawashima M, Tango T, Noguchi T, Inagi M, Nakagawa H, Harada S. Addition of fexofenadine to a topical corticosteroid reduces the pruritus associated with atopic dermatitis in a 1-week randomized, multicentre, double-blind, placebo-controlled, parallel-group study. Br J Dermatol. 2003;148(6):1212–21. http://www.ncbi.nlm.nih.gov/pubmed/12828751. Accessed 16 June 2017.
13. Simpson EL, Chalmers JR, Hanifin JM, et al. Emollient enhancement of the skin barrier from birth offers effective atopic dermatitis prevention. J Allergy Clin Immunol. 2014;134(4):818–23. doi:10.1016/j.jaci.2014.08.005.
14. Lodén M. Role of topical emollients and moisturizers in the treatment of dry skin barrier disorders. Am J Clin Dermatol. 2003;4(11):771–88. http://www.ncbi.nlm.nih.gov/pubmed/14572299. Accessed 15 June 2017.
15. Ghadially R, Halkier-Sorensen L, Elias PM. Effects of petrolatum on stratum corneum structure and function. J Am Acad Dermatol. 1992;26(3):387–96. doi:10.1016/0190-9622(92)70060-S.
16. Xu S, Immaneni S, Hazen GB, Silverberg JI, Paller AS, Lio PA. Cost-effectiveness of prophylactic moisturization for atopic dermatitis. JAMA Pediatr. 2017;171(2):e163909. doi:10.1001/jamapediatrics.2016.3909.
17. Lane AT, Drost SS. Effects of repeated application of emollient cream to premature neonates' skin. Pediatrics. 1993;92(3):415–9. http://www.ncbi.nlm.nih.gov/pubmed/8361795. Accessed 15 June 2017.
18. Imokawa G, Ishida K. Role of ceramide in the barrier function of the stratum corneum, implications for the pathogenesis of atopic dermatitis. J Clin Exp Dermatol Res. 2014;5(1) doi:10.4172/2155-9554.1000206.
19. Gupta MK. Sunflower oil and its applications. Lipid Technol. 2014;26(11–12):260–3. doi:10.1002/lite.201400068.
20. Eichenfield LF, McCollum A, Msika P. The benefits of Sunflower Oleodistillate (SOD) in pediatric dermatology. Pediatr Dermatol. 2009;26(6):669–75. doi:10.1111/j.1525-1470.2009.01042.x.
21. Danby SG, AlEnezi T, Sultan A, et al. Effect of olive and sunflower seed oil on the adult skin barrier: implications for neonatal skin care. Pediatr Dermatol. 2013;30(1):42–50. doi:10.1111/j.1525-1470.2012.01865.x.
22. Goddard AL, Lio PA. Alternative, complementary, and forgotten remedies for atopic dermatitis. Evid Based Complement Alternat Med. 2015;2015:676897. doi:10.1155/2015/676897.
23. Nevin KG, Rajamohan T. Wet and dry extraction of coconut oil: impact on lipid metabolic and antioxidant status in cholesterol coadministered rats. Can J Physiol Pharmacol. 2009;87(8):610–6. doi:10.1139/y09-045.
24. Evangelista MTP, Abad-Casintahan F, Lopez-Villafuerte L. The effect of topical virgin coconut oil on SCORAD index, transepidermal water loss, and skin capacitance in mild to moderate pediatric atopic dermatitis: a randomized, double-blind, clinical trial. Int J Dermatol. 2014;53(1):100–8. doi:10.1111/ijd.12339.
25. Bayles B, Usatine R. Evening primrose oil. Am Fam Physician. 2009;80(12):1405–8. http://www.ncbi.nlm.nih.gov/pubmed/20000302. Accessed 15 June 2017.
26. Schlichte MJ, Vandersall A, Katta R. Diet and eczema: a review of dietary supplements for the treatment of atopic dermatitis. Dermatol Pract Concept. 2016;6(3):23–9. doi:10.5826/dpc.0603a06.
27. Simon D, Eng PA, Borelli S, et al. Gamma-linolenic acid levels correlate with clinical efficacy of evening primrose oil in patients with atopic dermatitis. Adv Ther. 2014;31(2):180–8. doi:10.1007/s12325-014-0093-0.
28. Holleran WM, Feingold KR, Mao-Qiang M, Gao WN, Lee JM, Elias PM. Regulation of epidermal sphingolipid synthesis by permeability barrier function. J Lipid Res. 1991;32(7):1151–8. http://www.jlr.org/content/32/7/1151.full.pdf. Accessed 15 June 2017.
29. Imokawa G, Kuno H, Kawai M. Stratum Corneum Lipids Serve as a Bound-Water Modulator. J Invest Dermatol. 1990;96(6):845–51. doi:10.1111/1523-1747.ep12474562.
30. Jungersted JM, Scheer H, Mempel M, et al. Stratum corneum lipids, skin barrier function and filaggrin mutations in patients with atopic eczema. Allergy. 2010;65(7):911–8. doi:10.1111/j.1398-9995.2010.02326.x.

31. Umeda Y, Mizutani H, Imokawa G, Shimizu. Topical ceramide corrected epidermal cell hyperproliferation and stratum corneum dysmaturation in atopic eczema. In: New trends in allergy IV. Berlin: Springer; 1997. p. 237–9. doi:10.1007/978-3-642-60419-5_38.
32. Shaw TE, Currie GP, Koudelka CW, Simpson EL. Eczema prevalence in the United States: data from the 2003 National Survey of Children's Health. J Invest Dermatol. 2011;131(1):67–73. doi:10.1038/jid.2010.251.
33. Ellis CN, Drake LA, Prendergast MM, et al. Cost of atopic dermatitis and eczema in the United States. J Am Acad Dermatol. 2002;46(3):361–70. http://www.ncbi.nlm.nih.gov/pubmed/11862170. Accessed 15 June 2017.
34. Nankervis H, Thomas KS, Delamere FM, Barbarot S, Rogers NK, Williams HC. Scoping systematic review of treatments for eczema. Southampton: NIHR Journals Library; 2016. doi:10.3310/PGFAR04070.
35. Willemsen MG, van Valburg RWC, Dirven-Meijer PC, Oranje AP, van der Wouden JC, Moed H. Determining the severity of atopic dermatitis in children presenting in general practice: an easy and fast method. Dermatol Res Pract. 2009;2009:357046. doi:10.1155/2009/357046.
36. Garside R, Stein K, Castelnuovo E, et al. The effectiveness and cost-effectiveness of pimecrolimus and tacrolimus for atopic eczema: a systematic review and economic evaluation. Health Technol Assess. 2005;9(29):iii, xi–xiii,1–230. http://www.ncbi.nlm.nih.gov/pubmed/16022804. Accessed 15 June 2017.
37. Huang JT, Abrams M, Tlougan B, Rademaker A, Paller AS. Treatment of staphylococcus aureus colonization in atopic dermatitis decreases disease severity. Pediatrics. 2009;123(5):e808–14. http://pediatrics.aappublications.org/content/123/5/e808. Accessed 16 June 2017.
38. Wong S, Ng TG, Baba R. Efficacy and safety of sodium hypochlorite (bleach) baths in patients with moderate to severe atopic dermatitis in Malaysia. J Dermatol. 2013;40(11):874–80. doi:10.1111/1346-8138.12265.
39. Andersen R, Thyssen J, Maibach H. The role of wet wrap therapy in skin disorders-a literature review. Acta Derm Venereol. 2014;95(8):0. doi:10.2340/00015555-3134.
40. Hindley D, Galloway G, Murray J, Gardener LA. randomised study of "wet wraps" versus conventional treatment for atopic eczema. Arch Dis Child. 2006;91(2):164–8. doi:10.1136/adc.2004.050831.
41. Wiegand C, Hipler U-C, Boldt S, Strehle J, Wollina U. Skin-protective effects of a zinc oxide-functionalized textile and its relevance for atopic dermatitis. Clin Cosmet Investig Dermatol. 2013;6:115–121. http://doi.org/10.2147/CCID.S44865.
42. JC S, Dailey R, Zallmann M, et al. Determining Effects of Superfine Sheep wool in INfantile Eczema (DESSINE): a randomized paediatric crossover study. Br J Dermatol. 2017; doi:10.1111/bjd.15376.
43. Weber TM, Samarin F, Babcock MJ, Filbry A, Rippke F. Steroid-free over-the-counter eczema skin care formulations reduce risk of flare, prolong time to flare, and reduce eczema symptoms in pediatric subjects with atopic dermatitis. J Drugs Dermatol. 2015;14(5):478–85. http://www.ncbi.nlm.nih.gov/pubmed/25942666. Accessed 16 June 2017.

Chapter 12
Adherence in Atopic Dermatitis

Nupur Patel and Steven R. Feldman

Abstract Atopic dermatitis is a chronic dermatologic condition requiring extended treatment times with topical application of medications. While atopic dermatitis treatments can be highly effective when used as directed, oftentimes patients do not respond as expected, raising concern for non-adherence versus non-response. This chapter aims to describe what is currently known about adherence in atopic dermatitis and to discuss strategies to improve adherence in order to improve treatment outcomes. Whether intentional or unintentional, non-adherence to treatment can limit patient outcomes of this disease for a variety of reasons. These include frustration with medication efficacy, inconvenience, and fear of side effects. Other factors include forgetfulness, financial burden of treatment, lack of trust in the physician, dislike of prescribed medication, or lack of understanding of disease or treatment. Several interventions have been studied with the aim of improving adherence in atopic dermatitis—such as educational workshops for patients and caregivers, earlier follow-up visits, and text messages reminders—however these are often limited by sample size and power. Further research is needed to study both specific patterns of nonadherence in atopic dermatitis, as well as methods to improve them.

Keywords Adherence • Compliance • Atopic dermatitis • Eczema • Patient education

12.1 Introduction

Atopic dermatitis is a chronic relapsing skin condition that requires treatment over an extended period and can be difficult to treat. Poor adherence to treatment in atopic dermatitis can be a major limiting factor for the outcome of this disease [1,

N. Patel, M.S. (✉) • S.R. Feldman, M.D., Ph.D.
Department of Dermatology, Wake Forest University School of Medicine,
Winston Salem, NC, USA
e-mail: nupur.uma.patel@gmail.com

E.A. Fortson et al. (eds.), *Management of Atopic Dermatitis*, Advances in
Experimental Medicine and Biology 1027, DOI 10.1007/978-3-319-64804-0_12

2]. While atopic dermatitis treatments can be highly effective when used as directed, oftentimes patients do not respond as expected, raising concern for non-adherence versus non-response [1]. The potential for poor adherence to cause poor outcomes should not be underestimated in atopic dermatitis.

With chronic skin conditions, such as atopic dermatitis or psoriasis, some of the most important reasons patients are non-adherent to their treatment plans include frustration with medication efficacy, inconvenience, and fear of side effects. Other factors include forgetfulness, financial burden of treatment, lack of trust in the physician, dislike of prescribed medication, or lack of understanding of disease or treatment [2–4]. Lack of accountability may be a critical and underappreciated component. On occasion, when faced with atopic dermatitis that is not improving, clinicians assume medications are not effective and give patients increasingly potent or complicated regimens that further worsen adherence. This chapter describes what is currently known about adherence in atopic dermatitis and strategies to improve adherence and patients' treatment outcomes.

12.2 Background Terminology

The terminology used to understand adherence behavior is important. The term "compliance" has traditionally been used in clinical situations to describe the extent to which a patient takes their medications as prescribed [5]. Although originally used as a neutral alternative to describe whether patients followed clinician recommendations, the term has been more recently thought to suggest a one-sided relationship between physician and patient, in which the treatment is decided on by the clinical and the patient is expected to comply regardless of their perceptions about it [6]. In this context, patients' failure to comply may be attributed to the patient's inability to understand the benefits of the regimen or the regimen itself or is even considered a sign of maladaptive patient behavior [6].

Recently, the term "adherence" has become more commonly used, as it is considered to better recognize patients' autonomy and physicians' responsibility to encourage a therapeutic alliance with the patient. The term has generally been defined as "extent to which the patient's behavior matches agreed upon recommendations from the prescriber." [6] The concept of adherence emphasizes the process of the therapeutic relationship, in which treatment is discussed between clinician and patient and prescribed after mutual agreement. In this way, the concept of adherence focuses on an understanding between patient and clinician about the recommended treatment, and indicates that the patient is not obligated to accept the treatment regimen and will not be held solely responsible for its failure due to non-adherence [6]. The WHO project which examined treatment adherence defined the term as "the extent to which a person's behavior, taking medication, following a diet, and/or executing lifestyle changes, corresponds with agreed recommendations from a health care provider." [7] This definition focuses on active patient involvement in choosing treatments and emphasizes the need for both parties to participate [6].

Because the term adherence is more patient-centered than that of compliance, it has been suggested as a better way to define medication taking behavior. The term adherence also seems to facilitate description of a spectrum of behaviors rather than the dichotomy of compliance versus non-compliance to describe patient behavior [6]. Adherence can range from complete refusal of treatment regimen (termed fully non-adherent behavior), to partially following medication regimens (partially adherence behavior), to regular use of the precise treatment regimen (fully adherent behavior) [6, 8, 9].

Varying levels of adherence exist throughout the physician-patient interaction from conception of a treatment plan to the patient's use of the medication at home (Fig. 12.1) Primary adherence is the expectation that the patient will fill their initial prescription at a pharmacy, while secondary adherence describes the patient's correct use of the medication at home [10]. Acceptance of the treatment plan by the patient is seen when the patient fills a second prescription and continues using it as described, while persistence with the regimen is exhibited through the continued redemption and use of multiple subsequent prescriptions at regular intervals [10].

Various categories exist with regards to nonadherence (Table 12.1). These include non-initiation, poor execution (unintentional or intentional), or non-persistence

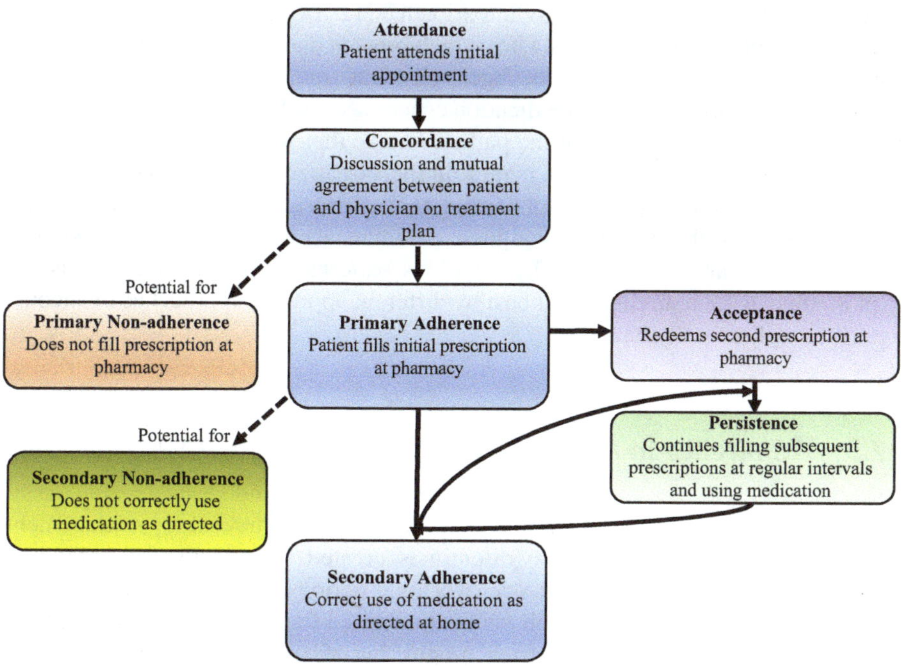

Fig. 12.1 Ideal adherence flowchart (*solid arrows, blue, purple, green boxes*); showing potential for non-adherence (*dashed arrows, orange, yellow boxes*)

Table 12.1 Defining terminology associated with non-adherence

Term	Defined
Primary non-adherence	Patient does not fill prescription at pharmacy to obtain medication
Secondary non-adherence	Patient does not correctly follow their treatment plan or use their medication as prescribed
Types of secondary non-adherence	
Non-initiation	Patient does not begin taking their treatment as recommended
Poor execution	Incorrect use of medications, incorrectly following treatment plan
Unintentional non-adherence	Non-adherence due to obstacles that prevent following clinician recommendations, such as age, physical or cognitive impairments, environmental barriers of medication cost, access to medication
Intentional non-adherence	Non-adherence due to unwillingness of the patient to take their medications as prescribed due to their personal preferences or views regarding their treatment
Non-persistence	Patient stops filling their repeated prescriptions at regular intervals and discontinues treatment
Early-termination	Patient discontinues maintenance of their treatment without regard for clinician recommendations

[11]. With non-initiation, the patient does not begin taking their medication as described. With poor execution of the treatment plan as prescribed, the non-adherence might be either "unintentional" or "intentional." [12–14] Unintentional non-adherence is thought to result from obstacles which prevent patients from following clinician recommendations, such as age, physical or mental impairments, or environmental barriers such as medication cost or access. Intentional non-adherence is attributed to unwillingness of the patient to take their medications as prescribed due to their preferences or views regarding their treatment [6]. Non-persistence is demonstrated when the patient stops filling their prescription, while early-termination occurs when the patient discontinues maintenance of their treatment without regard to medical advice [11]. These various patterns of non-adherence must be kept in mind as each might benefit best by different approach approaches to encourage better adherence behavior.

12.3 Adherence in Atopic Dermatitis

Because atopic dermatitis is a chronic skin condition, it requires daily management with treatment regimens that are oftentimes created specifically for individual patients. Maintaining good adherence over long periods of time can be a difficult hurdle. An estimated 30–40% of all medications used for chronic conditions are not taken as prescribed [15, 16]. Electronic monitoring of dermatologic patients reveals that patients are often poorly adherent to topical therapy and that patients may overstate their use of medication in treatment logs [16, 17].

Several studies have revealed varying degrees of nonadherence to therapy specifically for atopic dermatitis. Primary non-adherence describes the first stage of nonadherence by a patient, when they do not redeem their initial prescription at a pharmacy. Secondary non-adherence occurs at home when the patient does not correctly follow their treatment plan or use their medication as prescribed. In Denmark, the primary adherence behavior of 322 outpatient dermatology patients was analyzed through a national pharmacy register indicating their redemption of prescriptions within 4 weeks of their consultation appointment [10]. 31.8% of the atopic dermatitis patients did not redeem their prescriptions within 4 weeks, meaning that almost one-third of these patients exhibited primary non-adherence [10]. Although there is often greater focus on improving secondary non-adherence, primary non-adherence is equally as important and should not be discounted. If the medication is not filled, it is not likely to be effective.

If patients do fill the medication, secondary adherence can still be poor. Secondary adherence has been measured in studies in which patients are given the medication with electronic monitors. Often, patients overstate their use of treatment. The median daily adherence for 5 days of treatment with fluocinonide 0.1% cream was 40% per electronic monitoring, while subjects reported 100% adherence in medication diaries [18]. Adherence was better on day 1 of treatment with 6 of 9 patients using their treatment regimen, while on day 5 only 1 of 9 patients was adherent [18]. Of 41 adult patients with mild-to-moderate atopic dermatitis, mean adherence to twice-daily desonide hydrogel declined from 81% adherence on day 1 to 50% by day 27 over a 4-week period [19].

Electronic monitoring of 26 pediatric atopic dermatitis patients revealed overall adherence to topical triamcinolone to be 32% at the end of 8 weeks of treatment [16]. Adherence was highest at the date of initial visit then dropped rapidly, doubling before the return visit date, and decreasing again afterwards [16]. In Japan, adherence in atopic dermatitis patients was generally lower than patients with psoriasis or tinea [20]. Ninety-two percent of patients in a small pilot study of 25 patients reported they sometimes forgot to use their medications, 88% reported they often stopped their AD treatment when their skin symptoms improved, and 33.3% reported that they stopped their AD treatment when their skin symptoms worsened [21].

Multiple reasons may exist for the decreased adherence to treatment seen in atopic dermatitis. In parents of children with skin conditions, cost of medication and concern about side effects were the most common reported reasons for nonadherence [2, 22]. Yet adherence has been poor in studies of atopic dermatitis in which patients were given the medication and agreed to participate, suggesting that cost and concerns about side effects are not the only major limitations to adherence in atopic dermatitis. Other reasons include forgetfulness, complicated instructions, time burden for treatment application, phobia of corticosteroids, or lack of understanding about disease or treatment [1, 2, 22]. In a group of parents of children specifically with atopic dermatitis, parents' cooperation, resentment against treatment, reluctance to bathe, late bedtimes, lack of social support, worry about eczema, feelings of victimization, and perceived severity of disease were factors associated with adherence [23, 24]. Adherence may also be affected by factors such as patient expectations, previous experiences with therapies, and mode of drug administration, as topical treatments can be more troublesome for patients [10, 24]. Even short term use of topical application of fluorescent test cream is difficult [10, 25]. Adherence to topical medication may also be influenced by patients' preferences for specific vehicle formulations to others [2, 22].

While a multitude of treatments exist for atopic dermatitis and more are in the process of being developed, topical therapies such as corticosteroids remain the first line treatment for this disease. Adherence to these treatments can vary, with apprehension about corticosteroid use, also known as "steroid phobia" playing a role in patients' use of these medications. Patients commonly express fear and anxiety about topical steroid use despite their safety and efficacy in treating atopic dermatitis [26–28]. Patients or caregivers may also confuse topical corticosteroids with anabolic steroids, creating further misconception regarding use of these medications. This steroid phobia may also be propagated by the media (particularly social media), along with the common misconception that topical steroids can have the same side effects as oral or systemic steroids [2, 26, 29]. In France, 80.7% of 208 patients or parents of patients with atopic dermatitis reported having fears about topical steroids, and 36% admitted nonadherence to their treatment [28]. 47.8% of those surveyed were not aware of specific medication side effects, but still expressed fear about using these medications. In 300 Italian patients with atopic dermatitis, fear of topical corticosteroids was significantly associated with believing that treatment advantages do not overweigh disadvantages ($p = 0.011$) and believing that TCS may be dangerous independently from the specific side effect ($p < 0.001$) [30]. Similarly, of 200 atopic dermatitis patients surveyed in Britain, 72.5% stated concern about topical steroids, and 24% reported non-compliance with their treatment due to these worries [2, 31]. The most common concerns among patients include perceived skin thinning, systemic absorption, skin irritation, non-specific long-term effects, and a negative impact on growth and development [29, 31, 32].

In addition to misconceptions about steroid side effects, other misunderstandings about steroid use exist. Of 100 parents of atopic dermatitis patients, only 41% understood that hydrocortisone (the most commonly used topical steroid) is weakly potent, with 44% marking it as moderately potent [2, 33]. In a group of 200 atopic dermatitis patients or parents, 31% incorrectly graded hydrocortisone as strong, very strong, or unknown potency [2, 26]. While all subjects had used both hydrocortisone and clobetasol proprionate, only 62% correctly identified the more potent medication [2, 26]. Cultural beliefs and language barriers may also influence patients' beliefs about topical steroids. Over half of subjects from a Chinese patient population stated their belief that corticosteroids could kill bacteria [2, 29].

Other topical treatments for atopic dermatitis include topical calcineurin inhibitors, emollients, wet wraps, and antimicrobial treatments. Less information is available about adherence to these therapies due the very limited number of clinical trials in existence about them. Topical calcineurin inhibitors have been FDA-approved in the United States as second line therapy for short-term and intermittent long-term use in moderate to severe AD in children and adults [2]. They are available as ointments (tacrolimus 0.03%, 0.1%) and cream (pimecrolimus 0.1%). One randomized controlled trial evaluated patient adherence to twice daily application of 0.03% tacrolimus ointment. This study utilized MEMS (Medication Event Monitoring Systems) caps for monitoring; the mean adherence in the intervention group, who had an extra follow-up visit at 1 week, was 69% as compared to 54% in the standard-of care control group who were seen only at week 4 in follow up [34]. Although this result was not statistically significant and the study population was small, there was a strong trend toward improved adherence with the early follow-up visit [2]. The extended use of topical calcineurin inhibitors does not cause skin atrophy, and these are the preferred medications for atopic dermatitis of the face and eyelids or other sensitive areas of thin skin where local effects of corticosteroids is of concern [35]. Patients with recalcitrant disease or frequent flares may benefit from topical calcineurin inhibitors rather than continuous topical steroid use [2]. However, these medications also contain a black box warning about a theoretical risk for malignancy with their use, which could cause anxiety and fears similar to steroid phobia, adversely affecting both primary and secondary adherence. [2, 36] Topical calcineurin inhibitors can also cause stinging and irritation which may affect adherence. Although one method to help limit skin irritation is to combine topical calcineurin inhibitors with topical steroids, this combination complicates treatment plans with an increased potential for apprehension of the regimen and greater treatment burden, making good adherence more difficult [2].

Emollients are a cornerstone of atopic dermatitis treatment, and are often prescribed for daily topical use. Although emollient use is less controversial than topical steroids, patients and their parents also report having concerns about the long-term use of emollients, which can also influence adherence [2, 26]. Caregivers of atopic dermatitis patients reported that although they thought emollients helped the symptoms of atopic dermatitis in the short term, they held mixed beliefs about the utility of emollients in preventing long-term flare ups [2, 31]. In 20 surveyed patients, 2 of 20 expressed concern about emollients, moisturizers, or ointments and admitted to nonadherence because of these anxieties [16, 29]. Although emollients improve skin barrier dysfunction associated with atopic dermatitis, a higher prevalence of contact sensitization to emollients, fragrances, preservatives, and surfactants have been observed in atopic dermatitis patients [35]. Because these undesirable effects can be increased in this patient population, it may lead to decreased use of these medications and less adherence to the treatment regimen.

Wet wrap therapy is a less common but intensive treatment for severe atopic dermatitis or disease that is refractory to standard topical therapies [2]. Wet wrap therapy consists of a soaking bath followed by the application of topical emollients or medications onto lesions, which are then wrapped with a wet layer followed by a dry layer [2]. Nonadherence is thought to be the main cause for wet wrap therapy failure, evidenced by the rapid improvement with wet wrap treatment in patients hospitalized with severe atopic dermatitis. With this treatment, lack of patient education or incomplete training of healthcare professionals administering the treatment can contribute to nonadherence [2, 37]. Because wet wrap therapy must be monitored closely and applied with care, the treatment can become tedious for caregivers, patients, and their clinicians, leading to less frequent use despite efficacy [2].

Other reasons for disuse are also the time-intensive nature of the treatment as well as its high expense, along with dislike of the treatment by pediatric patients [37]. Due to the variable technique of the wet wrap application, along with the time burden and special training required for applying the treatment, providers must keep in mind the potential for nonadherence [2].

Although adherence rates to topical antimicrobial therapies for atopic dermatitis have not been formally assessed, patients may be nonadherent simply due to lack of knowledge about these complementary therapies [2]. Of 100 parents of pediatric patients, 53% of those whose children were using the steroid/antimicrobial combination clobetasone butyrate/nystatin/tetracycline assumed the medication was a potent topical steroid [33]. Forty-six percent believed that fusidic acid was a steroid ingredient rather than an antibiotic in another combination topical medication, and all combinations were perceived as being more potent than the steroid ingredient alone [33].

12.4 Interventions Studied for Adherence

There have been several interventions that have been studied for their ability to improve adherence specifically in atopic dermatitis. Of the interventions that have been studied, all except two increased adherence rates or decreased disease severity in patients [1]. The different methods studied to increase adherence included written eczema action plans, various educational methods, text message use, and increased office visits (Table 12.2). Many of these studies utilized the assumption that an improvement in disease severity was the reflection of an improvement in adherence to treatment [1, 2].

Written eczema action plans were studied by Rork et al. in 35 pediatric patients. The eczema action plan was given to patients at their initial visit and consisted of written instructions on daily treatment regimens as well as where and when to apply topical steroids [1]. Parents of the patients completed surveys at baseline, 3 months, and 12 months to assess their child's disease severity, treatment comfort level, and previous use of an action plan. At follow up, 80% of parents rated their child's eczema as improved, 86% found the action plan to be helpful, and 68% credited the action plan as a factor in improving their child's eczema [38]. The investigators concluded that better adherence was the cause of improved disease severity [1].

In a study utilizing educational eczema workshops, 99 atopic dermatitis patients attended one of two clinics, either a dermatologist-led clinic in which patients were given an action plan based on the standard protocol of the hospitals' eczema guidelines or the intervention, a nurse-led eczema workshop in which a plan, demonstrations of topical medication application, and take-home booklets were given [39]. After 4 weeks, disease severity was measured using the SCORAD index, revealing that 73% of children in the eczema workshop improved to mild eczema versus only 40% in the control group. Although this study did not directly measure adherence, it also concluded that better adherence resulted in the improved SCORAD index in the intervention group [1, 39].

Table 12.2 Studies of interventions to improve adherence in atopic dermatitis; grouped by category and by decreasing chronological order[a]

References	Year of study	Intervention	Sample size	Primary outcome measure	Direct measure of adherence?	Main findings
Written eczema action plan						
Rork et al. [38]	2012	Written eczema action plan	35	Survey of parents to assess disease severity, comfort level with treatment, and previous receipt of an action plan at baseline and follow-up 3–12 months	No	80% of the parents rated their child's eczema lower on the severity scale
						68% attributed improved severity due to the EAP
Technology: text messages						
Pena-Robichaux et al. [21]	2010	Daily text message reminder and educational information	25	SCORAD index—severity	Yes	Adherence—72% reported improved adherence with recall calendar and questionnaire
				7-day recall calendar—adherence		Disease Severity- SCORAD index improvement in 76% of participants
				Multiple-choice Questionnaire—adherence and preferences		Preferences—88% found text message reminders helpful and 92% found educational texts helpful
						84% stated desire to continue using the system; 72% willing to pay small fee for service
Early follow-up						
Sagransky et al. [34]	2010	Early follow-up visit at 1 week	20	EASI, VAS—severity	Yes—via MEMS caps	Adherence—mean adherence was 69% in the intervention group versus 54% in the control group
				MEMS cap—adherence		Disease Severity- Intervention group VAS and EASI scores improved 65% and 76%, respectively, vs. 36% and 45% in the control group (not statistically significant)

(continued)

Table 12.2 (continued)

References	Year of study	Intervention	Sample size	Primary outcome measure	Direct measure of adherence?	Main findings
Yentzer et al. [19]	2010	Follow-up phone call on day 3; early follow-up visit at 1 week, 2 weeks, and 4 weeks	39	EASI, VAS, BSA, IGA, TLA—severity	Yes- via MEMS caps	Disease Severity-Week 1—significant improvements in EASI (40%), VAS (42%), BSA (18%), IGA (15%), TLA (34%)
						Week 4—significant improvements in EASI (61%), VAS (60%), BSA (63%), IGA (30%), TLA (58%)
				MEMS caps—adherence		Adherence—mean adherence declined from 81% on day 1 to 50% on day 27
Educational workshops						
Moore et al. [39]	2009	Nurse-led eczema workshops	99	SCORAD index—severity	No	73% improvement in severity in the intervention group vs. 40% in the control group
Shaw et al. [40]	2008	15-min educational session by trained atopic dermatitis educator	106	SCORAD index—severity	No	Disease severity—Decrease in disease severity in 31% in the intervention group vs. 21% in the control group (results not statistically significant)
				IDQOL, CDLQI—quality of life		Quality of life—No significant difference in quality of life
Grillo et al. [41]	2006	2-h educational workshop	61	SCORAD index—severity	No	Disease severity –mean improvement in SCORAD of 45% at week 4 and 54% at week 12 in the intervention group vs. to 7% at week 4 and 16% at week 12 in the control group
				DFI—family impact		Other- no significant difference in DFI, IDQOL, and CDLQI scores between groups
				IDQOL, CDLQI—quality of life		

Staab et al. [42]	2002	Educational program of 6 group sessions, 2-h each	204	SCORAD index—severity	Yes	Disease severity- SCORAD index in intervention group decreased by 20 points vs. to 16 points in the control group (not statistically significant)
				Questionnaire- Treatment behavior, dietary restriction, indoor allergen reduction, quality of life, coping, and treatment costs		Adherence-1 year: 82% of the intervention group vs. 67% of the control group stated regular use of their skin care products vs. Baseline: 88% of the intervention group vs. 89% of the control group
Chinn et al. [39]	2002	30-min session with atopic dermatitis nurse	235	FDI—family impact	No	Family impact- marginal benefit in intervention group using the FDI only at 4 weeks
				IDQOL, CDLQI—quality of life		Quality of life—no significant difference seen between the groups

[a]SCORAD index (Scoring of Atopic Dermatitis); IDQOL (Infant's Dermatitis Quality of Life); CDLQI (Children's Dermatology Life Quality Index); EASI (Eczema and Severity Index); VAS (100 mm Visual Analog Scale); FDI (Family Dermatitis Impact); MEMS (Medication Event Monitoring Systems); BSA assessment (Body Surface Area); IGA (Investigator Global Assessments); TLA (Target Lesion Assessments)

A 2-h educational workshop was evaluated in a study of 61 pediatric patients with atopic dermatitis for its effect on disease severity, family impact, and quality of life without alteration to the patients' current treatment regimen [1, 41]. At weeks 4 and 12 after the workshop, multiple measures were used to assess outcomes, the SCORAD index, the Dermatitis Family Impact questionnaire, the IDQOL or CDLQI (Infant Dermatitis Quality of Life) and the CDLQI (Children's Dermatology Life Quality Index). At weeks 4 and 12, mean improvement in severity was 45% and 54%, respectively, in the intervention group, compared with 7% and 16% at weeks 4 and 12, respectively, in the control group [41]. There were no significant differences seen in family impact or quality of life between the two groups. In this study, improved adherence was inferred based on improved disease severity [1].

Another educational intervention utilizing an atopic dermatitis educator was evaluated in a clinical trial to determine the intervention's effectiveness in improving disease severity, quality of life, and resolution of disease in children [1, 40]. Subjects in the intervention group attended a 15 min education session about the proper use of emollients and bathing habits at their initial visit [40]. (Shaw, Bass) In this study, there was no significant difference seen in the SCORAD index or quality of life measures of the two groups, and the investigators concluded that the intervention did not improve adherence.

A similar study utilizing a single 30-min educational session with a dermatology nurse as an intervention yielded similar results [43]. After the session, which provided demonstrations of medicine application, as well as education and advice, family impact and quality of life were assessed at 4 and 12 weeks. No significant difference was appreciated in quality of life between the intervention and control groups, and of the 235 pediatric patients in the intervention group, only a marginal benefit on family impact was seen at 4 weeks [43]. Similar to the previously mentioned study utilizing a 15 min session, this study concluded that the intervention did not improve adherence based on the lack of difference in quality of life between the groups.

Another study of more intensive educational intervention assessed the effects of a parental training program on improving atopic dermatitis in pediatric patients. In this training program, parents attended 6 group sessions of 2 h duration, separate from their doctor's visits, with discussion of medical, psychological, and nutritional topics, along with personal experiences [42]. Severity, treatment habits, SCORAD index, and questionnaires in the intervention group were compared with the control group at baseline and 1 year. The change in SCORAD index or severity of disease was not statistically significant. However, in terms of treatment behavior after 1 year of intervention, 82% of the intervention group regularly used their treatment regimen versus 88% at baseline, compared with 67% of the control group versus 89% at baseline ($p = 0.041$) [42]. Completed parent questionnaires revealed that the intervention group demonstrated greater improvement in quality of life, dietary restriction, indoor allergen reduction, and coping strategies measured by the treatment costs compared to the control group [1, 42].

The use of technology through text messages has also been studied as a method for increasing adherence. Seventy-two percent of 25 patients receiving daily text message reminders and educational information reported improved adherence when using a 7-day recall calendar at the last study visit to remember when they were adherent during the last week as well as with a multiple-choice questionnaire [21]. Although adherence was self-reported, there was objective confirmation of improvement in disease severity with significant improvement in SCORAD scores for 76% of participants. Eighty-eight percent of participants reported that they found the TM reminders helpful, while 92% reported that they found the educational texts helpful. Eighty-four percent stated they would want to continue using the system if given a choice, and would recommend it to a friend [21]. Seventy-two percent of subjects stated that they would be willing to pay a small monthly fee for the service and all participants stated that they were willing to use technology to manage their health care. With regards to security issues, only 24% reported that they were worried about the security of sending health information by email or phone [21].

Other studies have used an increased frequency of follow-up contact to study adherence. One such study of desonide hydrogel utilized shorter follow-up visit intervals at weeks 1, 2, and 4, as well as follow-up phone calls on day 3 of treatment. Adherence was assessed using electronic monitoring, and although it decreased slowly over time, it was better than adherence to a historical control [19]. In a small pilot study, 20 patients with atopic dermatitis on a treatment regimen of tacrolimus ointment twice daily were scheduled for follow-up visit at weeks 1 and 4 in the intervention group, while a control group was scheduled only at 4 weeks [34]. Using the MEMS (Medication Event Monitoring Systems) cap, adherence was measured as the dates and times the tube was opened were recorded. Disease severity and pruritus were also evaluated clinically using the EASI (Eczema Area and Severity Index) and a VAS (100 mm visual analog scale) of itch intensity [1, 34]. Mean adherence in the intervention group was 69%, ranging from 39% to 114%, while in the control group mean adherence was 54%, ranging from 15 to 79% [34]. There was greater clinical improvement in the intervention group with EASI and VAS score improvement in 76% and 65% of patients, respectively, compared with 45% and 36% in the control group. However the improvements were not statistically significant, which the investigators concluded was due to the limited sample size [1].

12.5 Ethics of Adherence Monitoring

Most of the studies of adherence interventions formed their conclusions based on the idea that increased improvement in severity of disease reflects increased adherence to medications and not on a direct measure of adherence. Studies that measure adherence directly may use patients' self-reporting of adherence which is an unreliable method of gathering adherence data. In Yentzer et al., patients reported complete adherence throughout 4 weeks of treatment, although MEMS cap monitoring demonstrated that adherence slowly declined from 81% on day 1 to 50% by day 27 [19]. The use of electronic monitoring provides a more accurate and objective measure of adherence but raises ethical questions when adherence monitoring is not fully disclosed to the research subjects.

Adherence monitoring may use varying levels of nondisclosure by the clinician [44]. Full disclosure and partial disclosure are the most conservative methods of monitoring, in which patients are informed they will be monitored and are given full details or kept from knowing the extent of monitoring. Authorized deception is a form of monitoring in which the subject is informed of that some deception will be used but will not be revealed until the study is over [44]. Withholding and stealth monitoring are more radical forms of adherence monitoring. With withholding, patients are consented for the study but are not informed that adherence monitoring will be used until a debriefing session at the study conclusion. In stealth monitoring, which can be done with MEMS cap use, the study is conducted without informing patients they are being monitored and collecting data without patients knowing they are even enrolled in such a study [16, 44]. Although this method uses the highest levels of deception, the data that is acquired comes closest to resembling the adherence behavior of patients in a clinical setting [44]. Stealth monitoring raises concern for potential damage to the physician-patient relationship with regards to loss of trust. However, this potential risk could be mitigated by the potential gains of better understanding what patients do, unbiased by their participation in a clinical trial. Understanding and improving adherence is critically important for improving outcomes in dermatologic disorders [19, 45]. Having adherence data is important not only for atopic dermatitis and dermatologic disorders, but also for improving the outcomes of patients with all chronic diseases. The use of stealth monitoring can provide important insights that justify its use, though require careful consideration in balancing the benefits of deception with the benefits of obtaining such data to improve patient outcomes.

12.6 Practical Methods for Improving Adherence

Several themes are seen in the interventions studied for increasing adherence: education and increased contact between physician and patient, whether through more office visits or other means of increased communication. Strategies that focus on these themes may be used as the source for practical methods in the clinical setting to improve adherence [2].

Utilizing educational methods provide patients and their parents with detailed explanation of their disease, treatment plan, and side effects and can be an effective way for clinicians to improve adherence. Both atopic dermatitis patients and their caregivers are often seeking further explanation about the nature of eczema and how to use prescribed treatments [44, 46]. Workshops demonstrating topical application of medication and providing educational materials have been successful in improving adherence for atopic dermatitis patients [1, 39, 42]. A longer educational workshop of 2-h was more successful than 15 and 30-min sessions, either given by an atopic dermatitis educator or a single nurse consultation, suggesting that perhaps a longer more informative session might result in adherence improvement [40, 41, 43]. Following the receipt of educational information about emollients, caregivers expressed more positive views towards using these topical medications long-term, suggesting that reluctance in using emollients might be overcome with patient education [2, 47]. Parents who received more frequent education at every visit, with verbal and written treatment instructions as well as demonstrations of application technique from a dermatology specialist nurse, had greater use of emollients at target quantities and an 89% decrease in mean disease severity scores [2, 32, 48]. The success of using educational tools at every visit suggests that more frequent opportunities for patient and caregiver education may be more useful in achieving clinical improvement for atopic dermatitis [2]. More intensive educational opportunities such as 'atopic schools' are also becoming more common and positively correlate with better treatment results [2, 49]. These programs offer multi-disciplinary therapeutic patient education aimed at both parents and pediatric patients. Parents of children with atopic dermatitis who receive extra guidance and health education have increased knowledge of the disease, and this may improve adherence to treatment and the outcome of their child's eczema. Health care providers can consider providing this form of support, either in the form of separate educational sessions or at every visit by an atopic dermatitis educator [48, 50].

Another educational method that can be used by physicians is the written eczema action plan, a powerful tool that educates patients but makes more efficient use of physicians' time. The treatment of atopic dermatitis can be complicated by the use of multiple therapies at different stages of disease, leading to confusion and frustration for patients and their caregivers. The eczema action plan is a standardized set of written instructions for atopic dermatitis management—including everything from the daily skin care regimen to what to do for severe flares—and was helpful for 86% of parents and attributed as a factor in their child's disease improvement by 68% [1, 2, 38]. Not only does this tool simplify the treatment regimen for patients and their parents, it also serves as a means of educating them about the different medications and their importance. Written action plans can be tailored to allow for patient or parental input regarding their preferences. Taking vehicle preference into account can improve adherence by ensuring that patients do not dislike their prescribed medicine and that they find it easy to use. As an intervention to improve adherence, eczema action plans have the added effect of involving parents and patients in their healthcare, as utilizing parental input when creating a therapy plan can encourage adherence to the regimen [51].

Using early or more frequent follow-up visits is a practical method of improving adherence to implement(?) for atopic dermatitis patients. Just as piano students practice before lessons, patients tend to use their medications before their doctors' visits. (Feldman parable) "White coat adherence" is a term used to describe this tendency for patients to increase adherence before their follow-up appointments [1, 16, 52]. Piano teachers follow-up with their students on a weekly basis, creating accountability to ensure that their pupils practice. If piano instructors saw their pupils once every 8 weeks at the recital with the expectation that students would practice on their own, the recital would likely sound terrible, with students practicing for only a few days before the recital [2, 53]. Clinicians can harness the tendency of humans to use their medication prior to follow-up appointments, creating accountability for patients early in their treatment. By scheduling early return visits, such as within a week or two of the initial appointment, patients are held accountable for medication use [2]. By doing so, patients are more likely to fill their prescription and use their medication, see results earlier in their treatment course, create a habit of using treatment, get better long term outcomes and, potentially, *reduce* the overall number of visits needed.

Like early follow-up visits, increasing the frequency of follow-up visits overall may also play a role in improving adherence. In clinical trials which evaluate topical medications for atopic dermatitis and other skin conditions, follow-up visits are often scheduled at 1, 2, 4, 6 and 8 weeks after starting treatment [1, 2, 54, 55]. Although these follow-up visits may be intended to assess improvement in disease symptoms and severity over time, the visits also likely encourage and enhance adherence to treatment by creating accountability for patients thereby changing the outcomes that they are intended to measure [56]. These follow-up visits may explain the greater efficacy of drugs in clinical trials as compared to clinical practice [57]. One study utilizing frequent follow-up visits at 1, 2, and 4 weeks found that their rate of adherence declined at a much slower rate in comparison to similar studies without an increased frequency of visits [19]. The early return visit has only been evaluated for atopic dermatitis patients by Sagransky et al., using a 1-week follow-up interval [34]. By improving early adherence and, therefore, early outcomes of treatment, patients see the treatment working and may be encouraged to keep using the treatment.Thus, early follow-up apoointments during the start of treatment course can reduce the perception that treatment doesn't work (a perception that poisons adherence behavior) and help build a medication habit that could promote long-term adherence in diseases such as atopic dermatitis [2, 57]. There remains a clear need for further studies to investigate these strategies as a means of improving adherence and thereby improving patient outcomes and satisfaction.

Improving communication by increasing the frequency of contact between physician (or other members of the health care provider team) and patient may also serve as an important method for increasing adherence. Communication has been a major theme in the successful interventions that have been studied to improve adherence for not only atopic dermatitis, but other skin conditions as well. Increasing contact through a variety of communication methods such as e-mails, text messages, and phone calls have the potential to successfully increase adherence with atopic dermatitis patients as well as other dermatologic conditions [2, 45, 52]. For atopic dermatitis patients, daily text messages of reminders and educational tools led to significant improvement in disease severity and increased self-reported adherence. Of 25 patients, 88% reported that text message reminders were helpful, and 72% stated they would be willing to pay a small monthly fee for the service [21]. Text messages which integrate reminders with education provide a cost-effective way to deliver information to patients as an adjunct to conventional therapy. As automated text message platforms begin to support two-way communication, the use of this technology requires little additional effort from clinicians, and can contribute to the optimization of communication between patient and physicians [21]. Whether the benefit of these approaches is due to education or simply to the expectation of contact with the health care provider (and the resulting perception of accountability) remains unexplored.

Regular contact with patients or their caregivers directly after prescribing a new treatment regimen may also improve adherence. Steroid phobia has been strongly associated with a need for reassurance by the physician to patients or their parents [28]. Additionally, only half of patients state that they have discussed their concerns about steroids with their physician [2, 29]. Scheduling phone calls to "check-up" on a patient shortly after the initial visit can be an opportunity for patients to voice their concerns about new medications [2]. Maintaining open lines of communication can also optimize the relationship between physicians and their patients or caregivers. Some of the strongest predictors of adherence to topical atopic dermatitis treatment in pediatric disease were a good parent-doctor relationship and severity of disease, as perceived by the mother [58]. Parent-physician interactions play a critical role in shaping mothers' attitudes toward treatment, with physician communication skills contributing to a favorable experience [51]. When mothers perceive that physicians do not consider including parental input in the discussion and design of a treatment plans, there is decreased motivation for adherence [51]. Fostering a therapeutic alliance between patient and physician is one of the components of the definition of adherence. Strengthening this relationship with communication to foster mutual trust and respect, may ease patient concerns and serve to improve adherence [23, 51].

An alternative proposed method for increased communication that has been studied in atopic dermatitis is the use of e-health service portal [59]. After initial diagnosis and treatment visit, follow-up maintenance through these systems could provide a simple, cost-effective method for clinicians to have open communication with their patients, provide e-consultation and education, and ensure they are taking their medications as prescribed [59]. (van Os-Medendorp H) Other interventions for pediatric patients that have been proposed but not yet studied include creating games for treatment application, involving children in their treamtent, and distracting patients during treatment application [2, 60]. For pediatric patients especially, physicians should consider less frequent appliactions in order to avoid or minimize treatment fatigue from occuring [60].

Another practical (though not well studied) approach to combat nonadherence due to forgetfulness is to fit the medication into existing daily routine, such as applying topical medicaton just before brushing teeth [2, 60]. Sticker charts are another powerful tool that can be used to guide children's behavior [61]. For patients and parents desirous of an "all natural skincare routine," safe and effective "natural" products can be suggested. Individualizing treatment plans to best meet patients' personal preferences is another logical approach for enhancing adherence.

Research on adherence to medications in atopic dermatitis is essential, yet so far limited. Further studies are needed to assess the effectiveness of different interventions (ideally utilizing objective monitoring techniques) in clinical practice. By increasing the of study adherence in atopic dermatitis patients and caregivers, clinicians can develop new methods of improving adherence and begin implementing them in the clinical setting. By improving adherence, physicians can lessen the psychosocial and financial burden of this disease on patients and their families [2, 62]. Focusing on increasing adherence to effective treatments, rather than the development of novel agents, may be a more cost-effective method of improving outcomes for patients of atopic dermatitis [2].

12.7 Conclusion

As a chronic condition, atopic dermatitis requires long-term adherence, a long-term treatment burden for the patient. The burden is especially heavy because topical medications are difficult to apply and require more time and effort than just taking a pill. Adherence in atopic dermatitis is worse than in many other conditions. The strength of relationship and open communication between physician and patient is critical to improving and maintaining adherence throughout what may be years of different treatments and disease course. Clinicians can improve patient outcomes by improving adherence to treatment regimens through educational methods, earlier follow-up visits, and enhanced communication with patients and their caregivers. Practical measure such as frequent reminders and open lines of communication can combat nonadherence due to forgetfulness and alleviate patient concerns about their therapy plans. Physicians can work with patients and their caregivers to foster a strong therapeutic alliance to improve adherence to treatment regimens, and thus their patients; outcomes.

References

1. Bass AM, Anderson KL, Feldman SR. Interventions to increase treatment adherence in pediatric atopic dermatitis: a systematic review. J Clin Med. 2015;4(2):231–42. doi:10.3390/jcm4020231.
2. Patel NU, D'Ambra V, Feldman SR. Increasing adherence with topical agents for atopic dermatitis. Am J Clin Dermatol. 2017;8(3):323–32. doi:10.1007/s40257-017-0261-5.
3. Brown KK, Rehmus WE, Kimball AB. Determining the relative importance of patient motivations for nonadherence to topical corticosteroid therapy in psoriasis. J Am Acad Dermatol. 2006;55(4):607–13. doi:10.1016/j.jaad.2005.12.021.
4. Kelsay K, Klinnert M, Bender B. Addressing psychosocial aspects of atopic dermatitis. Immunol Allergy Clin N Am. 2010;30(3):385–96. doi:10.1016/j.iac.2010.05.003.
5. Fawcett J. Compliance: definitions and key issues. J Clin Psychiatry. 1995;56(Suppl 1):4–8; discussion 9–10. http://www.ncbi.nlm.nih.gov/pubmed/7836349. Accessed 13 Sept 2016.
6. Chakrabarti S. What's in a name? Compliance, adherence and concordance in chronic psychiatric disorders. World J Psychiatry. 2014;4(2):30–6. doi:10.5498/wjp.v4.i2.30.
7. Burkhart PV, Sabaté E. Adherence to long-term therapies: evidence for action. J Nurs Scholarsh. 2003;35(3):207. http://www.ncbi.nlm.nih.gov/pubmed/14562485. Accessed 18 Jan 2017.

8. Julius RJ, Novitsky MA, Dubin WR. Medication adherence: a review of the literature and implications for clinical practice. J Psychiatr Pract. 2009;15(1):34–44. doi:10.1097/01.pra.0000344917.43780.77.
9. Velligan DI, Weiden PJ, Sajatovic M, et al. The expert consensus guideline series: adherence problems in patients with serious and persistent mental illness. J Clin Psychiatry. 2009;70(Suppl 4):1–46; quiz 47–8. http://www.ncbi.nlm.nih.gov/pubmed/19686636. Accessed 16 Mar 2017.
10. Storm A, Andersen SE, Benfeldt E, Serup J. One in 3 prescriptions are never redeemed: primary nonadherence in an outpatient clinic. J Am Acad Dermatol. 2008;59(1):27–33. doi:10.1016/j.jaad.2008.03.045.
11. Brodtkorb E, Samsonsen C, Sund JK, Bråthen G, Helde G, Reimers A. Treatment non-adherence in pseudo-refractory epilepsy. Epilepsy Res. 2016;122:1–6. doi:10.1016/j.eplepsyres.2016.02.001.
12. Horne R, Weinman J, Barber N, Elliott R. Concordance, adherence and compliance in medicine taking. Report for the National Co-ordinating Centre for NHS Service Delivery and Organisation R & D (NCCSDO). 2005:1–331. doi:10.1007/SpringerReference_64584.
13. Clifford S, Barber N, Horne R. Understanding different beliefs held by adherers, unintentional nonadherers, and intentional nonadherers: application of the necessity–concerns framework. J Psychosom Res. 2008;64(1):41–6. doi:10.1016/j.jpsychores.2007.05.004.
14. Gadkari AS, McHorney CA. Unintentional non-adherence to chronic prescription medications: how unintentional is it really? BMC Health Serv Res. 2012;12(1):98. doi:10.1186/1472-6963-12-98.
15. Richards HL, Fortune DG, O'Sullivan TM, Main CJ, Griffiths CE. Patients with psoriasis and their compliance with medication. J Am Acad Dermatol. 1999;41(4):581–3. http://www.ncbi.nlm.nih.gov/pubmed/10495380. Accessed 16 Mar 2017.
16. Krejci-Manwaring J, Tusa MG, Carroll C, et al. Stealth monitoring of adherence to topical medication: adherence is very poor in children with atopic dermatitis. J Am Acad Dermatol. 2007;56(2):211–6. doi:10.1016/j.jaad.2006.05.073.
17. Carroll CL, Feldman SR, Camacho FT, Manuel JC, Balkrishnan R. Adherence to topical therapy decreases during the course of an 8-week psoriasis clinical trial: commonly used methods of measuring adherence to topical therapy overestimate actual use. J Am Acad Dermatol. 2004;51(2):212–6. doi:10.1016/j.jaad.2004.01.052.
18. Hix E, Gustafson CJ, O'Neill JL, et al. Adherence to a five day treatment course of topical fluocinonide 0.1% cream in atopic dermatitis. Dermatol Online J. 2013;19(10):20029.
19. Yentzer BA, Camacho FT, Young T, Fountain JM, Clark AR, Feldman SR. Good adherence and early efficacy using desonide hydrogel for atopic dermatitis: results from a program addressing patient compliance. J Drugs Dermatol. 2010;9(4):324–9. http://www.ncbi.nlm.nih.gov/pubmed/20514788. Accessed 20 Oct 2016.
20. Furue M, Onozuka D, Takeuchi S, et al. Poor adherence to oral and topical medication in 3096 dermatological patients as assessed by the Morisky Medication Adherence Scale-8. Br J Dermatol. 2015;172(1):272–5. doi:10.1111/bjd.13377.
21. Pena-Robichaux V, Kvedar JC, Watson AJ. Text messages as a reminder aid and educational tool in adults and adolescents with atopic dermatitis: a pilot study. Dermatol Res Pract. 2010;2010 doi:10.1155/2010/894258.
22. Ellis RM, Koch LH, McGuire E, Williams JV. Potential barriers to adherence in pediatric dermatology. Pediatr Dermatol. 2011;28(3):242–4. doi:10.1111/j.1525-1470.2011.01493.x.
23. Ohya Y, Williams H, Steptoe A, et al. Psychosocial factors and adherence to treatment advice in childhood atopic dermatitis. J Invest Dermatol. 2001;117(4):852–7. doi:10.1046/j.0022-202x.2001.01475.x.
24. Serup J, Lindblad AK, Maroti M, et al. To follow or not to follow dermatological treatment. Acta Derm Venereol. 2006;86(3):193–7. doi:10.2340/00015555-0073.
25. Ulff E, Maroti M, Kettis-Lindblad Å, et al. Single application of a fluorescent test cream by healthy volunteers: assessment of treated and neglected body sites. Br J Dermatol. 2007;156(5):974–8. doi:10.1111/j.1365-2133.2007.07754.x.

26. Charman C, Williams H. The use of corticosteroids and corticosteroid phobia in atopic dermatitis. Clin Dermatol. 2003;21(3):193–200. http://www.ncbi.nlm.nih.gov/pubmed/12781437. Accessed 20 Oct 2016.
27. Surber C, Itin PH, Bircher AJ, Maibach HI. Topical corticosteroids. J Am Acad Dermatol. 1995;32(6):1025–30. http://www.ncbi.nlm.nih.gov/pubmed/7751447. Accessed 20 Oct 2016.
28. Aubert-Wastiaux H, Moret L, Le Rhun A, et al. Topical corticosteroid phobia in atopic dermatitis: a study of its nature, origins and frequency. Br J Dermatol. 2011;165(4):808–14. doi:10.1111/j.1365-2133.2011.10449.x.
29. Hon K-LE, Kam W-YC, Leung T-F, et al. Steroid fears in children with eczema. Acta Paediatr. 2006;95(11):1451–5. doi:10.1080/08035250600612298.
30. El Hachem M, Gesualdo F, Ricci G, et al. Topical corticosteroid phobia in parents of pediatric patients with atopic dermatitis: a multicentre survey. Ital J Pediatr. 2017;43(1):22. doi:10.1186/s13052-017-0330-7.
31. Charman CR, Morris AD, Williams HC. Topical corticosteroid phobia in patients with atopic eczema. Br J Dermatol. 2000;142(5):931–6. doi:10.1046/j.1365-2133.2000.03473.x.
32. Lee JY, Her Y, Kim CW, Kim SS. Topical corticosteroid phobia among parents of children with atopic eczema in Korea. Ann Dermatol. 2015;27(5):499–506. doi:10.5021/ad.2015.27.5.499.
33. Beattie PE, Lewis-Jones MS. Parental knowledge of topical therapies in the treatment of childhood atopic dermatitis. Clin Exp Dermatol. 2003;28(5):549–53. doi:10.1046/j.1365-2230.2003.01357.x.
34. Sagransky MJ, Yentzer BA, Williams LL, Clark AR, Taylor SL, Feldman SRA. randomized controlled pilot study of the effects of an extra office visit on adherence and outcomes in atopic dermatitis. Arch Dermatol. 2010;146(12):1428–30. doi:10.1001/archdermatol.2010.368.
35. Halling-Overgaard A-S, Kezic S, Jakasa I, Engebretsen KA, Maibach H, Thyssen JP. Skin absorption through atopic dermatitis skin: a systematic review. Br J Dermatol. 2016; doi:10.1111/bjd.15065.
36. Siegfried EC, Jaworski JC, Kaiser JD, Hebert AA. Systematic review of published trials: long-term safety of topical corticosteroids and topical calcineurin inhibitors in pediatric patients with atopic dermatitis. BMC Pediatr. 2016;16:75. doi:10.1186/s12887-016-0607-9.
37. Oranje A, Devillers A, Kunz B, et al. Treatment of patients with atopic dermatitis using wet-wrap dressings with diluted steroids and/or emollients. An expert panel's opinion and review of the literature. J Eur Acad Dermatol Venereol. 2006;20(10):1277–86. doi:10.1111/j.1468-3083.2006.01790.x.
38. Rork JF, Sheehan WJ, Gaffin JM, et al. Parental response to written eczema action plans in children with eczema. Arch Dermatol. 2012;148(3):391–2. doi:10.1001/archdermatol.2011.2267.
39. Moore EJ, Williams A, Manias E, Varigos G, Donath S. Eczema workshops reduce severity of childhood atopic eczema. Australas J Dermatol. 2009;50(2):100–6. doi:10.1111/j.1440-0960.2009.00515.x.
40. Shaw M, Morrell DS, Goldsmith LA. A study of targeted enhanced patient care for pediatric atopic dermatitis (STEP PAD). Pediatr Dermatol. 2008;25(1):19–24. doi:10.1111/j.1525-1470.2007.00575.x.
41. Grillo M, Gassner L, Marshman G, Dunn S, Hudson P. Pediatric atopic eczema: the impact of an educational intervention. Pediatr Dermatol. 2006;23(5):428–36. doi:10.1111/j.1525-1470.2006.00277.x.
42. Staab D, von Rueden U, Kehrt R, et al. Evaluation of a parental training program for the management of childhood atopic dermatitis. Pediatr Allergy Immunol. 2002;13(2):84–90. http://www.ncbi.nlm.nih.gov/pubmed/12000479. Accessed 18 Oct 2016.
43. Chinn DJ, Poyner T, Sibley G. Randomized controlled trial of a single dermatology nurse consultation in primary care on the quality of life of children with atopic eczema. Br J Dermatol. 2002;146(3):432–9. http://www.ncbi.nlm.nih.gov/pubmed/11952543. Accessed 18 Oct 2016.
44. Patel NU, Moore BA, Craver RF, Feldman SR. Ethical considerations in adherence research. Patient Prefer Adherence. 2016;10:2429–35. doi:10.2147/PPA.S117802.
45. Balato N, Megna M, Di Costanzo L, Balato A, Ayala F. Educational and motivational support service: a pilot study for mobile-phone-based interventions in patients with psoriasis. Br J Dermatol. 2013;168(1):201–5. doi:10.1111/j.1365-2133.2012.11205.x.

46. Long CC, Funnell CM, Collard R, Finlay AY. What do members of the National Eczema Society really want? Clin Exp Dermatol. 1993;18(6):516–22. doi:10.1111/j.1365-2230.1993.tb01020.x.
47. Santer M, Muller I, Yardley L, Lewis-Jones S, Ersser S, Little P. Parents' and carers' views about emollients for childhood eczema: qualitative interview study. BMJ Open. 2016;6(8):e011887. doi:10.1136/bmjopen-2016-011887.
48. Cork MJ, Britton J, Butler L, Young S, Murphy R, Keohane SG. Comparison of parent knowledge, therapy utilization and severity of atopic eczema before and after explanation and demonstration of topical therapies by a specialist dermatology nurse. Br J Dermatol. 2003;149(3):582–9. doi:10.1046/j.1365-2133.2003.05595.x.
49. Ersser SJ, Cowdell F, Latter S, et al. Psychological and educational interventions for atopic eczema in children. Cochrane Database Syst Rev. 2014;1:CD004054. doi:10.1002/14651858.CD004054.pub3.
50. Broberg A, Kalimo K, Lindblad B, Swanbeck G. Parental education in the treatment of childhood atopic eczema. Acta Derm Venereol. 1990;70(6):495–9. http://www.ncbi.nlm.nih.gov/pubmed/1981422. Accessed 21 Oct 2016.
51. Fenerty SD, O'Neill JL, Gustafson CJ, et al. Maternal adherence factors in the treatment of pediatric atopic dermatitis. JAMA Dermatol. 2013;149(2):229. doi:10.1001/2013.jamadermatol.253.
52. Feldman SR, Camacho FT, Krejci-Manwaring J, Carroll CL, Balkrishnan R. Adherence to topical therapy increases around the time of office visits. J Am Acad Dermatol. 2007;57(1):81–3. doi:10.1016/j.jaad.2007.04.005.
53. Feldman SR. The parable of the piano teacher. The Dermatologist. 2007;15(8). http://www.the-dermatologist.com/article/7570.
54. Evangelista MTP, Abad-Casintahan F, Lopez-Villafuerte L. The effect of topical virgin coconut oil on SCORAD index, transepidermal water loss, and skin capacitance in mild to moderate pediatric atopic dermatitis: a randomized, double-blind, clinical trial. Int J Dermatol. 2014;53(1):100–8. doi:10.1111/ijd.12339.
55. Canpolat F, Erkoçoğlu M, Tezer H, Kocabaş CN, Kandi B. Hydrocortisone acetate alone or combined with mupirocin for atopic dermatitis in infants under two years of age—a randomized double blind pilot trial. Eur Rev Med Pharmacol Sci. 2012;16(14):1989–93. http://www.ncbi.nlm.nih.gov/pubmed/23242727. Accessed 25 Oct 2016.
56. Glenn C, McMichael A, Feldman SR. Measuring patient satisfaction changes patient satisfaction. J Dermatolog Treat. 2012;23(2):81–2. doi:10.3109/09546634.2012.666883.
57. Feldman SR. Tachyphylaxis to topical corticosteroids: the more you use them, the less they work? Clin Dermatol. 2006;24:229–30.
58. Kojima R, Fujiwara T, Matsuda A, et al. Factors associated with steroid phobia in caregivers of children with atopic dermatitis. Pediatr Dermatol. 2013;30(1):29–35. doi:10.1111/j.1525-1470.2012.01808.x.
59. van Os-Medendorp H, Koffijberg H, Eland-de Kok PCM, et al. E-health in caring for patients with atopic dermatitis: a randomized controlled cost-effectiveness study of internet-guided monitoring and online self-management training. Br J Dermatol. 2012;166(5):1060–8. doi:10.1111/j.1365-2133.2012.10829.x.
60. Santer M, Burgess H, Yardley L, et al. Managing childhood eczema: qualitative study exploring carers' experiences of barriers and facilitators to treatment adherence. J Adv Nurs. 2013;69(11):2493–501. doi:10.1111/jan.12133.
61. Luersen K, Davis SA, Kaplan SG, Abel TD, Winchester WW, Feldman SR. Sticker charts: a method for improving adherence to treatment of chronic diseases in children. Pediatr Dermatol. 2012;29(4):403–8. doi:10.1111/j.1525-1470.2012.01741.x.
62. Carroll CL, Balkrishnan R, Feldman SR, Fleischer AB, Manuel JC. The burden of atopic dermatitis: impact on the patient, family, and society. Pediatr Dermatol. 2005;22(3):192–9. doi:10.1111/j.1525-1470.2005.22303.x.

Chapter 13
Atopic Dermatitis: Managing the Itch

William S. Farmer and Kalyani S. Marathe

Abstract Atopic dermatitis has a substantial impact on sleep, appearance, psychological well-being, and other qualities of life. The visual appearance of lichenification, cheilitis, hyperpigmentation, ichthyosis, and erythema can be socially stigmatizing, and treatment of these symptoms is challenging. In managing pruritus in patients, practitioners should assess and document pruritus through questionnaires at each routine visit. Initially, practitioners should advise patients to employ non-pharmaceutical treatments such as emollients with wet wraps, elimination of triggers, changing scratching habits, and psychological interventions. If these methods of treatment are not successful or if the disease presentation is severe, pharmacological therapies should be employed. This chapter describes the therapeutic ladder for pruritus in atopic dermatitis and discusses each treatment modality in further detail for practitioners to advise their patients.

First-line topical pharmaceutical agents include topical glucocorticoids and topical calcineurin inhibitors. Second-line topical agents include coal tar, menthol, capsaicin, or doxepin. After the use of topical agents has been exhausted, primary systemic agents can be applied. These include sedating antihistamines, non-sedating antihistamines, oral glucocorticoids, or cyclosporine A. Finally, neuromodulating or immunomodulating agents can be attempted, including SSRI/SNRIs, TCAs, immunosuppressants, neural modulators, and opioid receptor modulators. Outside of pharmacological treatments, phototherapy has been shown to provide a dramatic improvement of pruritus in atopic dermatitis and can be used at any stage of treatment including as a first-line agent.

Keywords Pruritus • Treatment • Anti-Puritus therapeutic ladder

---

W.S. Farmer, B.S.
Georgetown University School of Medicine, Washington, DC, USA

K.S. Marathe, M.D., M.P.H. (✉)
Department of Dermatology, George Washington University, Washington, DC, USA

Department of Dermatology, Children's National Medical Center, Washington, DC, USA
e-mail: kalyanimarathe@gmail.com

E.A. Fortson et al. (eds.), *Management of Atopic Dermatitis*, Advances in Experimental Medicine and Biology 1027, DOI 10.1007/978-3-319-64804-0_13

13.1 Introduction

Atopic dermatitis is referred to as "the itch that rashes" due to the extensive pruritus involved in the disease [1]. The disease has a significant impact on major aspects of quality of life including sleep, appearance, and psychological well-being. Nocturnal pruritus often hinders sleep which causes anxiety and daytime somnolence. The visual appearance of lichenification, cheilitis, hyperpigmentation, ichthyosis, and erythema can be socially stigmatizing. Social isolation and embarrassment can occur in children as well as adults. The disease impacts care takers, demanding money, time, and energy. While the pathophysiology of pruritus in atopic dermatitis is incompletely characterized, some molecular mechanisms are known to play a role, as demonstrated in Fig. 13.1. These mechanisms include: histamine 1/4 receptors (H1R, H4R), protease-activated receptor 2 (PAR 2), interleukin 31 receptor (IL31R), and transient receptor potential cation channel subfamily V member 1 (TRPV1).

13.2 Pathophysiology of Pruritus

Complement and immunoglobulin deposits have been discovered in patients with atopic dermatitis within the dermal-epidermal junctions [2]. The highest density of thin, unmyelinated C-fibers that mediate pruritus are located in this same junction [3, 4]. For this reason, patients may scratch their skin until it bleeds because erosion of the dermal-epidermal junction is thought to provide relief [5].

Histamine is also thought to play a role in the development of itch. Basophils and mast cells release histamine which binds to central and peripheral receptors. Histamine is an autocasoid that has been found to be increased in atopic dermatitis

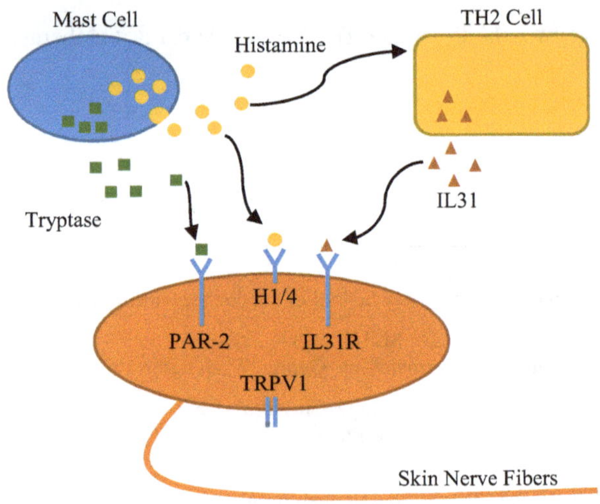

Fig. 13.1 Proposed pathophysiology of pruritus in atopic dermatitis with H1/4, PAR-2, IL31R, and TRPV1

lesions [5, 6]. The histamine 4 receptor specifically has been shown to play a role in atopic dermatitis pruritus and is believed to be activated on Th2 cells leading to IL-31 production [5–9]. Although studies suggest a role of both H1R and H4R in pruritus, only H1R antagonists are available to treat pruritus [5]. Within the class of H1R antagonists, efficacy of non-sedating antihistamines has been limited in the treatment of atopic dermatitis, suggesting the lack of a significant role of peripheral histamine 1 receptors for atopic dermatitis [9]. In addition to histamine, mast cells are thought to release tryptase which binds to specific receptors on nociceptive afferent nerves known as PAR-2 [10]. Atopic dermatitis lesions have been found to demonstrate enhanced immunostaining for PAR-2. Thus, another proposed mediator for atopic dermatitis pruritus is PAR-2.

Several therapies for pruritus in atopic dermatitis utilize transient receptor potential (TRPV1) ion channels on C fibers which activate pain neurons. These ion channels respond to heat and cold temperatures, to protons via pH changes, and to biological mediators such as prostanoids. It is thought that phosphorylation and desensitization of these ion channels work to counteract pruritus.

13.3 Assessment of Severity of Pruritus

Assessment of the severity of the pruritus is important so that improvement can be monitored over time. Particular features of the disease are important to characterize: the severity of the excoriations, distribution of the pruritus, lesion morphology, presence of alloknesis (itch produced by gentle touch), color, history of skin infections, presence of urticaria, intensity of the pruritus, duration, frequency, location, and quality of the pruritus, aggravating and palliative factors, current treatments, quality of life, degree of disability, coping strategies, and scratch response. Other medical history components are important as well: patient age, current medications, presence of diabetes or malignancy, triggers (heat, cold, change in weather, water, chemicals, haptens). These features allow the practitioner to assess the severity of the pruritus to help determine what type of treatment would be best suited for the patient. Symptoms concerning for systemic involvement that should be investigated include: anemia, cholestasis, immunosuppression, infections, jaundice, presence of other skin diagnoses, signs of neoplasia, signs of psychiatric disease, and weight loss [11]. The presence of these factors may be cause for a more comprehensive workup with blood testing, including: a complete blood count, ferritin, folates, total iron binding capacity with iron, reticulocyte count, vitamin B12, folic acid, and liver function tests.

Because pruritus can be subjective, a questionnaire can be used to determine the severity of the pruritus at each office visit. Table 13.1 lists assessment question topics to document pruritus in patients. The Eppendorf Itch Questionnaire, shown in Fig. 13.2, is a short survey that rates the severity of the symptoms and assesses the temporal nature of the pruritus, location of the itch, and palliation [12]. It is helpful in assessing a patient's symptoms in a more objective manner.

Table 13.1 Assessment of pruritus

Age of patient	Localization of the pruritus
Aggravating factors	Morphology of the lesions
Color of the lesions	Other medications used
Coping strategy	Palliating factors
Current treatment regiment	Presence of alloknesis
Dimensions of the lesions	Presence of urticaria
Disabilities due to the pruritus	Quality of life
Distribution of the pruritus	Quality of the pruritus
Duration of pruritus	Scratch response
Frequency of pruritus	Severity of the excoriations
History of skin infections	Triggers of pruritus
Intensity of the pruritus	

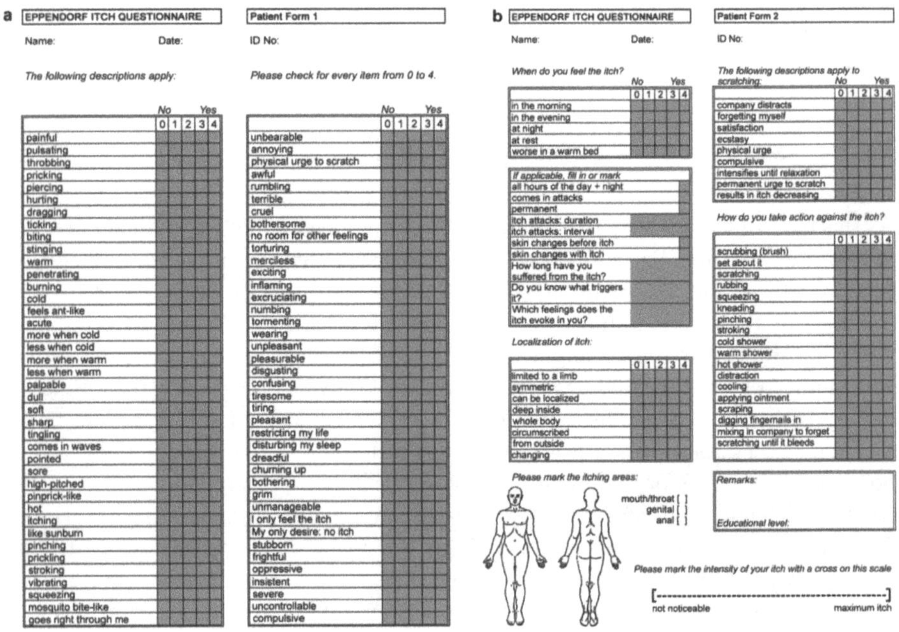

Fig. 13.2 Eppendorf Itch Questionnaire used for assessment of pruritus in atopic dermatitis (Darsow et al. [12])

In certain populations such as children and the elderly, it may not be possible for the patient to fully communicate the extent of pruritus. In these patients, the physical exam as well as direct observation of behaviors during the office visit may be more helpful indicators.

13.4 Interventions

Identification and elimination of pruritic triggers can improve quality of life in patients with atopic dermatitis. Patients should be educated on possible triggers so that they can keep track of potential exposures. Common factors that can induce pruritus include: animals, cigarette smoke, cosmetics, detergents, dry air, wool clothing, dust mites, food allergens, humidity, jewelry, long and hot baths/showers, non-cotton clothing, pollen, polyester, and sweat. Infections including *Staphylococcus aureus*, Herpes simplex, *Trichophyton* species, and *Malassezia (pityrosporum)* can also trigger pruritus. Emotional stress has been known to trigger pruritus as well [13].

Patients should be advised to wear 100% cotton clothing. Silver-based textiles have been produced for additional clothing options outside of cotton due to their antiseptic nature, suppressing *S. aureus* colonization & toxin formation [14]. Patients should bathe regularly with fragrance-free detergents. The patient should be advised to avoid smoking and second-hand smoke exposure. Ideally, patients should keep their homes clean and free of dust, mold, and pollen to minimize allergen exposure. Humidifiers and dehumidifiers can be purchased to improve air quality; however, these should be thoroughly cleaned regularly to prevent microorganism contamination.

13.5 Non-pharmacological Interventions for Pruritus

Patients can perform certain measures to minimize pruritus and skin damage from excoriations. These nonpharmacological interventions for pruritus are listed in Table 13.2. Cutting fingernails and keeping them well-filed can minimize trauma caused by excoriation. If tolerated, wearing soft cotton gloves at night can be especially helpful for younger patients. Practitioners should advise skin rubbing and cooling rather than scratching. Soaking the skin in a cool water bath has been found

Table 13.2 Nonpharmacological interventions for pruritus

Chinese herbal therapy
Cool water baths
Cutting fingernails
Elimination of triggers
Emollients
Psychological coping strategies
Rubbing & cooling
Tepid water baths
Wearing gloves at night
Wet wraps

to reduce pruritus in patients with atopic dermatitis [13]; moreover, tepid baths may also be helpful to alleviate pruritus. Bathing should be immediately followed by use of bland emollients such as fragrance-free ointments and humectants.

Wet wraps are a commonly used therapy for controlling active eczema and associated pruritus. The practitioner should instruct the patient to apply warm wet cotton bandages over the lesion and then to apply a dry dressing over top. Not only can this reduce pruritus, but it can also alleviate erythema and crusting. Covering skin lesions limit access to the skin preventing further excoriation especially at night. Emollients can be placed under the wet wraps to reduce symptoms. Topical medication placement under wet wraps should not be used as first line but can be used for unresponsive and recalcitrant lesions [13]. An alternative method of wet wrapping involves the use of generous bland ointments to moisturize the skin, followed by the application of petroleum jelly impregnated gauze, then covering with a dry rolled gauze dressing.

Traditional Chinese herbal therapy has been shown to have some success compared to placebo in reducing pruritus and improving sleep quality when compared to placebo in randomized controlled trials. Reported adverse effects include: dizziness, headache, abdominal distention, and nausea. It is thought that herbal remedies may have an inhibitory role in monocytes expression of CD23 [13]. St John's wort, licorice, mahonia, hypnotherapy, biofeedback, and massage therapy are other homeopathic therapies used to alleviate pruritus. There is insufficient evidence regarding published controlled trials on homeopathic remedies in atopic dermatitis [13].

Randomized controlled trials with patients receiving cognitive-behavioral treatment and relaxation therapy after 1 year have shown significantly decreased pruritus and scratching episodes when compared to standard dermatologic care. Not only do psychological factors exacerbate pruritus, but the itch-scratch cycle of atopic dermatitis causes anxiety. Specifically for managing pruritus, studies have demonstrated that habit reversal therapy alongside topical corticosteroids has shown significant reductions in scratching when compared with steroids alone [15]. Practitioners should assess and help manage patients' stress and anxiety at each appointment in order to prevent exacerbation of pruritus.

13.6 Topical Therapies for Pruritus

Once elimination of triggers, emollients, wet wraps, habit modification, psychological support, and other non-pharmacologic therapies have been tried, topical therapies should be initiated. Topical therapies may also be used for extensive lesions that are unlikely to respond without pharmacotherapy. Due to the risk of side effects, topical therapies should be tried prior to initiating systemic therapies. The vehicle of topical therapies should be heavily considered. For acute care, lotions, foams, and creams can be considered, although when applied to open or excoriated skin, these can cause burning and pain. For chronic care, ointments and ceramide-containing creams should be used. Based on the location of the lesion, particular

Table 13.3 Topical pharmacological interventions for pruritus in atopic dermatitis

Calcineurin Inhibitors	Pimecrlimus 1% cream; tacrolimus 0.03, 0.1% ointments	Transient burning, erythema, pruritus
Capsaicin	Start 0.025% cream 4–5× daily, gradually increase as needed up to 0.1%; 0.006% cream on sensitive skin	Burning, erythema, pruritus
Coal tar	20% coal tar + petrolatum (gold tar); 3–5% coal tar + unguentum leniens, (cool cream)	Burning, contact dermatitis, folliculitis, irritation, phototoxicity
Doxepin	5% cream	allergic contact dermatitis, burning, eczema exacerbation, and pruritus, somnolence, stinging, xerostomia
Glucocorticoids	Clobetasol proprionate 0.05% lotion; desonide hydrogel 0.05%; fluticasone proprionate 0.05% cream; hydrocortisone 1%; methylprednisolone aceponate 0.1% cream; prednicarbate 0.25% ointment	Adrenal suppression, chills, infection, skin atrophy
Lidocaine	3% cream; 5% patch	Erythema, edema, hypersensitivity
Menthol	1–3% cream increase up to 16%	Contact dermatitis
PEA	0.3% cream	Burning, erythema, pruritus

vehicles may be more ideal. Foams are an elegant vehicle for hair-bearing sites such as the scalp [11]. The main topical therapies used for pruritus that will be discussed are listed in Table 13.3 and include: coal tar, menthol, capsaicin, doxepin, naltrexone, PEA, and lidocaine. Topical corticosteroids and calcineurin inhibitors will be discussed in the chapter on atopic dermatitis management.

13.6.1 Coal Tar

The exact mechanism of coal tar is not understood; however, it has been shown to have antimicrobial, anti-inflammatory, and antipruritic effects. It comes in a variety of formulations which are often compounded with glucocorticoids. As an alternative to glucocorticoids, 20% coal tar can be compounded with petrolatum known as gold tar or 3–5% coal tar compounded with unguentum leniens can be used, which is known as cool cream. Three percent menthol is added to reduce odor [16]. There are few randomized controlled trials on coal tar for patients with atopic dermatitis, and it remains a second line agent. Reported trials have shown significant improvement with excoriation [13]. The main adverse effects of coal tar include burning, contact dermatitis, folliculitis, irritation, and phototoxicit [17]. Publications have shown no increased risk of cancers with topical coal tar [18].

13.6.2 Menthol

Menthol is a cyclic terpene alcohol antipruritic agent whose mechanism of action is not understood. It is thought to act on A-delta fibers, κ-opioid, and C-fiber TRPM8 channels that are thermally sensitive to cold temperatures [13]. Over the counter external use is approved up to 16% by the Food and Drug Administration as a cream, foam, gel, or ointment. Menthol is considered safe with the main adverse effect of menthol being contact dermatitis. It should be noted that because menthol can cause increased transepidermal water loss, it should not be substituted for emollient [19].

13.6.3 Capsaicin

Capsaicin is an alkaloid (8-methyl-N-vanillyl-6 nonenamide) made from hot chili peppers which induces neurogenic inflammation likely by depletion and desensitization of the transient receptor potential (TRPV1) ion channels C fiber [20]. These ion channels respond to physical and biological mediators such as heat, cold, pH changes, and prostanoids to counteract pruritus via activating pain neurons [11]. The stimulation of neuropeptide release that occurs upon applying capsaicin produces an intense burning sensation for usually half an hour; however, in most cases these symptoms resolve after 2–3 weeks. Although case-control studies are lacking and its overall efficacy has been questioned in systematic review for atopic dermatitis, there have been reports of topical capsaicin ointment in atopic dermatitis reducing pruritus within 12 days [21]. Adverse effects of capsaicin are burning, erythema, and pruritus. It is recommended to start at capsaicin 0.025% topical four to five times daily and gradually increase the dose as needed. The exception to this is sensitive skin areas such as face, axillae, or groin in which case 0.006% capsaicin should be used. Lidocaine gel, cream, or patch can be applied 20–60 min prior to capsaicin application to reduce burning and increase compliance [19].

13.6.4 Doxepin

Topical antihistamines are not considered effective for pruritus associated with atopic dermatitis; however, clinical trials have found that topical doxepin was the only anti-histamine with efficacy for chronic pruritus [11]. Doxepin is a tricyclic antidepressant with anti-adrenergic and anti-serotoninergic properties as well as potent H1 and H2 blocking properties. Doxepin is a second or third line agent for atopic dermatitis and is approved by the Food and Drug Administration as a 5% cream for up to 8 days of treatment for adults [22]. Randomized controlled trials have shown a significant reduction in pruritus relief after a week of use compared to a vehicle [23]. Doxepin combined with 2.5% hydrocortisone or with 0.1% triamcinolone provided faster and greater pruritus relief than either corticosteroid alone

[24]. It is relatively safe with a long history of use; adverse effects of doxepin include allergic contact dermatitis, burning, eczema exacerbation, and pruritus, somnolence, stinging, and xerostomia [25]. Short duration of therapy limits use.

13.6.5 Topical N-Palmitoylethanolamine (PEA)

PEA (N-palmitoylethanolamine) is a cannabinoid agonist that has been shown to have analgesic and anti-inflammatory effects likely by downregulating mast cell degranulation. Activation of the cannabinoid receptor has been found to prevent pruritus from escalating [11]. PEA 0.3% cream has been found to improve pruritus and excoriation in patients with moderate atopic dermatitis [26]. One study that lacked a control group showed a 45% reduction in pruritus based on a visual analog scale after 6 days, and after 4–6 weeks there was a 60% scale reduction in pruritus. Due to lack of data, PEA is not commonly used for atopic dermatitis. Adverse effects include burning, erythema, and pruritus [13].

13.6.6 Lidocaine

Lidocaine is amide local anesthetic, anti-arrhythmic, and sodium channel blocker also used for the management of neuropathic pain. There are only a few studies showing topical lidocaine's effectiveness for pruritus; however, the anti-pruritic nature of lidocaine has been established in mice [13, 27].

13.6.7 Naltrexone

Some patients with atopic dermatitis have been shown to have biopsies with a decreased number of μ-opiate receptors in the skin. Opioid receptor modulators are more thoroughly discussed later in the systemic therapies for pruritus. In one study, topical naltrexone was found to have a 29.4% improvement on pruritus and faster time to relief than placebo [24]; however, naltrexone remains understudied for pruritus. For this reason, naltrexone is not commonly used as a first-line agent for pruritus.

13.7 Phototherapy

Ultraviolet A, ultraviolet A1, broad-band ultraviolet B, narrow-band ultraviolet B, psoralen ultraviolet light, and excimer 308-nm laser have been found to be effective in reducing pruritus in patients with atopic dermatitis. It is considered a safe first or second-line treatment, especially for wide-spread and generalized atopic dermatitis and for those who do not tolerate other systemic therapies. Phototherapy is a good therapy for topical antihistamine and steroid resistant pruritus in pregnant patients. The exact mechanism of the direct role of ultraviolet therapy on cutaneous cell release of anti-pruritic mediators is not well understood. Several mechanisms of action have been proposed including: inhibition of pro-inflammatory mediators (IL-1 and tumor necrosis factor alpha), inhibition of anti-inflammatory neuropeptides release, inhibition of immunoglobulin E binding, reduction of mast cell numbers, inhibition of Langerhans cell epidermal migration, reduction of the number of HLADR+ T cells, and destruction of epidermal cutaneous nerves [11, 13]. Longer wavelengths of phototherapy penetrate farther into the skin. Ultraviolet A can reach the superficial to mid-dermis, whereas ultraviolet B remains in the epidermis. Because neurons associated with pruritus are thought to be at the dermal-epidermal junction, phototherapy applied deeper than the epidermis is more effective in reducing pruritus. Patients receiving high-dose ultraviolet A1, which is less commonly available than ultraviolet B, have been shown to be more effective than topical corticosteroids on reducing the severity of pruritus in patients with atopic dermatitis [28]. Combining oral psoralen with ultraviolet light therapy (pUVA) has been found to relieve all symptoms of pruritus within the first 2 weeks of treatment [29]. Twice weekly 308 nm laser UVB therapy has been shown to have an 81% reduction from baseline pruritus scores after 1 month [30]. Moreover, 308 nm laser has shown equivalence to clobetasol propionate 0.05% ointment for pruritus in atopic dermatitis [41]. Narrow-band ultraviolet B has shown success when combined with steroids/antihistamines or cyclosporine [11, 13]. The combination of phototherapy with crude coal tar is known as Goeckerman therapy, first described by William Goeckerman in 1925. While most studies have been limited to psoriasis, Goeckerman therapy is safely used for atopic dermatitis in children and adults, especially those requiring systemic medication [42].

Adverse effects of phototherapy are based on the depth of the UV ray penetration. Adverse effects of ultraviolet B include erythema, skin aging, and tanning, with no or only slightly increased risk of non-melanoma skin cancer. Adverse effects of psoralen ultraviolet light include erythema, burning, headache, itching, lentigines, and nausea, with some risk of non-melanoma skin cancer, particularly squamous cell carcinoma. Adverse effects of 308 nm laser include burning, edema, erythema, hyperpigmentation, pruritus, and vesicles [13].

13.8 Systemic Therapies for Pruritus

Systemic therapies for pruritus should be saved for after topical pharmaceutical therapies have been attempted due to higher risk of adverse effects. There have been no randomized controlled trials finding one systemic medication to be safer or more effective than all the others [11]. The main systemic therapies for pruritus described here are listed in Table 13.4 and include: glucocorticoids, cyclosporine A, Ketotifen, antihistamines, opioid receptor modulators, lidocaine, SSRIs, TCAs, and neural

Table 13.4 Systemic pharmacological interventions for pruritus in atopic dermatitis

Antihistamines	Cetirizine 20 mg; cyproheptadine 4 mg; hydroxyzine 25 mg; diphenhydramine 25–50 mg	Anti-muscarinergic effects, sedation, anti-motion effects, arrhythmia, renal dysfunction
Cyclosporine A	2.5–4 mg/kg/day twice a day	Gingival hyperplasia, gout, headache, hyperlipidemia, hypertension, hypertrichosis, paresthesia, renal dysfunction; rarely infections and malignancies
Doxepin	Start at 10 mg at bedtime, increase every third day until the sedation is not tolerable	Anti-adrenergic, anti-serotoninergic, anti-histaminic, arrhythmia
Glucocorticoids	Beclomethasone; flunisolide	Suppression of the hypothalamic-pituitary adrenal axis
Opioid receptor modulators	Start at naltrexone 25 mg daily, increase every 3–7 days	Cramping, diarrhea, headaches, nausea, vomiting
SSRIs, SNRIs neural modulators	Fluvoxamine 25–150 mg daily; mirtazapine 7.5–15 mg daily; paroxetine10–40 mg daily; sertraline 75–50 mg daily	Appetite loss, insomnia, sexual dysfunction, weight loss, weight gain

modulators. It is important to consider the age of patient, arrhythmia risk, drug interactions, renal function, and sedation when selecting the proper systemic agent [11].

13.8.1 Antihistamines

Histamine is not known to be a chief mediator of pruritus in atopic dermatitis [31]. Large, randomized, controlled studies have not been conducted for the antipruritic effects of systemic antihistamines in atopic dermatitis; however, they are widely used as an adjunct therapy [32]. The soporific effect of antihistamines may reduce scratching during the night, thereby reducing the scratch-itch cycle of atopic dermatitis [33]. Thus, sedating antihistamines (cyproheptadine, hydroxyzine, diphenhydramine) may be more effective by improving sleep quality [32]. Normal doses of non-sedating antihistamines are not usually considered useful for the pruritus in atopic dermatitis unless urticaria or allergic rhinoconjunctivitis are present. Higher doses of non-sedating antihistamines have shown improvement in pruritus. One study has found 20 mg of cetirizine used daily for 4 weeks to be more effective than placebo in reducing pruritus [34]. If systemic anti-histamines are used, it is recommended to start with a higher dose of a non-sedating antihistamine in the daytime and a sedating antihistamine at night [11]. At higher doses, typically three to four times greater than recommended dosing for allergic rhinitis, non-sedating antihistamines are well tolerated and function as an anti-pruritic agent. For this reason, systemic antihistamines are considered first line of the systemic treatments for adjuvant treatment before other systemic medications. Systemic antihistamines are not recommended without concurrent topical anti-inflammatory and anti-xerotic therapy. Antihistamines should be used with caution in the elderly due to potential for sedation and anti-cholinergic effects [11].

13.8.2 Glucocorticoids

Glucocorticoids have numerous anti-inflammatory effects including decreasing edema, inhibiting leukocyte migration, hindering phagocytosis, and blocking T lymphocyte cytokine release, which are all thought to suppress pruritus in patients with atopic dermatitis [11, 13]. Randomized controlled trials are limited on systemic glucocorticoid use for atopic dermatitis; however, one randomized controlled trial has found that 4 weeks of combined nasal and oral beclomethasone showed significantly decreased pruritus compared to placebo in patients with atopic dermatitis [34]. Another showed that 2 weeks of flunisolide nasal spray use in children with severe atopic dermatitis significantly reduced pruritus compared to placebo [35]. Glucocorticoids should be used with caution due to potential suppression of the hypothalamic-pituitary adrenal axis and rebound flares after tapering [11].

13.8.3 Cyclosporine A (CyA) & Immunosuppressants

Cyclosporine A binds intracellular cyclophilin receptor causing a decrease in T-lymphocyte activation and transcription of interleukin 2, which is thought to play a key role in pruritus [33]. It can be used off-label for the treatment of pruritus in patients with atopic dermatitis. Patients receiving cyclosporine A show a 55% reduction in pruritus after 6–8 weeks. The medication has been shown to be efficacious in both adults and children; however, pruritus returned after the medication was discontinued in 50% of patients [13]. Adverse effects of cyclosporine A are gingival hyperplasia, gout, headache, hyperlipidemia, hypertension, hypertrichosis, paresthesias, and renal dysfunction; infection and malignancies are rare [11].

Animal models have shown both tacrolimus and cyclosporine A may be better antipruritic agents than systemic glucocorticoids [11]. Additional studies have shown montelukast, mepolizumab, thymopentin, and rIFN-γ significantly reduce pruritus of atopic dermatitis by 12% compared to placebo [23]. The use of other systemic immunosuppressants including azathioprine, cyclophosphamide, and mycophenolate mofetil have not been well studied for pruritus in atopic dermatitis. Case series of the successful use of mycophenolate mofetil as an antipruritic drug for atopic dermatitis have been reported but without a control group [11]. Moreover, azathioprine may have potential use for photodermatitis-associated pruritus in adults and children with severe atopic dermatitis; however, hepatotoxicity and hepatitis have been observed with its use [11].

13.8.4 SSRIs, TCAs, and Neural Modulators

Selective serotonin reuptake inhibitors (SSRIs) block the reuptake of serotonin and thus increase the concentration of serotonin within the synaptic cleft. The mechanism of action in relation to pruritus is not understood, but SSRIs have been used to treat the pruritus associated with atopic dermatitis. Effectiveness has been documented with fluvoxamine, paroxetine, and sertraline for atopic dermatitis [11]. Adverse effects include appetite loss, insomnia, sexual dysfunction, and weight loss [11]. Serotonin-norepinephrine reuptake inhibitors (SNRIs) have not been thoroughly studied in atopic dermatitis [11].

TCAs block the serotonin transporter and the norepinephrine transporter, increasing the concentration of both serotonin and norepinephrine in the neural cleft. The difference among TCAs are their effects on adrenergic receptors, calcium channels, histamine receptors, N-Methyl-D-aspartate receptors, serotonin receptors, and sodium channels. Doxepin is a tricyclic antidepressant with anti-adrenergic and anti-serotoninergic properties as well as potent H1 and H2 blocking properties. Low-dose doxepin is used in patients with atopic dermatitis [13]. However, the effectiveness of doxepin is not predictable. Adult patients should start at 10 mg of doxepin at bedtime, and then the dose should be gradually titrated upwards until itch control is achieved or the medication becomes too sedating. Because of their side effects, oral TCAs should be second or third-line therapy. No large controlled studies have compared the effects of TCAs, SSRIs or SNRIs [11].

Systemic neural modulators directly interact with nerves to reduce pruritus; however, their efficacy is not well established and there have been no randomized-controlled studies. This class of drugs includes amitriptyline, gabapentin, mirtazapine, paroxetine and pregabalin. These drugs are understudied; however, mirtazapine, paroxetine, and fluvoxamine have been reported to improve nocturnal pruritus in atopic dermatitis [36, 37]. The role of aprepitant, an anti-emetic which works as an antagonist of Substance P on neurokinin-1 receptors, has been studied in Sezary syndrome and prurigo nodularis but has not been studied in atopic dermatitis [13].

13.8.5 Opioid Receptor Modulators

Spinal μ and δ opioid receptors are activated by opioids providing analgesia, but they also cause or exacerbate pruritus [38]. The μ opioid receptor is found in the epidermis and dermis which can be blocked by opioid receptor modulators such as naltrexone and nalmefene. Studies with naltrexone and nalmefene for atopic dermatitis have shown variable results as anti-pruritic agents. Some studies have shown naltrexone and nalmefene to be superior to placebo in reducing pruritus, however others have shown no significant difference [13]. It is recommended to start the patient at a low dose of 10 mg of nalmefene daily or 25 mg of naltrexone daily, and increase the dose every 3–7 days to minimize adverse effects. Typical adverse effects are cramping, diarrhea, headaches, nausea, and vomiting which are dose dependent and usually limited to the first 2 weeks of treatment [39]. Opioid receptor modulators should be considered second or third line agents due to mixed results and potential for tachyphylaxis. Kappa opioid receptor agonists such as butorphanol and nalfurafine (TRK-820) are thought to have the potential to be anti-pruritic agents but have not yet been formally investigated for atopic dermatitis [11, 13].

13.9 Immunosuppressants

Dupilumab is a fully human monoclonal antibody which binds to the IL-4α receptor subunit, thereby inhibiting IL-4 and IL-13 signaling which are two primary cytokines necessary for Th2 response. In recent studies, the drug's deployment resulted in significant improvement in pruritus and visible disease state and is undergoing further testing in pediatric and adult patients for FDA approval. Using a Numerical Rating Scale, patients in one study on dupilumab monotherapy reported a statistically-significant 56% reduction in pruritus as compared to a 15% reduction seen in placebo at 12 weeks. Another study showed similar results with dupilumab monotherapy: a 53% reduction in pruritus on a Numerical Rating Scale versus 8% reduction for placebo at 12 weeks [40].

The use of other immunosuppressants as therapeutic agents including tested thymopentin, montelukast, mepolizumab, and rIFN-γ, significantly reduced the pruritus of AD by 12% in patients compared to placebo [23]. Tumor necrosis factor alpha antagonists, immunoglobulin E (omalizumab) receptor antagonists, interleukin 5 (mepolizumab) and CD20 (rituximab) antagonists have not demonstrated efficacy in atopic dermatitis [13]. Ketotifen is a mast cell stabilizer that has not shown to efficacy in treating pruritus in atopic dermatitis [11].

13.10 Summary of Recommendations for Anti-Pruritus Therapeutic Ladder

Pruritus has a significant impact on the quality of life in patients with atopic dermatitis. It is important that practitioners assess and record pruritus through questionnaires such as the Eppendorf Itch Questionnaire at each routine visit. Patients should employ non-pharmaceutical treatments such as emollients with wet wraps, elimination of triggers, changing scratching habits, and psychological interventions. If these methods of treatment are not successful or if the disease presentation is severe, patients should be treated based on the therapeutic ladder for treatment of pruritus shown in Fig. 13.3. First-line topical pharmaceutical agents should be prescribed, namely topical glucocorticoids and topical calcineurin inhibitors. Second-line topical agents can be used including coal tar, menthol, capsaicin, or doxepin. After the use of topical agents has been exhausted, primary systemic agents can be applied, such as sedating antihistamines, non-sedating antihistamines, oral glucocorticoids,

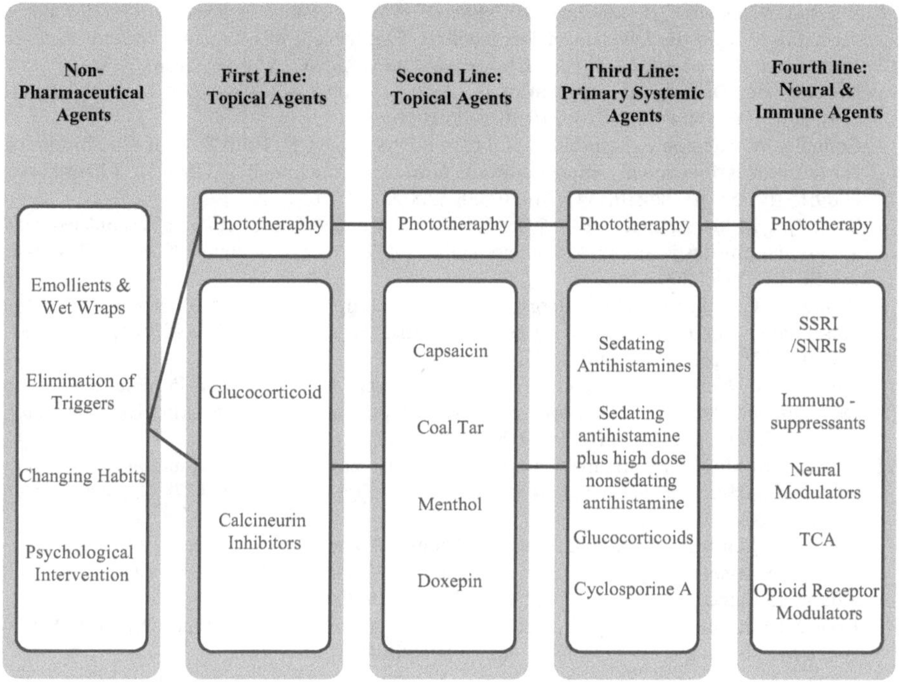

Fig. 13.3 Therapeutic ladder for treatment of pruritus in atopic dermatitis

or cyclosporine A. If primary systemic agents are found to be ineffective, neuromodulating or immunomodulating agents can be used, including SSRI/SNRIs, TCAs, immunosuppressants, neural modulators, and opioid receptor modulators. Phototherapy has been shown to provide a dramatic improvement of pruritus in atopic dermatitis and can be used at any stage of treatment including as a first-line agent. Other agents include topical naltrexone, topical PEA, topical lidocaine, systemic Kappa opioid agonists, and immunosuppressants.

References

1. Romeo S. Atopic dermatitis: the itch that rashes. Pediatr Nurs. 1995;21(2):157–63.
2. Ring J, Senter T, Cornell R, Arroyave C, TAN E. Complement and immunoglobulin deposits in the skin of patients with atopic dermatitis. Br J Dermatol. 1978;99(5):495–501. doi:10.1111/j.1365-2133.1978.tb02016.x.
3. Shelley W. The neurohistology and neurophysiology of the itch sensation in man. Arch Dermatol. 1957;76(3):296. doi:10.1001/archderm.1957.01550210020004.
4. Ständer S, Gunzer M, Metze D, Luger T, Steinhoff M. Localization of μ-opioid receptor 1A on sensory nerve fibers in human skin. Regul Pept. 2002;110(1):75–83. doi:10.1016/s0167-0115(02)00159-3.
5. Bastian B, van der Piepen U, Römisch J, Pâques E, Bröcker E. Localization of annexins in normal and diseased human skin. J Dermatol Sci. 1993;6(3):225–34. doi:10.1016/0923-1811(93)90043-o.

6. Johnson H, DeOreo G, Lascheid W, Mitchell F. Skin histamine levels in chronic atopic dermatitis**From the Division of Dermatology, Department of Medicine, Western Reserve University, School of Medicine, Cleveland, Ohio.(Aided by grant from Research and Development Division, Department of the Army, Contract #DA-49-007-MD-573). J Invest Dermatol. 1960;34(4):237–8. doi:10.1038/jid.1960.38.
7. Connelly W, Shenton F, Lethbridge N, Leurs R, Waldvogel H, Faull R, et al. The histamine H4 receptor is functionally expressed on neurons in the mammalian CNS. Br J Pharmacol. 2009;157(1):55–63. doi:10.1111/j.1476-5381.2009.00227.x.
8. Sonkoly E, Muller A, Lauerma A, Pivarcsi A, Soto H, Kemeny L, et al. IL-31: a new link between T cells and pruritus in atopic skin inflammation. J Allergy Clin Immunol. 2006;117(2):411–7. doi:10.1016/j.jaci.2005.10.033.
9. Wahlgren C, Hagermark O, Bergstrom R. The antipruritic effect of a sedative and a non-sedative antihistamine in atopic dermatitis. Br J Dermatol. 1990;122(4):545–51. doi:10.1111/j.1365-2133.1990.tb14732.x.
10. Steinhoff M, Neisius U, Ikoma A, Fartasch M, Heyer G, Skov P, et al. Proteinase-activated receptor-2 mediates itch: a novel pathway for pruritus in human skin. Exp Dermatol. 2008;13(9):591. doi:10.1111/j.0906-6705.2004.0212co.x.
11. Steinhoff M, Cevikbas F, Ikoma A, Berger T. Pruritus: management algorithms and experimental therapies. Seminars in Cutaneous Medicine and Surgery. 2011;30(2):127–37. doi:10.1016/j.sder.2011.05.001.
12. Darsow U, Scharein E, Simon D, Walter G, Bromm B, Ring J. New aspects of itch pathophysiology: component analysis of atopic itch using the 'Eppendorf Itch Questionnaire'. Int Arch Allergy Immunol. 2012;124(1–3):326–31. doi:10.1159/000053748.
13. Hong J, Buddenkotte J, Berger T, Steinhoff M. Management of itch in atopic dermatitis. Semin Cutan Med Surg. 2011;30(2):71–86. doi:10.1016/j.sder.2011.05.002.
14. Juenger M, Ladwig A, Staecker S, Arnold A, Kramer A, Daeschlein G, et al. Efficacy and safety of silver textile in the treatment of atopic dermatitis (AD). Curr Med Res Opin. 2006;22(4):739–50. doi:10.1185/030079906x99990.
15. Noren P, Melin L. The effect of combined topical steroids and habit-reversal treatment in patients with atopic dermatitis. Br J Dermatol. 1989;121(3):359–66. doi:10.1111/j.1365-2133.1989.tb01430.x.
16. Arnold W. Tar. Clin Dermatol. 1997;15(5):739–44. doi:10.1016/s0738-081x(97)00018-7.
17. Niordson A, Stahl D. Treatment of psoriasis with clinitar cream. A controlled clinical trial. Br J Clin Pract. 1985;39:67–8.
18. Roelofzen J, Aben K, Oldenhof U, Coenraads P, Alkemade H, van de Kerkhof P, et al. No increased risk of cancer after coal tar treatment in patients with psoriasis or eczema. J Investig Dermatol. 2010;130(4):953–61. doi:10.1038/jid.2009.389.
19. Yosipovitch G, Szolar C, Hui X, Maibach H. Effect of topically applied menthol on thermal, pain and itch sensations and biophysical properties of the skin. Arch Dermatol Res. 1996;288(5–6):245–8. doi:10.1007/s004030050053.
20. Dray A. Neuropharmacological mechanisms of capsaicin and related substances. Biochem Pharmacol. 1992;44(4):611–5. doi:10.1016/0006-2952(92)90393-w.
21. Zhang W, Li Wan Po A. The effectiveness of topically applied capsaicin. Eur J Clin Pharmacol. 1994;46(6):517–22. doi:10.1007/bf00196108.
22. Bonnel R, La Grenade L, Karwoski C, Beitz J. Allergic contact dermatitis from topical doxepin: food and drug administration's postmarketing surveillance experience. J Am Acad Dermatol. 2003;48(2):294–6. doi:10.1067/mjd.2003.46.
23. Sher L, Chang J, Patel I, Balkrishnan R, Fleischer A. PSS1 relieving the pruritus of atopic dermatitis: a meta-analysis. Value Health. 2012;15(4):A249–50. doi:10.1016/j.jval.2012.03.1345.
24. Berberian B, Breneman D, Drake L, Gratton D, Raimir S, Phillips S, et al. The addition of topical doxepin to corticosteroid therapy: an improved treatment regimen for atopic dermatitis. Int J Dermatol. 1999;38(2):145–7. doi:10.1046/j.1365-4362.1999.00505.x.

25. Drake L, Fallon J, Sober A. Relief of pruritus in patients with atopic dermatitis after treatment with topical doxepin cream. J Am Acad Dermatol. 1994;31(4):613–6. doi:10.1016/s0190-9622(94)70225-x.
26. Eberlein B, Eicke C, Reinhardt H, Ring J. Adjuvant treatment of atopic eczema: assessment of an emollient containing N-palmitoylethanolamine (ATOPA study). J Eur Acad Dermatol Venereol. 2007;22(1):73–82. doi:10.1111/j.1468-3083.2007.02351.x.
27. Inan S, Dun N, Cowan A. Inhibitory effect of lidocaine on pain and itch using formalin-induced nociception and 5′-guanidinonaltrindole-induced scratching models in mice: behavioral and neuroanatomical evidence. Eur J Pharmacol. 2009;616(1–3):141–6. doi:10.1016/j.ejphar.2009.06.026.
28. Krutmann J, Diepgen T, Luger T, Grabbe S, Meffert H, Sönnichsen N, et al. High-dose UVA1 therapy for atopic dermatitis: results of a multicenter trial. J Am Acad Dermatol. 1998;38(4):589–93. doi:10.1016/s0190-9622(98)70123-9.
29. Der-Petrossian M, Seeber A, Hönigsmann H, Tanew A. Half-side comparison study on the efficacy of 8-methoxypsoralen bath-PUVA versus narrow-band ultraviolet B phototherapy in patients with severe chronic atopic dermatitis. Br J Dermatol. 2000;142(1):39–43. doi:10.1046/j.1365-2133.2000.03239.x.
30. Nisticò S, Saraceno R, Capriotti E, Felice C, Chimenti S. Efficacy of monochromatic excimer light (308 nm) in the treatment of atopic dermatitis in adults and children. Photomed Laser Surg. 2008;26(1):14–8. doi:10.1089/pho.2007.2116.
31. Lewis T. The blood vessels of the human skin and their responses. Arch Dermatol. 1928;18(6):991. doi:10.1001/archderm.1928.02380180188023.
32. Klein P, Clark R. An evidence-based review of the efficacy of antihistamines in relieving pruritus in atopic dermatitis. Arch Dermatol. 1999;135(12):1522–5. doi:10.1001/archderm.135.12.1522.
33. Eichenfield L, Hanifin J, Luger T, Stevens S, Pride H. Consensus conference on pediatric atopic dermatitis. J Am Acad Dermatol. 2003;49(6):1088–95. doi:10.1016/s0190-9622(03)02539-8.
34. Heddle R, Soothill J, Bulpitt C, Atherton D. Combined oral and nasal beclomethasone dipropionate in children with atopic eczema: a randomised controlled trial. BMJ. 1984;289(6446):651–4. doi:10.1136/bmj.289.6446.651.
35. La Rosa M, Musarra I, Ranno C, Maiello N, Negri L, del Giudice M, et al. A randomized, double-blind, placebo-controlled, crossover trial of systemic flunisolide in the treatment of children with severe atopic dermatitis. Curr Ther Res. 1995;56(7):720–6. doi:10.1016/0011-393x(95)85143-7.
36. Hundley J, Yosipovitch G. Mirtazapine for reducing nocturnal itch in patients with chronic pruritus: a pilot study. J Am Acad Dermatol. 2004;50(6):889–91. doi:10.1016/j.jaad.2004.01.045.
37. Ständer S, Böckenholt B, Schürmeyer-Horst F, Weishaupt C, Heuft G, Schneider T. Treatment of chronic pruritus with the selective serotonin re-uptake inhibitors paroxetine and fluvoxamine: results of an open-labelled, two-arm proof-of-concept study. Acta Derm Venereol. 2009;89(1):45–51. doi:10.2340/00015555-0553.
38. Ständer S, Schmelz M. Chronic itch and pain-similarities and differences. Eur J Pain. 2006;10(5):473–8. doi:10.1016/j.ejpain.2006.03.005.
39. Phan N, Bernhard J, Luger T, Ständer S. Antipruritic treatment with systemic μ-opioid receptor antagonists: a review. J Am Acad Dermatol. 2010;63(4):680–8. doi:10.1016/j.jaad.2009.08.052.
40. Blakely K, Gooderham M, Papp K. Dupilumab, a monoclonal antibody for atopic dermatitis: a review of current literature. Skin Therapy. 2016;21(2):1–5.
41. Brenninkmeijer E, Spuls P, Lindeboom R, Van Der Wal A, Bos J, Wolkerstorfer A. Excimer laser vs. clobetasol propionate 0·05% ointment in prurigo form of atopic dermatitis: a randomized controlled trial, a pilot. Br J Dermatol. 2010;163(4):823–31. doi:10.1111/j.1365-2133.2010.09858.x.
42 Goeckerman W. The treatment of psoriasis. Northwest Med. 1925;24:229–31, 211.

Chapter 14
Atopic Dermatitis Disease Education

Wayne Sy and Angela J. Lamb

Abstract Atopic dermatitis is a skin condition that is increasing burdensome to patient's lives. Patients require effective strategies to cope with the condition as well as the vast amount of new research that is coming to the forefront. This chapter discusses the patient education aspect of atopic dermatitis. We drew from various sources—such as peer-reviewed academic journals, online groups, and organizational websites—to provide a brief survey of the available types of patient educational resources. We discuss educational materials and interventions, such as workshops and support groups. In addition to the content of the workshops, we also explore the importance of their facilitators. We also review organizations in the US that pertain to atopic dermatitis and eczema care, such as the National Eczema Association and the American Academy of Dermatology. Lastly, we survey the role of technology—such as social media, web-based applications and teledermatology—in facilitating patient education. Despite the promising impacts of these technological interventions in the way patients consume educational materials, we also acknowledge that they are not widely used.

Keywords Atopic dermatitis • Dermatology • Eczema • Patient education • Social media • Teledermatology

14.1 Introduction

Patient education is a critical aspect of health care delivery. This is particularly true in the long-term management of chronic diseases such as atopic dermatitis. Much of the treatment regimen can be highly demanding, resulting in low compliance to therapy [1]. Patient education can take on many forms, varying from a simple

W. Sy, M.S., M.P.H. • A.J. Lamb, M.D. (✉)
Department of Dermatology, The Mount Sinai Hospital, New York, NY, USA
e-mail: angela_lamb@hotmail.com

E.A. Fortson et al. (eds.), *Management of Atopic Dermatitis*, Advances in Experimental Medicine and Biology 1027, DOI 10.1007/978-3-319-64804-0_14

informational pamphlet that a primary care physician gives to their patient to classes on weight management. The type or format of patient education may also determine the extent to which it is effective. This chapter seeks to discuss different types of educational materials and interventions for the management of atopic dermatitis by patients and their families.

14.2 Educational Materials and Interventions

Educational workshops seek to give comprehensive information on the disease itself, including symptoms, treatments, and disease management. Moore et al.'s [2] "eczema workshop" trial showed that a 90-min, nurse-led eczema workshop was more effective in reducing pediatric atopic dermatitis severity when compared to the standard, shorter, dermatologist-led clinic. They suggest the intervention was effective because there was more time for the nurses to educate the patients and their caregivers, and perform demonstrations on how to use available treatment [2]. A later study by Ersser et al. [3] added that pediatric eczema patients in similar, nurse-led eczema workshops had an improved quality of life in addition to decreased disease severity. Across the different workshop interventions, there were common themes in content: understanding the disease, understanding symptoms, eczema triggers, and information about coping with the disease [1, 3].

In conducting educational programs, it is important to consider the role of the facilitators or teachers that are leading the workshop. According to Lebovidge et al. [4], effective management of atopic dermatitis should utilize a multidisciplinary team to address the interactions of biological, psychological, behavioral and dietary factors in the disease course. These multidisciplinary providers include AD specialists, nurses, psychologists, and dietitians. The specialist—which is often an allergist or dermatologist—is in charge of the diagnosis, developing a comprehensive treatment plan, and integrating information from the rest of the multidisciplinary team. Psychologists address the psychological and behavioral aspects of atopic dermatitis, such as picking behaviors and stress management. Dietitians are important for teaching patients and caregivers about adequate nutrition and managing food allergies that may trigger symptoms [4]. A trial on atopic dermatitis education utilized a senior medical student as the main educator, which showed non-significant differences in disease severity and quality of life in a pediatric population [5]. Shaw, Morrell & Goldsmith [5] discussed multiple possible reasons for why the intervention failed such as a high dropout rate (30%), inconsistent caregivers for follow-up visits, and the possibility that the trained medical student was not as knowledgeable or thorough as a trained nurse.

The delivery of the patient education materials distributed within these educational interventions is an additional important consideration. Armstrong et al. [6] found that in adults with atopic dermatitis, improvement in knowledge about the disease was significantly higher in those who used a video-based education module when compared to those who used a written pamphlet. The inherent benefit in learning through audio-visual presentation combined with ease of distribution and accessibility were cited as reasons for this increased effectiveness [6].

14.2.1 Support Groups

Support groups are seen as particularly beneficial given that atopic dermatitis has significant psychosocial impacts in patients' lives [7]. A study by Weber et al. [8] found that children placed in a support group intervention—led by a child psychiatrist and volunteer medical students every 2 weeks for 6 months—had improvements in their pruritus symptoms, mood, and quality of life. In addition to group therapy techniques, the support group included educational segments as well [8]. This suggests that social support received from group settings may be helpful in patient comprehension of techniques to manage atopic dermatitis.

In group settings, a study by Staab et al. [9] showed that separate, age-related group education workshops for children and adolescents with atopic dermatitis yielded improvements in disease severity and quality of life. Education workshops and support groups that focus on a specific age group allow the materials to be tailored to the needs of that particular group of patients. A comparison between the effectiveness of separate, age-related group education and non-separate group education has not been studied.

14.3 Organizational Resources in the US

The two main organizations that pertain to atopic dermatitis in the United States are the National Eczema Association (NEA) and the American Academy of Dermatology (AAD).

Established in 1988, the NEA is a non-profit national organization that supports the health and quality of life for individuals with eczema through research, support, and education [11]. They are funded through individual donations, fee for service programs, and corporate contributions. The organization creates, distributes, and presents educational materials online and in medical conferences for both patients and physicians. On their website (https://nationaleczema.org), users can access free information on atopic dermatitis symptoms, treatments, triggers, and other related information. The NEA provides information on support groups for patients with eczema and their families. Although there is no research specific to this organization's impact on patients, anecdotally, it is a frequently referenced on-line resource and given to patients as a source of information.

Founded in 1938, the AAD is the largest dermatologist collective in the United States [10]. Although the content of their website largely caters to dermatologists and other medical professionals, there are patient education materials for those with atopic dermatitis (https://www.aad.org). Aside from basic information about atopic dermatitis, the website houses a video library that is accessible to patients.

14.4 Role of Technology

Technology is an efficient way to disseminate information to patients in a variety of ways. This section discusses the roles of two aspects of technology in patient education for the management of atopic dermatitis: social media and smartphones.

Social media websites allow patients to form online support communities, rapidly exchange information, and engage in meaningful discussion with fellow users among their networks. These websites can have different purposes, ranging from casual (e.g. Facebook, Twitter) to professional (LinkedIn); however, their contents vary because they are user-driven. In addition to patient users, scientific journals and professional organizations also use social media websites to communicate and provide forums for health-related discussion. Although dermatology journals and organizations have some social media presence, they lag behind their general medicine counterparts [12]. These information sources could reach a wider audience by utilizing popular social media platforms, such as Facebook, Instagram, and Pinterest [13–16]. Conversely, it is possible for certain users to influence the dissemination of false information by dominating the comments section of posts made by professional organizations, such as the National Eczema Association's Facebook page [16].

The availability of unregulated information and discussion from social media websites can have profound effects on eczema patients—particularly concerning the use of topical corticosteroids. Teasdale, Muller and Santer [17] argue that despite a professional consensus on the safety of correctly-used topical-corticosteroids for eczema, there is still "steroid phobia" that persists in the community of eczema patients and their caregivers. This uncertainty and fear among eczema patients and their caregivers are further amplified by input from online forum users that are perceived to have experiential expertise on topical corticosteroid use [17]. There may be a diverse set of beliefs propagated in these forums—both positive or negative—about the usage and effects of topical corticosteroids for the treatment of eczema but these beliefs may contain unverifiable information, which could potentially be dangerous.

Web-based interventions are convenient for patients and caregivers because they can be accessed at home. According to a pilot study by Santer et al. [18], a web-based intervention that had educational modules, including printable materials and instructional videos, was well-received by users as evidenced by preliminary qualitative interviews. The participants were families of children with eczema. Some themes that were derived from the interviews included increased confidence in eczema management, increased awareness of different treatments, and satisfaction with available instructional videos [18]. Although there are not many web-based interventions for eczema, patient response seems to be consistent with the experience of in-person, educational workshops.

14.4.1 Teledermatology and Mobile Health

Teledermatology—defined as the use of telecommunications technology to exchange clinical information between provider and patient—has been used in patient education settings [19]. These include smartphone apps, such as Eczema Doc or Eczema Care, which provide access to advice and information on symptoms and treatments for eczema via a mobile device. These appear promising though it is difficult to comment on the effectiveness of these apps due to the lack of empirical studies.

Conceptually introduced in the 1990s, teledermatology is a relatively new field. Advances in imaging quality and increased dermatologists confidence in using the systems has improved platform quality [20]. Landow et al. [21] argue that in recent years, the value of teledermatology lies in providing "better, cheaper, and faster" dermatologic care, however, this is only true when face-to-face appointments after teleconsultations are minimized. A review by Bashshur et al. [20] found that there is a high correlation between diagnoses and treatment plans in teledermatology appointments and face-to-face care from dermatologists. The content and style of physician communication in teledermatology settings compared to in-person visits were found to be similar, including in small talk, clinical assessment, psychosocial issues, patient compliance, patient treatment, and administrative issues [22]. These findings suggest teledermatology is as effective as in-person appointments. However, this data is not specific for atopic dermatitis care and that more research is needed to discern effectiveness in this specific patient population.

References

1. Bostoen J, Bracke S, De Keyser S, Lambert J. An educational programme for patients with psoriasis and atopic dermatitis: a prospective randomized controlled trial. Br J Dermatol. 2012;167(5):1025–31. doi:10.1111/j.1365-2133.2012.11113.x.
2. Moore EJ, Williams A, Manias E, Varigos G, Donath S. Eczema workshops reduce severity of childhood atopic eczema. Australas J Dermatol. 2009;50(2):100–6. doi:10.1111/j.1440-0960.2009.00515.x.
3. Ersser SJ, Farasat H, Jackson K, Dennis H, Sheppard ZA, More A. A service evaluation of the Eczema Education Programme: an analysis of child, parent and service impact outcomes. Br J Dermatol. 2013;169(3):629–636
4. LeBovidge JS, Elverson W, Timmons KG, Hawryluk EB, Rea C, Lee M, Schneider LC. Multidisciplinary interventions in the management of atopic dermatitis. J Allergy Clin Immunol. 2016;138(2):325–34. doi:10.1016/j.jaci.2016.04.003.
5. Shaw M, Morrell DS, Goldsmith LA. A study of targeted enhanced patient care for pediatric atopic dermatitis (STEP PAD). Pediatr Dermatol. 2008;25(1):19–24. doi:10.1111/j.1525-1470.2007.00575.x.
6. Armstrong AW, Kim RH, Idriss NZ, Larsen LN, Lio PA. Online video improves clinical outcomes in adults with atopic dermatitis: a randomized controlled trial. J Am Acad Dermatol. 2011;64(3):502–7. doi:10.1016/j.jaad.2010.01.051.
7. Tuckman A. The potential psychological impact of skin conditions. Dermatol Ther. 2017;7(Suppl 1):53–7. doi:10.1007/s13555-016-0169-7.

8. Weber MB, Neto F, Pde T, Prati C, Soirefman M, Mazzotti NG, Barzenski B, Cestari TF. Improvement of pruritus and quality of life of children with atopic dermatitis and their families after joining support groups. J Eur Acad Dermatol Venereol. 2008;22(8):992–7. doi:10.1111/j.1468-3083.2008.02697.x.
9. Staab D, Diepgen TL, Fartasch M, Kupfer J, Lob-Corzilius T, Ring J, Gieler U. Age-related, structured educational programmes for the management of atopic dermatitis in children and adolescents: multicentre, randomised controlled trial. BMJ. 2006;332(7547):933–8. doi:10.1136/bmj.332.7547.933.
10. American Academy of Dermatology. (n.d.). About the AAD | American Academy of Dermatology. https://www.aad.org/about. Accessed 14 Jan 2017
11. National Eczema Association. (2013, August 28). About NEA. https://nationaleczema.org/about-nea/. Accessed 14 January 2017
12. Amir M, Sampson BP, Endly D, Tamai JM, Henley J, Brewer AC, Dunn JH, Dunnick CA, Dellavalle RP. Social networking sites: emerging and essential tools for communication in dermatology. JAMA Dermatol. 2014;150(1):56–60. doi:10.1001/jamadermatol.2013.6340.
13. Fogel AL, Teng JMC. Social media use in pediatric dermatology. Pediatric Dermatol. 2016;33(2):e131–3. doi:10.1111/pde.12763.
14. Whitsitt, Jacob; Mattis, Daiva; Hernandez, Melia; Kollipara, Ramya; & Dellavalle, Robert P. (2015). Dermatology on Pinterest. Dermatology Online Journal, 21(1). doj_25442. Retrieved from: http://escholarship.org/uc/item/7dj4267p
15. Karimkhani, Chante; Connett, Jessica; Boyers, Lindsay; Quest, Tyler; & Dellavalle, Robert P. (2014). Dermatology on Instagram. Dermatology Online Journal, 20(7). doj_23129. Retrieved from: http://escholarship.org/uc/item/71g178w9
16. Savas, J. A., Huang, K. E., Tuchayi, S. M., & Feldman, S. R. (2014). Understanding the influence of social media in medicine: lesson learned from facebook. Dermatol Online J, 20(9). http://escholarship.org/uc/item/2099j0z1.
17. Teasdale E, Muller I, Santer M. Carers' views of topical-corticosteroid use in childhood eczema: a qualitative study of online discussion forums. Br J Dermatol. 2017;176(6):1500–7. doi:10.1111/bjd.15130.
18. Santer M, Muller I, Yardley L, Burgess H, Selinger H, Stuart BL, Little P. Supporting self-care for families of children with eczema with a web-based intervention plus health care professional support: pilot randomized controlled trial. J Med Internet Res. 2014;16(3):e70. doi:10.2196/jmir.3035.
19. Coates SJ, Kvedar J, Granstein RD. Teledermatology: from historical perspective to emerging techniques of the modern era: part I: history, rationale, and current practice. J Am Acad Dermatol. 2015;72(4):563–74. doi:10.1016/j.jaad.2014.07.061.
20. Bashshur RL, Shannon GW, Tejasvi T, Kvedar JC, Gates M. The empirical foundations of teledermatology: a review of the research evidence. Telemed J E Health. 2015;21(12):953–79. doi:10.1089/tmj.2015.0146.
21. Landow SM, Mateus A, Korgavkar K, Nightingale D, Weinstock MA. Teledermatology: key factors associated with reducing face-to-face dermatology visits. J Am Acad Dermatol. 2014;71(3):570–6. doi:10.1016/j.jaad.2014.02.021.
22. Edison KE, Fleming DA, Nieman EL, Stine K, Chance L, Demiris G. Content and style comparison of physician communication in teledermatology and in-person visits. Telemed J E Health. 2013;19(7):509–14. doi:10.1089/tmj.2012.0227.

Chapter 15
The Future of Atopic Dermatitis Treatment

Nupur Patel and Lindsay C. Strowd

Abstract In recent years, there has been a growing movement towards the use of targeted therapies in treating of atopic dermatitis (AD), parallel to that which has occurred in psoriasis. Among the systemic medications being studied are subcutaneous or intravenously administered biologic drugs targeting specific molecules such as IL4, IL13, IL17, and IgE. Non-biologic oral therapies are also being developed for AD and include small molecule drugs targeting phosphodiesterase type IV (PDE4) inhibition or Janus Kinase (JAK) inhibition. Numerous topical formulations are also being studied, with some formulations that are novel therapies that act as topical biologic or small molecule agents with mechanisms of action similar to systemic treatments. Others are being developed as skin barrier repair therapies for reduction of AD symptoms. This chapter will discuss new advances in AD treatment from medications in the initial stages of development to those nearing FDA approval.

Keywords Atopic dermatitis • Future therapeutics • Advances in treatment • Targeted therapies • Systemic treatment • Topical treatment

15.1 Introduction

Current management of AD includes moisturizers, antibiotics, anti-pruritics, and anti-inflammatory therapies. Although this combination of therapies aims to combat the variety of pathologic processes that define AD, there remain gaps in the understanding of the pathogenesis. In recent years, there has been a growing movement towards the use of targeted therapies in treating of AD, parallel to that which has occurred in psoriasis. This chapter will discuss new advances in AD treatment from medications in the initial stages of development to those nearing FDA approval.

N. Patel, M.S. (✉) • L.C. Strowd, M.D.
Department of Dermatology, Wake Forest University School of Medicine, Winston Salem, NC, USA
e-mail: nupur.uma.patel@gmail.com

E.A. Fortson et al. (eds.), *Management of Atopic Dermatitis*, Advances in Experimental Medicine and Biology 1027, DOI 10.1007/978-3-319-64804-0_15

15.2 Systemic Medications

There is a growing trend in dermatology towards using target-specific therapy. Similar to the development of biologics in psoriasis, researchers are examining the use of similar biologics in AD and developing new therapies with specific immune targets relevant to AD (Table 15.1).

15.2.1 Subcutaneous and Intravenous Medications by Target

Of the novel systemic therapies being studied, the furthest developed is Dupilumab, a fully human monoclonal antibody directed against the interlukin-4 receptor alpha subunit (IL-4Ra). IL-4 is the cytokine responsible for stimulating T helper type 2 cell (Th2) cell differentiation, and the secondary production of IL-4 and IL-13 which are promoters of IgE production by B lymphocytes [1–3]. The predominance of the Th2 cellular response in the pathogenesis of AD has been well documented [3]. A significant increase in gene expression of IL-4, IL-13, and IL-31 has been demonstrated in the biopsies of acute lesions of AD patients [4].

Two randomized placebo-controlled phase 3 trials of identical design (SOLO1 and SOLO2 trials) have been completed with promising results. Of the 671 patients in the SOLO1 trial and 708 patients in the SOLO2 trial, 36–38% of patients receiving the achieved the primary outcome of having clear or almost clear skin on the Investigator's Global Assessment (IGA) and a reduction of 2 or more points in their score from baseline at 16 weeks [5]. Patients receiving drug were significantly more likely to achieve study end-point compared to 8% of participants who received placebo ($P < 0.001$ for all comparisons). Significantly more patients receiving dupilumab achieved a 75% improvement on the Eczema Area and Severity Index (EASI) and had reduction of symptoms of anxiety and depression, pruritus, and an improvement in quality of life [5].

Another study examining adults with moderate-to-severe atopic dermatitis found that 100% of patients treated with duplilumab and topical glucocorticoids met the criteria for a 50% reduction in EASI score (EASI-50) compared to only 50% of those who received topical glucocorticoids with placebo injections ($P = 0.002$) [6]. The most frequent adverse events reported were nasopharyngitis and headache, occurring equally in treatment and placebo groups [6]. The most common serious adverse events were skin infections and flare of AD, both of which were more common in the placebo group [6].

Three additional clinical trials examining dupilumab are ongoing. The first trial is an open label study examining the efficacy and safety of dupilumab as a monotherapy in patients who previously participated in dupilumab studies (NCT01949311). The other two studies examine the long-term safety and efficacy of dupilumab alone or a combination therapy of dupilumab and topical corticosteroids (NCT02277743,

Table 15.1 Emerging systemic treatments for atopic dermatitis[a]

Drug candidate	Phase	Mechanism	Route	Clinicaltrials.gov identifier
Biologics				
Dupilumab	3	IL-4R antibody	SC	NCT01949311
				NCT02277743
				NCT02260986
	2		SC	NCT02407756
Tralokinumab	2	IL-13 antibody	SC	NCT02347176
Lebrikizumab	2	IL-13 antibody	SC	NCT02340234
BMS-981164	1	IL-31 antibody	SC	NCT01614756
CIM331 (Nemolizumab)	2	IL-31RA	SC	NCT01986933
ILV-094	2	IgGIA antibody	SC	NCT01941537
Secukinumab	2	IL-17 antibody	SC	NCT02594098
Ustekinumab	2	anti-IL12/23	SC	NCT01806662
CNTO 7160	1	IL-33R antibody	SC	NCT02345928
XmAb7195	1	IgE Antibody	IV	NCT02148744
	1			NCT02881853
Omalizumab	2	IgE Antibody	SC	NCT02300701
Ligelizumab (QGE031)	2	IgE Antibody	SC	NCT01552629
MEDI4212	1	IgE Antibody	SC/IV	NCT01544348
AMG 157 (MEDI9929)	2	TSLP Antibody	SC	NCT02525094
Mesenchymal Stem Cells				
FURESTEM-AD	1/2	Mesenchymal stem cells	SC	NCT01927705
	1		SC	NCT02888704
Small Molecules				
Apremilast	2	PDE4 Inhibitor	Oral	NCT0139315
	2			NCT00931242
	2			NCT02087943
Baricitinib (LY3009104)	2	JAK 1/2 inhibitor	Oral	NCT02576938
Tofacitinib		JAK 1/3 inhibitor	Oral	Levy 2015
PF-0496582	2	JAK 1 inhibitor	Oral	NCT02780167
ABT-494	2	JAK 1 inhibitor	Oral	NCT02925117
AQX-1125	2	SHIP-1 activator	Oral	NCT02324972
Fevipiprant (QAW039)	2	CRTH2-R antagonist	Oral	NCT01785602
OC459 (OC000459)	2	CRTH2-R antagonist	Oral	NCT02002208
BBI-5000	1	CRTH2-R antagonist	Oral	NCT02590289
KHK4577	2	Unknown	Oral	NCT02004119

[a]*IL* Interleukin, *IL-17A* subtype A of IL-17, *IL-31RA* IL-31 receptor A, *IL-4Rα* IL-4 receptor alpha subunit, *IV* intravenous, *SC* subcutaneous, *JAK* Janus kinase, *PDE* phosphodiesterase, *SHIP* SH2-containing inositol-5′-phosphatase, *sPLA2* secretory phospholipase A2, *TSLP* thymic stromal lymphopoietin, *5-HT2BR* 5-hydroxytryptamine (2B) receptor, *CRTH2* chemoattractant receptor-homologous molecule expressed on Th2 cell, *Ig* immunoglobulin

NCT02260986) [3]. Recently dupilumab has received the United States Food and Drug Administration (US FDA) breakthrough therapy designation for AD, and is expected to be available in the United States for treatment of severe atopic dermatitis in the next 12 months [7].

The IL-13 specific monoclonal antibodies Tralokinumab and Lebrikizumab were originally developed for the treatment of asthma and other inflammatory conditions, as IL-13 is a potent promoter of type 1 IgE-mediated inflammation. Both drugs recently completed phase 2 trials for evaluation in AD patients. For Tralokinumab, results show a significant improvement from baseline in EASI score in the two highest dosage groups when compared with placebo. Significant improvements in the Dermatology Life Quality Index (DLQI) were also seen (NCT02347176) [8].

TREBLE was a Phase 2 double-blind, dose-ranging study involved 209 adults with moderate-to-severe AD who had failed topical corticosteroids. All patients continued topical corticosteroid treatment and were randomized to either a single 125 mg subcutaneous dose of lebrikizumab at week 0, a single 250 mg, 125 mg every 4 weeks, or placebo injections (NCT02340234) [9]. A dose-response effect was demonstrated, as the primary endpoint of EASI50 rate was 69.2% with a single 125-mg dose of lebrikizumab, 69.8% with a single 250-mg dose, and 82.4% with 125 mg of lebrikizumab at weeks 0, 4, 8, and 12, compared with 62.3% in the placebo group. Only the group with monthly dosing had an EASI 50 response rate significantly better than the placebo group. The EASI75 rate was significantly greater in the monthly dosing group than placebo group. The EASI 50 and 75 response rates in the monthly dosing group continued to increase when the trial ended at 12 weeks. With regards to safety, the total number of adverse and serious adverse events were similar across all treatment arms. Herpes infection occurred in 2–6% of lebrikizumab subjects but none of the control group subjects [9]. The results of both studies suggest that further study of anti- IL-13 therapies in AD are warranted, and they have the potential to provide a valuable treatment option in the future.

IL-31 has been shown to cause continuous itch-associated scratching behavior in mice, and its overexpression causes severe pruritus, alopecia, and skin lesions in transgenic mice [10, 11]. IL31 has shown to induce late-onset itch in human AD patients and is thought to be involved in promoting the pathophysiology of AD and pruritus via the “scratch-itch cycle.” [12, 13].

BMS-981164 is an anti-IL31 monoclonal antibody against the IL-31 receptor that can be administered subcutaneously or intravenously (IV). A placebo-controlled dose-escalation phase 1 trial of BMS-981164 sponsored by Bristol-Myers Squibb was completed in April 2015 with unpublished results (NCT01614756).

Another drug targeting IL31 is CIM331, also known as nemolizumab, a humanized monoclonal antibody that competitively blocks binding to the IL31 alpha-receptor (IL-31RA). It is administered as an injectable medication and is being evaluated primarily for improvement of pruritus. Results of a randomized, double-blind, placebo-controlled phase 2 trial showed that CIM331 rapidly and consistently improved AD, pruritus, and sleep disturbance in patients with previously uncontrolled moderate-to-severe AD (NCT01986933) [14, 15]. Using a pruritus visual analog scale (VAS) patients treated with nemolizumab reported dose-dependent reductions in pruritus compared to placebo ($P < 0.01$ for all comparisons). Significant reductions in pruritus began as early as week 1 in the group treated with 2 mg/kg of nemolizumab. Patients treated with the 0.5 mg/kg dosing showed the most improvement in EASI scores from baseline to week 12. The average sleep onset latency in the study groups was improved by 15–20 min at 4 weeks. The total sleep time increased significantly across all nemolizumab groups. The drug was generally well tolerated with the most common adverse events being exacerbation of AD and nasopharyngitis, with no significant difference between the treatment and placebo groups [15].

ILV-094 is a novel antibody which targets the cytokine IL-22. AD is associated with activation of Th2 pathway and the more recently discovered T-helper 22 cell (Th22) subset. The Th22 cell subset has been shown to be responsible for majority of the IL-22 production in AD skin lesions [16]. The primary component of the immune infiltrates of chronic AD lesions are Th22 and Th2 T-cells, although some Th1 and Th17 cells are also present [16, 17]. The production of IL-22 has been hypothesized to play a key pathogenic role in AD by promoting epidermal hyperplasia, contributing to epidermal barrier dysfunction, and inhibiting epidermal differentiation [4, 16, 18, 19].

ILV-094 is a human IgGIA antibody that binds with high specificity to IL-22 and is a potent neutralizer of IL22 activity [20]. After initial studies found ILV-094 has favorable pharmacokinetics and toxicity profiles, ILV-094 is now being studied as an intravenous drug in a phase 2 trial (NCT01941537). Because IL-22 is a potential key cytokine in AD, its inhibition may provide advantages over other available treatments through potentially increased safety and specific targeting compared with other immunosuppressants [20].

While IL-17 production by Th17 cells is thought to play a more dominant role in the pathogenesis of psoriasis, it has also present in smaller amounts in the skin lesions of AD [16, 17, 21]. In psoriasis, neutralization of IL-17 through IL-17a antibodies have led to disease reversal in 80% or more of treated subjects [22]. The success of targeting known cytokine signaling pathways (such as IL-17, IL-23, or p40) with these medications advocates for an upstream effect of reduced gene expression and suggests a feed forward inflammatory loop that amplifies drug effects [17, 21]. Because of the anti-inflammatory success that these biologic medications have had in multiple clinical trials of psoriasis patients, some are currently being studied as a means of treatment for AD [22–24].

A phase 2 clinical trial of secukinumab, an IL-17 antibody, is currently recruiting patients with moderate-to-severe AD (NCT02594098). The study aims to study the effect of a 300 mg injection of secukinumab on lesional skin epidermal thickness, and changes in SCORAD, EASI, and static IGA scores as secondary outcomes.

Ustekinumab is an anti-IL12/23 biologic medication that has had success in treating psoriasis patients. Ustekinumab acts by binding to the p-40 subunit of both IL-12 and IL-23 to prevent binding to their receptors, thus suppressing Th1, Th17/Th22 activation [25]. This medication may be effective in AD as mRNA expressions of IL-12 and IL-23 are up-regulated and even higher in AD than in psoriatic skin [17, 26]. While several case reports have demonstrated successful treatment of AD with ustekinumab, others have demonstrated partial or no response. Similarly to secukinumab, there is only one clinical trial evaluating ustekinumab in AD patients. The recently published results of this randomized placebo-controlled double-blinded single-center, cross-over study revealed higher SCORAD50 responses in the treatment group compared with the placebo group, but the difference was not significant (NCT01806662) [27]. Distinct modulation of Th1, Th17 and Th22 but also Th2-related AD genes (i.e. MMP12, IL-22, IL-13, IFN-γ, elafin/PI3, CXCL1 and CCL17) was seen after 4 weeks of ustekinumab treatment [27]. These results indicate IL12 and 23 contribute to the inflammatory pathways of AD, however they highlight the need for future studies to further examine the pharmacokinetics of ustekinumab in patients with AD [27].

There are two injectable medications in phase 1 development for the treatment of AD as well as asthma. The first is the biological therapy CNTO 7160, an IL-33 receptor (IL-33R) monoclonal antibody that prevents IL-33 from binding to its receptor. IL-33 is part of the IL-1 cytokine family and is also a promoter of Th2 inflammation [28]. Recent data suggest that IL-33 is involved in the pathogenesis of various allergic diseases, including asthma, allergic rhinitis and AD [28, 29]. Serum levels of IL-33 were significantly higher in AD patients compared to patients with urticaria, psoriasis, and healthy control patients, and correlated to AD disease severity [28]. Currently there is an ongoing phase 1 study evaluating intravenous CNTO 7160 in subjects with asthma and atopic dermatitis (NCT02345928).

XmAb7195 is a monoclonal antibody that targets IgE and acts an immune inhibitor to target FcγRIIB, a receptor that inhibits B cell function [30]. IgE is a known mediator of allergic symptoms and has been shown to be increased in the circulation of AD patients. Per Xencor, XmAB7195 has been shown to rapidly reduce free and total IgE as well as block production of IgE by immune cells in animal models. There is a phase 1 study (NCT02148744) of this drug in patients with elevated IgE levels (phase1a) and with atopic dermatitis, and/or allergic rhinitis, and/or allergic conjunctivitis (phase 1b). The phase 1a results show 90% of patients have a reduction of free IgE levels below the detectable limit of the assay (<10 ng/mL) at the end of the XmAb7195 intravenous infusion with reduction lasting for at least 1 week following a single infusion [30]. Total IgE was reduced to below the limit of detection (<2.0 IU/mL) in 26 of 30 (87%) subjects with detectable total IgE pre-dose. Another phase 1 trial is currently recruiting patients for evaluation of the safety, tolerability and bioavailabilty of the drug via subcutaneous administration in patients with atopic disease (NCT02881853). While more clinical studies are needed to further assess XmAb7195, these preliminary phase 1 results indicate that the drug may have promising potential as a future therapy for the treatment of AD.

Omalizumab is a humanized anti-IgE monoclonal antibody that downregulates the expression of FcεRI on basophils, eosinophils, mast, cells, and dendritic cells by binding to free IgE and decreasing its levels [7]. The drug has not shown efficacy for AD in clinical studies, however has had conflicting results based on several case reports. There is one phase 2 study currently enrolling patients to evaluate the efficacy and safety of omalizumab in children ages 4–19 years old with severe AD

(NCT02300701). Omalizumab has been associated with rare but serious adverse events such as cardiovascular events, cerebrovascular events, and anaphylaxis, along with a potential risk of cancer. These adverse effects along with the drug's unclear efficacy may limit its future as a treatment for AD.

Ligelizumab (QGE031) is an anti-IgE monoclonal antibody that has demonstrated a higher affinity for IgE when compared with omalizumab, and demonstrates greater reductions in free IgE in atopic patients along with greater attenuation of skin prick test response to allergens [7, 31]. A phase 2 trial evaluating the drug compared with placebo and cyclosporine in adult patients with moderate to severe AD has completed enrollment (NCT01552629).

Medi4212 is another anti-IgE monocloncal antibody thought to have a higher affinity for IgE compared with omalizumab. The drug has an enhanced affinity for the Ig receptor FcγRIIIa, which helps it eliminate IgE expressing B cells through antibody-dependent cell-mediated cytotoxicity [7]. One phase 1 safety trial comparing MEDI4212 with omalizumab and placebo has been completed, with preliminary results demonstrating that a single dose of MEDI4212 (5–300 mg) reduces serum free IgE at rates similar or better than those for omalizumab (NCT01544348) [7]. However at these concentrations MEDI4212 caused more non-serious adverse events than omalizumab. Since the completion of this study, the status of the future development of MEDI4212 is unknown.

Medi9929, also known as AMG 157, is a monoclonal antibody targeting human thymic stromal lymphopoietin (TSLP). MEDI9929 binds to and inhibits TSLP from interacting with its receptor. TSLP is an epithelial cytokine that is thought to play a critical role in causing allergic inflammation and is produced in response to skin barrier disruption or innate signals [7]. Its actions are mediated through its effects on a number of cells, including dendritic cells [32]. Medi9929 has recently completed a phase 2a trial to evaluate the safety and efficacy of MEDI9929 administered subcutaneously to adult subjects with moderate to severe AD (NCT02525094). The results of this randomized double-blinded multi-center placebo-controlled study are not yet available.

15.2.2 Mesenchymal Stem Cells

Several proof-of-concept studies have shown mesenchymal stem cells (MSC) to be a promising alternative therapy for diseases such as macular degeneration, refractory Crohn's disease, amyotrophic lateral sclerosis, and multiple sclerosis [33–36]. MSCs have been used for the treatment of immune disorders, such as graft-vs.-host disease and systemic lupus erythematous [37, 38]. Two recent studies demonstrated MSCs efficacy for the treatment of AD [39, 40]. One study used mouse models to reveal that subcutaneous administration of human umbilical cord blood-derived MSCs (hUCB-MSCs) can efficiently improve AD through the production of multiple factors in response to AD-specific biomarkers such as IL-4, one of the dominant cytokines produced by Th2 cells during active AD [39]. In this study, higher levels of serum IgE induced by AD and mast cell degranulation were suppressed by the administration of hUCB-MSCs [39].

These findings were applied to a phase1/2a clinical trial, which aimed to evaluate the safety and therapeutic efficacy of FURESTEM-AD, a stem cell therapy derived from hUCB to improve moderate-to-severe AD (NCT01927705) [39]. Thirty-four patients were enrolled and randomly allocated to receive low dose (2.5×10^7 cells) or high dose (5.0×10^7 cells) of FURESTEM-AD injection subcutaneously. EASI, IGA and SCORAD scores were evaluated as endpoints along with adverse effect assessments and serum biomarker levels [41]. A single treatment of the hUCB-MSCs resulted in dose-dependent improvements in AD. Fifty-five percent of the high dose infusion group achieved EASI50 score at week 12, while the IGA score and SCORAD score were decreased by 33% and 50%, respectively in this group. Thirty-six percent of patients in the low dose treated group achieved an EASI-50 response. The high dose hUCB-MSCs exerted a continuous, gradual therapeutic effect until week 12, resulting in a greater significant reduction in EASI score by the end of study compared to week 2 ($p = .0016$) [41]. No serious adverse events occurred. All dosages of FURESTEM-AD administration downregulated levels of serum total IgE and blood eosinophil counts with a statistically significant decrease in blood eosinophil number in the high dose group when compared with baseline ($p = 0.452$, $p = 0.0041$) [41]. Another phase 1 study is currently recruiting patients to assess efficacy of autologous adult human mesenchymal stem cells (ADSTEM) injections (NCT02888704).

15.3 Oral Therapies by Target

In addition to the target-specific injectable systemic medications, there are numerous non-biologic oral therapies that are currently undergoing clinical trials (Table 15.1). One such class of drug can be referred to as small molecules, which can modulate proinflammatory cytokines through targeting select signaling pathways and cytokines within immune cells, suggesting the potential to treat inflammatory diseases [42, 43].

Apremilast is a novel oral agent that acts as a small molecule drug to moderate multiple inflammatory pathways by targeting phosphodiesterase type IV (PDE4) inhibition [43]. The drug binds to the catalytic site of PDE4, blocking intracellular cyclic adenosine monophosphate (cAMP) degradation, thus increasing cAMP levels. The increase in cAMP activates protein kinase A and other downstream molecules, resulting in inhibition of pro-inflammatory cytokine production (TNF-α, IFN-γ, IL-2, IL-8, IL-12p70, leukotriene B4, adhesion molecules) and other cellular responses such as neutrophil chemotaxis, degranulation, and adhesion [44, 45]. Topical PDE4 inhibitors have shown promising clinical benefits for AD patients, however none are currently available in the United States [45–48]. Apremilast has been studied for the treatment of multiple immune-related disorders such as asthma, chronic obstructive pulmonary disease, psoriasis, and psoriatic arthritis [49]. It was approved by the United States Food and Drug Administration (US FDA) in 2014 for the treatment of active psoriatic arthritis in adults and of moderate-to-severe plaque psoriasis in patients who are candidates for phototherapy or systemic therapy [43, 50].

Several phase 2 trials provide limited data on apremilast efficacy in adult AD patients. One open-label pilot study evaluated 16 adult patients with moderate-to-severe AD who received 20 mg of apremilast twice daily for 3 months or 30 mg twice daily for 6 months (NCT0139315). The results showed significant reduction of EASI score at 3 months, with an average of 19% in the 20 mg treatment group and 39% in the 30 mg group [45]. Nausea was the most common side effect reported, followed by diarrhea [45]. Another open-label phase 2 study examined 10 patients with AD and/or allergic contact dermatitis who received 20 mg apremilast twice daily for 12 weeks (NCT00931242). EASI-75 was achieved by 10% of subjects and EASI50 by another 10%, and 20% had improvement in IGA score by 2 or more points [51]. Another phase II trial of apremilast was designed as double-blind, placebo-controlled study of 185 patients receiving either 30 mg or 40 mg of apremilast twice daily for 12 weeks versus placebo (NCT02087943). The results showed the primary endpoint of EASI score reduction was achieved with a −25.99% reduction in the 30 mg group and a −31.57% reduction in the 40 mg group, compared with the −10.98% reduction in the placebo group. Only the reduction of the 40 mg group was statistically significant when compared with placebo ($p = 0.03$). Although these results and the safety profile of apremilast are promising, further studies are needed to evaluate the efficacy and appropriate dosing of apremilast for the treatment of moderate-to-severe AD.

Another category of small molecule therapies show promise in the treatment of AD are the janus kinase (JAK) inhibitors. There are four JAK inhibitors now in phase II clinical trials for AD in human patients: oral baricitinib, oral tofacitinib, topical tofacitinib, PF-0496582, and ABT-494. Tofacitinib is a JAK 1 and 3 inhibitor that is currently FDA approved for the treatment of moderate to severely active rheumatoid arthritis in adult patients who have had an inadequate response or intolerance to methotrexate [52]. Oral tofacitinib was assessed in one study of 6 moderate-to-severe AD patients as add-on therapy to topical treatment, which found the SCORAD index decreased by 66.6% from 36.6 to 12.12 ($p < 0.05$) from week 8 to week 29 of treatment [53]. Clinical improvements such as decreased body surface area involvements, decreased erythema, edema/papulation, lichenification, and excoriations were observed in all patients [53].

Baricitinib (also known as LY3009104) is an oral JAK 1 and 2 inhibitor that is undergoing an active phase II AD clinical trial (NCT02576938). Baricitinib has shown efficacy for rheumatoid arthritis patients who are unresponsive to methotrexate in phase II trials and may be efficacious for alopecia areata. [54, 55] The drug is currently in phase III trials for RA (NCT02265705), phase II trials for diabetic kidney disease (NCT01683409), and several compassionate use trials [7]. PF-04965842 is a selective JAK1 inhibitor that has completed phase I studies and is currently recruiting for a phase 2 study of AD patients (NCT02780167). Research of this drug for treatment of patients with moderate to severe psoriasis or subjects with lupus vulgaris has been discontinued [7]. ABT-494 is an oral selective JAK1 inhibitor that is currently being evaluated in a phase 2b study for moderate-to severe AD adults (NCT02925117).

SH2-containing inositol-5′-phosphatase (SHIP)-1 is an endogenous inhibitor of the phosphoinositide-3-kinase (PI3 K) pathway, which is involved in the activation and chemotaxis of cellular inflammation [7, 56]. SHIP1 is predominantly expressed in hemapoietic cells, and it is thought that activation of SHIP1 would selectively induce down-regulation of the PI3 K pathway [7]. AQX-1125 is an oral SHIP1 activator currently being studied in a phase II trial for adults with mild to moderate AD (NCT02324972). The drug has been studied in adults asthma with small decreases in allergic responses and no statistically significant reduction in sputum leukocytes [57].

Another small molecule currently being studied for use in AD is chemoattractant receptor-homologous molecule expressed on Th2 cells (CRTH2, also known as DP_2). As one of the two receptors bound by prostaglandin D_2 (PGD_2), CRTH2 mediates the biological actions of PGD_2 [7]. PGD_2 is produced through the conversion of arachidonic acid (AA) into cyclic endoperoxidases, including PGD_2, through the actions of cyclooxygenase (COX)-1 or COX2 [7]. The major cellular source of PGD_2 is IgE-activated mast cells, but dendritic cells and Th2 cells also act as sources of the molecule [58]. PGD_2 is made in high concentrations as a response to allergen exposure and when bound to CRTH2 it activates and induces the chemotaxis of basophils, eosinophils, and Th2 cells. Experimental research suggests that CRTH2 may play a significant role in recruiting allergic cells and promoting Th2 cytokine production [7].

There are three small-molecule oral CRTH2 receptor antagonists currently in development for AD and allergic diseases. Fevipiprant, also known as QAW039, has completed a phase II trial of adults with moderate to severe AD (NCT01785602). In this 12-week trial subjects were treated with fevipiprant 450 g daily or placebo. Results showed minimal effect on the primary endpoint of change in EASI score from baseline as compared with placebo (mean $-8.65 \pm$ standard error of the mean [SEM] 0.01 for QAW039 and -6.95 ± 0.01 for placebo, no statistics provided) [7]. OC459 (also known as OC000459) is another oral CRTH2 receptor antagonist that is completing a phase II trial for adult patients with moderate-to-severe AD (NCT02002208). The last drug, BBI-5000, has completed phase I trials in healthy adults, with its first indication expected to be AD (NCT02590289) [7].

A final small-molecule drug that is being studied as an oral treatment for AD is KHK4577. The specific target of this drug is unknown. It has completed a phase II trial for adult patients with AD, however the results of this study are not yet available (NCT02004119).

15.4 Topical Medications

Numerous topical formulations are being studied for the treatment of AD. Some of these medications are novel therapies that act as topical biologic or small molecule agents with mechanisms of action similar to systemic treatments. Others are being developed as skin barrier repair therapies for reduction of AD symptoms (Table 15.2).

Table 15.2 Topical agents for atopic dermatitis[a]

Drug candidate	Phase	Mechanism	Route	Clinicaltrials.gov identifier
Target-specific topical agents				
Crisaborole (AN-2728)	3	PDE-4 inhibitor	Topical	NCT02118766
				NCT02118792
E6005	1/2	PDE-4 inhibitor	Topical	NCT02094235
				NCT01179880
	2			NCT01461941
OPA-15406	2	PDE-4 inhibitor	Topical	NCT02068352
Roflumilast	2	PDE-4 inhibitor	Topical	NCT01856764
DRM-02	2	PDE-4 inhibitor	Topical	NCT01993420
LEO29102	2	PDE-4 inhibitor	Topical	NCT01037881
Tofacitinib	2	JAK 1/3 Inhibitor	Topical	NCT02001181
INCB018424 (Ruxolitinib)	2	JAK 1/2 Inhibitor		NCT03011892
DMT210 (Sig990)	2	Isoprenylcysteine analog	Topical	NCT02949960
AM1030	1/2	5-HT Inhibitor	Topical	NCT02379910
SB011	2	DNAzyme	Topical	NCT02079688
MRX-6	2	sPLA2s Inhibitor	Topical	NCT02031445 (recently terminated)
Miscellaneous topical agents				
Cis-urocanic acid	2	Restoration of pH	Topical	NCT01320579
BPR277	1	Kallikrein-related peptidase	Topical	NCT01428297
HL-009	2	Adenosylcobalamin liposomal gel	Topical	NCT01568489
GSK2894512 (WBI-1001)	1	Anti-inflammatory	Topical	NCT02466152
	2			NCT02564055
VTP-38543	1/2	Liver X Receptor agonist	Topical	NCT02655679
Q301	2	Unknown	Topical	NCT02426359
LEO32731	1	Unknown	Topical	NCT02496546
LEO39652	1	Unknown	Topical	NCT02219633
BRT-FC-83C	2	Unknown	Topical	NCT00883311
PDI-192	2	Unknown	Topical	NCT01826461
DPK-060	1/2	Cationic anti-microbial peptide	Topical	NCT01522391
Omiganan	2	Cationic anti-microbial peptide	Topical	NCT02456480
Moisturizer + Subject's own antimicrobial bacteria	2	Anti-microbial	Topical	NCT02144142

[a]*JAK* Janus kinase, *PDE* phosphodiesterase, *5-HT* serotonin, *DNAzyme* deoxyribozyme, *sPLA2s* secretory Phospholipase A2s

Multiple small molecule topical PDE-4 inhibitors are currently under development. The furthest along in development is Crisaborole (also known as AN-2728) which was recently approved in December 2016 by the FDA as a topical treatment for children and adults with mild to moderate AD and is available for prescription use. The unique configuration of boron within the crisaborole molecule enables the selective targeting and inhibition of PDE4, thus increasing cAMP levels and controlling inflammation. The boron atom binds to the activated water in the bimetal center of the active site of PDE4 [59]. The use of novel boron chemistry enables synthesis of a low-molecular-weight compound (251 daltons) that facilitates effective penetration through human skin [59].

Results from the largest clinical trial reported twice-daily crisaborole 2% ointment resulted in total or partial clearance of target lesions in 62% of subjects after 29 days of treatment and 71% reduction in Atopic Dermatitis Severity Index Score (ADSI) score [60]. The most common adverse effects were application site reactions, nasopharyngitis, and upper respiratory tract infections, while the common side effects of systemic PDE4 inhibitors, such as nausea, vomiting, and headache, were not observed. Serum drug concentration studies reveal crisaborole is not absorbed systemically [7]. In two phase 3 studies (AD-301: NCT02118766; AD-302: NCT02118792), more crisaborole treated patients achieved ISGA score success of clear/almost clear with ≥2-grade improvement compared with vehicle group (AD-301: 32.8% vs. 25.4%, $P = .038$; AD-302: 31.4% vs. 18.0%, $P < .001$) [61]. Crisaborole-treated patients achieved success in ISGA score and improvement in pruritus earlier than those treated with vehicle (both $P \leq .001$). Treatment-related adverse events in both studies were infrequent and mild to moderate in severity [61].

E6005 is another novel topical PDE4 inhibitor that has shown efficacy in patients with AD. The drug has completed two phase 1/2 trials, with pediatric and adult study populations, and one phase 2 trial of adult AD patients (NCT02094235, NCT01179880, NCT01461941). Data from the adult trial showed clinical improvement after ointment application twice-daily for 4 weeks, but none were statistically significant. In an 8-week extension, statistically significant improvements in EASI and SCORAD scores from baseline were observed [62]. Low concentrations of an E6005 metabolite were seen in 47% of subjects, however plasma E6005 was undetectable in all subjects [7]. Although no serious adverse events were reported, some patients experienced increased alanine amino transferase levels and application site irritation [63].

OPA-15406 is a topical PDE4 inhibitor with high selectivity for PDE4-B. The drug recently completed a double-blind, vehicle-controlled phase 2 trial of subjects aged 10–70 years with mild to moderate AD (NCT02068352). The subjects were randomized to receive topical OPA-15406 0.3% ($n = 41$), 1% ($n = 43$), or vehicle ointment. IGA score of 0 or 1 with ≥2-grade reduction (primary endpoint) was achieved at week 4 by the 1% group, and mean percentage improvement in baseline EASI 1% was seen as soon as week 1 (31.4% versus 6.0% for vehicle; $P = .0005$), was even larger in week 2 (39.0% versus 3.0%; $P = .0001$), and persisted for 8 weeks [64]. During the first week, visual analog scores of pruritus were also improved in the 1% treatment group. Adverse events thought to be related to OPA-15406 treatment included worsening of AD, application site reactions, and vulvovaginal yeast infections [7].

The topical PDE4 inhibitor roflumilast has completed a phase 2a trial of adult patients with AD, with its results on clinicaltrials.gov revealing the only statistically significant outcome to be a reduction in pruritus [7]. However, results demonstrate trends towards improvement in SCORAD values and Transepidermal Water Loss (TEWL) values (NCT01856764).

Two additional topical PDE4 inhibitors, DRM-02 and LEO29102, have also completed phase 2 trials in AD patients, however these study results are not yet available (NCT01993420, NCT01037881). DRM-02 is a topical gel that is also being studied in rosacea and psoriasis, while LEO29102 is a cream that is also being studied for psoriasis [7].

Among other small molecule topical treatments for AD is a topical formulation of tofacitinib. This JAK1/3 inhibitor has completed a 4-week phase 2 study evaluating its efficacy and tolerability as a 2% ointment (20 mg tofacitinib/g) given twice daily to subjects with mild to moderate AD compared to vehicle (NCT02001181). The preliminary results published on clinicaltrials.gov of 69 adult patients demonstrate an 81.7% reduction in EASI score after 4 weeks, compared to 29.9% in the placebo group ($p < 0.0001$). INCB018424, also known as Ruxolitinib, is an inhibitor of both JAK1 and JAK2. In preclinical studies, the drug caused a decrease in levels of inflammatory cytokines IL-6 and TNF-alpha [65]. A topical phosphate cream formulation of INCB018424 is currently being studied in a recently initiated phase 2 trial for safety and efficacy compared with triamcinolone 0.1% cream and vehicle in adult AD patients (NCT03011892).

DMT210 (formerly known as Sig990) is a small molecule analog of isoprenylcysteine that inhibits toll-like receptor (TLR) and GPCR signaling to downregulate proinflammatory cytokines. A phase 2 trial of 5% DMT210 topical aqueous gel is currently recruiting patients age 12 and above (NCT02949960).

AM1030 is a topical cream that inhibits the biological actions of the neurotransmitter serotonin (5-HT). 5-HT is not only a neurotransmitter, but is also involved in pruritus, vasodilation, immunomodulation, induction of epithelial proliferation, and can act as a growth factor [7, 66]. Seven families of membrane-bound receptors mediate the biological actions of 5-HT, and AM1030 antagonizes one of these receptors, 5-HT2BR. In pre-clinical in vivo and in vitro models, AM1030 significantly reduced both T cell-dependent and T cell-independent inflammatory responses [67]. The drug has also been studied in a phase 1/2 clinical trial for its efficacy in suppression of inflammation and itching in adult AD patients (NCT02379910). The results of this study have not yet been made available.

SB011 is a topical formulation of deoxyribozyme (DNAzyme) hgd40, that cleaves GATA-3 messenger RNA (mRNA). The transcription factor GATA-3 acts a key regulatory factor of the Th2-driven immune response. It induces the differentiation and activates the expression of the Th2 cytokine pathway by binding to several sites that upregulate the expression of IL-4, IL-5, and IL-13 [7, 68]. By cleaving GATA-3 mRNA, hgd40 in SB011 is thought to reduce this cytokine production, reducing inflammation. DNAzymes differ from biologics in that they are completely generated by chemical synthesis and are not created using living organisms. SB011 has completed one phase 2 study of 2% emulsion in adults with mild to moderate AD (NCT02079688).

MRX-6 is a topical cream that acts a Secretory Phospholipase A2s (sPLA2s) inhibitor. sPLAs are a family of enzymes that generate lysophospholipids and release arachidonic acid from membrane phospholipids [7, 56]. They have recently been shown to have proinflammatory and antibacterial activities. MRX-6 was being studied as a treatment for AD, however the pediatric phase 2 study was recently terminated due to lack of efficacy in interim analysis (NCT02031445).

15.5 Miscellaneous Topical Therapies

Other topical therapies that are being studied for the treatment of AD in clinical trials have a wide array of different mechanisms of action and can act as barrier-repair therapies or have anti-microbial properties.

Cis-urocanic acid is another topical cream being developed for AD. Urocanic acid (UCA) is an endogenous molecule of the skin that forms a large component of pH-regulating materials known as natural moisturizing factors of the skin [69]. Epidermal UCA concentrations strongly correlate negatively with AD severity [69, 70]. Cis-UCA cream formulation is thought to improve skin barrier function through suppression of inflammation and restoration of acidic pH in atopic skin [67]. In a study of AD patients, overall results indicated superiority of the 5% cis-UCA emulsion cream over control vehicle in improving skin barrier function (measured as TEWL) and in decreasing skin redness in subjects with mild to moderate AD, with significant improvement observed within10 days of starting cis-UCA treatment. While improvement in PGA and EASI in the treatment area was also observed, it was not statistically significant [69]. There is one registered phase 2 trial evaluating 2.5% and 5% cis-UCA in comparison to placebo and active comparator in the treatment of adult patients with moderate or severe chronic AD that has been completed (NCT01320579). The results of this trial have not yet been published.

The kallikrein-related peptidase inhibitor BPR277 is a topical ointment that completed a three-part phase 1 first-in-human proof of concept study to evaluate its safety and efficacy as in adult AD patients, healthy patients, and patients with Netherton syndrome (NCT01428297).

HL-009 is an adenosylcobalamin liposomal gel thought to have anti-inflammatory properties. The drug has completed a phase 2 trial in adult patients with mild to moderate AD, however the results have not yet been published online (NCT01568489).

GSK2894512 (also known as WBI-1001) is a novel topical anti-inflammatory molecule being developed for the treatment of AD. Bissonette et al. reported significant decreases in IGA scores in WBI-1001 0.5% and 1.0% treated groups compared with placebo in their results from a 12-week, multicenter, randomized, placebo-controlled, double-blind trial, published in 2012 [71]. The drug has more recently completed a phase 1 clinical trial (NCT02466152) for adults with AD and is currently being studied in a phase 2 clinical trial (NCT02564055). This study will evaluate the efficacy and safety of two concentrations (0.5% and 1%) and two application frequencies (once a day and twice a day) of GSK2894512 cream for treatment in adolescent and adult subjects with atopic dermatitis.

VTP-38543 is a Liver X Receptor (LXR) selective agonist that is thought to improve barrier function and decrease inflammation in damaged skin tissue. Ligand-mediated activation of LXRs leads to keratinocyte differentiation, induction of key genes involved in lipid synthesis and cholesterol transport, and improved barrier function in animal models and exerts anti-inflammatory effects in vitro and in mouse models of dermatitis [72]. In preclinical studies, topical formulation of VTP-38543 was found decrease inflammation in human macrophages and in a chemically induced dermatitis mouse model with equal efficacy of potent glucocorticoids [72]. VTP-38543 in topical cream formulation has completed a phase 1/2 trial in adult patients with mild to moderate AD, without published results (NCT02655679).

Several topical agents that are currently being developed for the treatment of AD have unknown mechanisms of action. Q301 is a topical agent with unknown mechanism for which a phase 2 study has recently been completed in moderate to severe AD patients, however no results have been published (NCT02426359). LEO32731 is a topical drug thought to inhibit the secretion of TNF-alpha, Interferon (IFN)-gamma, and IL-5 while increasing levels of the anti-inflammatory cytokine IL-10, however its exact mechanism of action is unknown [73]. The drug recently completed a 3-week phase 1 exploratory study as a cream formulation in adults with mild to moderate AD without published results (NCT02496546). Another topical treatment with an unknown mechanism of action is LEO39652, which also recently completed a phase 1 clinical trial in adults with mild to moderate AD (NCT02219633).

Two additional topical treatments with unknown mechanisms of action are BRT-FC-83C topical cream and PDI-192 topical foam. Both drugs have completed phase 2 trials, with PDI-192 being studied for AD in children and adolescents (NCT01826461), and the older BRT-FC-83C studied for as skin barrier repair therapy for adults with AD (NCT00883311). Although both trials have been updated as complete on clinicaltrials.gov, their results have not been published.

There are several topical agents with anti-microbial properties that are being developed for the treatment of AD. DPK-060 and Omiganan (CLS001) are cationic antimicrobial peptides, molecules that are released primarily by neutrophils, monocytes, and macrophages by secretion or during degranulation [74]. Antimicrobial peptides target invading bacteria through initial electrostatic contact at the anionic bacterial surface and have the potential to reduce length of antibiotic treatment as well as inflammation induced by killed microbes and microbial product [74, 75]. DPK-060 has been studied as a topical ointment in a phase 1/2 trial (NCT01522391), while Omiganan has completed a phase 2 trial evaluating its safety and efficacy in a gel formulation for adults with AD (NCT02456480). Neither study has published results.

A phase 2 clinical trial examining moisturizer containing each subjects' own anti-microbial bacteria remains registered on clinicaltrials.gov with an unknown status (NCT02144142).

15.6 Anti-Pruritic Agents

Pruritus, or "itch," can be one of the most debilitating symptoms of AD. There are several medications currently undergoing clinical trials for specifically for the treatment of pruritus in AD (Table 15.3).

There are two oral medications that act as neurokinin 1 (NK1) receptor antagonists which have completed phase 2 trials for pruritus. There are number of pro-inflammatory neuropeptides that have been implicated in the pathogenesis of neurogenic inflammation, such as tachykinins. Tachykinins are involved in promot-

Table 15.3 Anti-pruritic agents[a]

Drug candidate	Phase	Mechanism	Route	Clinicaltrials.gov identifier
Tradipitant (VLY-686)	2	NK1-R antagonist	Oral	NCT02004041 NCT02651714
DNK333	2	NK1/NK2-R antagonist	Oral	NCT01033097
ZPL-3893787 (ZPL-389)	2	Histamine H4 receptor antagonist	Oral	NCT02424253
Clonidine and Naltrexone	1	Clonidine: reduces sympathetic system outflow. Naltrexone: opioid receptor antagonist	Oral	NCT02268448
Asimadoline (EMD-61753)	2	kappa-Opioid receptor agonist	Oral	NCT02475447
WOL0701–007	1	kappa-Opioid receptor agonist	Topical	NCT02576093
Serlopitant (VPD-737) for Prurigo Nodularis	1	NK1-R antagonist	Oral	NCT02196324
CT327	2	TrkA Inhibitor	Topical	NCT01808157
PAC-14028	2	TRPV1 channel antagonist	Topical	NCT02583022
				NCT02052531
				NCT02565134
	1/2			NCT02748993
	3			NCT02965118
TS-022	2	DP-1 receptor agonist	Topical	NCT00914186 (development since discontinued)

[a]*NK* neurokinin, *R* receptor, *TrkA* tropomyosin receptor kinase A, *TPRV1* transient receptor potential cation channel subfamily V member 1, *DP1-R* prostaglandin D2 receptor 1

ing numerous biological actions, including inflammation, pain transmission, vasodilatation, platelet function, smooth muscle contraction, activation of the immune and endocrine systems, and depression-like behavior [7, 76]. Local release of tachykinins leads to the sensitization of peripheral nerve endings and the activation of inflammatory and immune cells, which contribute to the neurogenic inflammatory process. These pro-inflammatory tachykinins, such as neurokinin A (NKA) and neurokinin B (NKB) activate the G protein-coupled tachykinin receptors, NK1, NK2, and NK3 [76, 77]. The development of antagonists acting on these receptors provides a targeted approach to anti-inflammatory pharmacotherapy [76].

The first of these oral medications is tradipitant, also known as VLY-686, an NK1-receptor (NK1-R) antagonist. Tradipitant has completed a phase 2 trial to determine its efficacy in reducing chronic treatment-resistant pruritus in subjects with atopic dermatitis (NCT02004041). The results of this study have not yet been published. The drug is undergoing another phase 2 multicenter, randomized, double-blind, placebo-controlled study being conducted in the United States that is currently recruiting subjects with treatment-resistant pruritus diagnosed with atopic dermatitis (NCT02651714).

DNK333 is a dual tachykinin NK1/NK2 receptor antagonist that has completed a phase 2 trial in patients with AD suffering from pruritus who require systemic treatment of the disease (NCT01033097). The results of this trial have not been published. In a previous study of asthma patients, DNK333 was shown to block against NKA-induced bronchoconstriction [78].

ZPL-3893787 (ZPL-389) is an oral histamine H4 receptor antagonist that recently completed phase 2 trial examining the effects of 8 weeks of daily oral treatment (30 mg dose) on pruritus in approximately 90 adults with moderate to severe AD (NCT02424253). The results showed a clinically and statistically significant reduction in signs and symptoms of moderate to severe AD [79]. After 8 weeks of treatment, ZPL-389 reduced EASI scores by 50% as compared to 27% of placebo patients ($p = 0.01$). There was also a statistically significant improvement on SCORAD, with ZPL-389 reducing SCORAD by 43% compared to 26% for placebo ($p = 0.004$) [79]. Both the EASI and SCORAD sub-scores associated with pruritus showed improvement and a statistically significant decrease in sleep loss in the ZPL-389 treatment group [79].

Two well-known medications, oral clonidine and oral naltrexone, are currently being studied for novel use in treating cutaneous nerve CNS itch. Clonidine reduces sympathetic system outflow while naltrexone acts an opioid receptor antagonist [7]. A phase 1 study is currently recruiting eight patients with symptomatic AD who will be treated with either oral clonidine or oral naltrexone (NCT02268448).

Other drugs being developed for pruritus in AD patients are kappa-opioid receptor (κ-opioid-R) agonists. Kappa-opioid receptors mediate the sensation of itch in animals and humans [80]. These receptors are expressed in the peripheral nervous system as well as in the central nervous system (CNS), and activation of these receptors at both sites has been shown to result in a reduction in pain and inflammation in preclinical models [80, 81]. These receptors are involved in the pathogenesis of pruritus not only because of their expression in the CNS, but also due to their presence in the skin. Previous research has demonstrated kappa-opioid receptors are down-regulated in the epidermis of atopic dermatitis patients [82]. Application of a peripherally acting kappa-opioid receptor agonist inhibits chloroquine-induced pruritus in mice, suggesting a possible peripheral pathway in itch suppression [83].

Asimadoline (also called EMD-61753) is an orally active, selective kappa-opioid receptor agonist that has demonstrated efficacy in several preclinical pruritus models [80]. A phase 2 clinical trial is currently recruiting patients to evaluate the safety, tolerability and clinical efficacy of asimadoline in patients with pruritus that is associated with AD (NCT02475447). WOL0701-007 is a novel kappa-opioid receptor agonist administered as a topical cream. It has completed a phase 1 trial examining the efficacy, safety, and tolerability of three different concentrations of WOL071-007 formulations in AD patients (NCT02576093). Serlopitant, or VPD-737, is an oral NK-1 receptor antagonist that has completed a phase 2 trial for the treatment of prurigo nodularis (NCT02196324).

Among other topical medications currently being studied for pruritus, is a tropomyosin-receptor kinase A (TrkA) inhibitor called CT327. This drug is thought to inhibit the TrkA receptor for Nerve Growth Factor (NGF), which is implicated in the pathogenesis of chronic pruritus by up-regulating the sensitivity and expression of specific TRPV1 (transient receptor potential cation channel subfamily V member 1) channels of sensory nerve terminals in the skin [84]. CT327 ointment has completed a phase 2 study evaluating pruritus reduction in patients with mild to moderate AD accompanied by moderate pruritus (NCT01808157). Although these results have not been published, results of study evaluating the drug for treatment of pruritus in psoriasis patients have shown significant reductions in patient-reported pruritus [84].

PAC-14028 is a topical cream that acts a TRPV1 channel antagonist. Initial studies demonstrated the efficacy of PAC-14028 in the attenuation of inflammation and pruritus associated with atopic dermatitis in mice [85]. PAC-14028 has also been shown to prevent barrier damages and accelerate skin barrier recovery [85, 86]. This drug has completed multiple phase 2 trials in determining efficacy in reducing pruritus associated with AD, severity of AD, and skin pruritus alone (NCT02583022, NCT02052531, NCT02565134). The drug is currently undergoing separate trials to examine its efficacy and safety in children with atopic dermatitis (NCT02748993, NCT02965118).

TS-022 is a prostanoid-1 (DP-1) receptor agonist, originally developed as topical anti-pruritic drug for atopic dermatitis. Although the drug completed phase 2 clinical trial, its development has since been discontinued due to lack of efficacy (NCT00914186).

15.7 Unconventional Therapies

Among the more unconventional therapies being developed for the treatment of AD is a device designed for removal of IgE from the circulation through adsorption of IgE on a specially designed column after apheresis of the blood (Table 15.4).

Table 15.4 Unconventional therapies

Drug candidate	Phase	Mechanism	Route	Clinicaltrials.gov identifier
IgE-specific adsorption column	2	Immunoadsorption: removal of IgE after apheresis of blood	Device	NCT02365246
Acupuncture	n/a[a]	Alternative medicine	Needle insertion	NCT02844452
D107G	2	Dihomo-gamma-linolenic acid (DLGA) derivative	Oral	NCT02211417
				NCT02864498
	2		Topical	NCT02925793
Lactobacillus reuteri DSM 17938 + vitamin D3	n/a	Probiotics	Oral	NCT02945683
Omega-3 long chain polyunsaturated fatty acid (LCPUFA)	n/a	Dietary supplement	Oral	NCT01473823
Ganoderma tea	1 and 2	Unknown	Oral	NCT02533635
Vitamin D	n/a	Cathelicidin production	Oral	NCT02058186
KM110329	2	Herbal compound	Oral	NCT01692093
Holly Mangrove shower gel	3	Barrier repair therapy	Topical	NCT02178215
SAN007	2	5% East Indian sandalwood oil	Topical	NCT02178215
			Topical	NCT03000595
Indigo naturalis	2	Traditional Chinese Medicine	Topical	NCT02669888
Oregano ointment	2	Anti-microbial/ anti-inflammatory	Topical	NCT02289989
Sodium hypochlorite (bleach bath) alteration of skin microbiome	n/a	Bathing additive	Topical	NCT01996150
Acetic acid vs. Sodium hypocholorite (bleach bath)	n/a	Bathing additive	Topical	NCT02582788

[a]Non-pharmaceutical or natural products are exempt from the phases of drug development

A phase 2 trial for the device is currently recruiting adult patients with severe AD (NCT02365246).

Acupuncture treatment is regarded in traditional Chinese medicine as having a curative effect on symptoms of AD. There is one clinical trial currently recruiting AD patients to evaluate the therapeutic effect of acupuncture on AD symptoms, including quality of life and pruritus. This trial is a randomized, sham-controlled, pilot trial with different visit frequencies. The main outcome measures are VAS for itch, SCORAD, EASI, DLQI, and the Patient Oriented Eczema Measure (POEM).

There are numerous dietary supplements that are being investigated for the treatment of AD in clinical trials. D107G is an oral formulation of a semi-synthetic derivative of dihomo-gamma-linolenic acid (DLGA), an omega-6 fatty acid. This drug has completed one phase 2 trial evaluating for the efficacy of a 2 gram dose for moderate to severe AD patients (NCT02211417). Another phase 2b trial is currently recruiting patients to determine the efficacy of D107G (NCT02864498). There is also a topical cream formulation of DS107 that is registered for a trial that will evaluate DS107 1% and 5% versus vehicle (NCT02925793).

Multiple clinical trials evaluating the efficacy of oral probiotics in improving AD symptoms have been completed, with one currently recruiting patients. This clinical trial aims to evaluate the efficacy of a combination of Lactobacillus reuteri DSM 17938 and vitamin D3 (Reuterin® D3) in improving the SCORAD in pediatric patients with mild to moderate AD (NCT02945683).

Omega-3 long chain polyunsaturated fatty acid (LCPUFA) is a dietary supplement theorized to have anti-inflammatory properties. It is currently being evaluated via clinical trial, however as a non-pharmaceutical product, it does not require FDA-approval before marketing and is exempt from the required phases of drug development [7]. The trial supplies infants with early development of IgE associated eczema and food allergy with omega-3 LCPUFA and assesses the effect of the supplementation on the future development of skin symptoms, food allergy, allergen sensitization and asthma (NCT01473823).

Ganoderma tea, a Master Ganoderma Detox Tea with an unknown mechanism of action, is being evaluated in single-blind, cross-over pilot study to observe its safety and efficacy on eczema patients. This phase 1/2 study is currently recruiting patients and aims to enroll 30 subjects for a study period of 16 weeks (NCT02533635).

Oral Vitamin D has been studied in AD patients (NCT02058186). An increase in skin colonization of Staphylococcus aureus (S. aureus) in AD patients from the reduction of cathelicidin production may play an important role in the pathogenesis of disease. In vivo studies have shown Vitamin D can stimulate cathelicidin production. Results of this clinical trial have not been published.

An older dietary supplement titled KM110329 has also been registered for a randomized, double-blind, placebo-controlled, multi-center phase 2 trial (NCT01692093). KM110329 is a functional food consisting of four herbal compounds found in Rubi Fructus, Houttuyniae Herba, Rehmanniae Radix, and Betulae Platyphyllae Cortex [87].

Multiple novel non-pharmaceutical topical barrier repair treatments are under development as adjunctive therapy for AD. One such treatment is called Holly Mangrove shower gel, which is currently undergoing phase 3 trials (NCT02178215) at Mahidol University. Another botanical drug product being studied for AD is called SAN007, a 5% East Indian sandalwood oil in a cream formulation. SAN007 has been registered for two phase 2 trials (NCT02178215, NCT03000595) which are not yet recruiting. Indigo Naturalis ointment is another topical formulation that has very recently completed a phase 2 trial in February 2017 (NCT02669888). Indigo naturalis is an alternative traditional Chinese medicine that has been used to treat various infectious and inflammatory skin diseases for hundreds of years.

Oregano ointment is also a non-pharmaceutical topical product being studied for its antimicrobial and anti-inflammatory properties. A phase 2 study is currently recruiting pediatric patients to evaluate and compare the efficacy of 3% oregano extract ointment versus 1% hydrocortisone ointment (NCT02289989).

Bleach baths have been used for decades in the treatment of AD. A current clinical trial is recruiting patients to assess whether bleach baths used for adult subjects with AD will significantly alter their skin microbiome (including S. aureus) (NCT01996150). Another study, currently recruiting pediatric patients, is being conducted at the Mayo Clinic to examine the use of dilute acetic acid (vinegar) baths compared to bleach baths (NCT02582788). While dilute acetic acid has been recommended for decades to treat patients hospitalized for AD, this practice has not been widely adopted in the pediatric dermatology community.

References

1. Harskamp CT, Armstrong AW. Immunology of atopic dermatitis: novel insights into mechanisms and immunomodulatory therapies. Semin Cutan Med Surg. 2013;32(3):132–9. http://www.ncbi.nlm.nih.gov/pubmed/24175400. Accessed 13 Feb 2017.
2. Vatrella A, Fabozzi I, Calabrese C, Maselli R, Pelaia G. Dupilumab: a novel treatment for asthma. J Asthma Allergy. 2014;7:123–30. doi:10.2147/JAA.S52387.
3. Montes-Torres A, Llamas-Velasco M, Pérez-Plaza A, Solano-López G, Sánchez-Pérez J. Biological treatments in atopic dermatitis. J Clin Med. 2015;4(4):593–613. doi:10.3390/jcm4040593.
4. Gittler JK, Shemer A, Suárez-Fariñas M, et al. Progressive activation of TH2/TH22 cytokines and selective epidermal proteins characterizes acute and chronic atopic dermatitis. J Allergy Clin Immunol. 2012;130(6):1344–54. doi:10.1016/j.jaci.2012.07.012.
5. Simpson EL, Bieber T, Guttman-Yassky E, et al. Two phase 3 trials of dupilumab versus placebo in atopic dermatitis. N Engl J Med. 2016;375(24):2335–48. doi:10.1056/NEJMoa1610020.
6. Beck LA, Thaci D, Hamilton JD, et al. Dupilumab treatment in adults with moderate-to-severe atopic dermatitis. N Engl J Med. 2014;371(2):130–9. doi:10.1056/NEJMoa1314768.
7. Wang D, Beck LA. Immunologic targets in atopic dermatitis and emerging therapies: an update. Am J Clin Dermatol. 2016;17(5):425–43. doi:10.1007/s40257-016-0205-5.
8. MedImmune LLC. Phase 2 study to evaluate the efficacy and safety of tralokinumab in adults with atopic dermatitis (D2213C00001). https://clinicaltrials.gov/ct2/show/NCT02347176.
9. Jancin B. Conference Coverage: Lebrikizumab opens new door in atopic dermatitis therapy. Dermatology News. http://www.mdedge.com/edermatologynews/article/115736/atopic-dermatitis/lebrikizumab-opens-new-door-atopic-dermatitis. Published 2016. Accessed 13 Feb 2017.
10. Arai I, Tsuji M, Takeda H, Akiyama N, Saito SA. single dose of interleukin-31 (IL-31) causes continuous itch-associated scratching behaviour in mice. Exp Dermatol. 2013;22(10):669–71. doi:10.1111/exd.12222.
11. Dillon SR, Sprecher C, Hammond A, et al. Interleukin 31, a cytokine produced by activated T cells, induces dermatitis in mice. Nat Immunol. 2004;5(7):752–60. doi:10.1038/ni1084.
12. Hawro T, Saluja R, Weller K, Altrichter S, Metz M, Maurer M. Interleukin-31 does not induce immediate itch in atopic dermatitis patients and healthy controls after skin challenge. Allergy. 2014;69(1):113–7. doi:10.1111/all.12316.
13. Kasutani K, Fujii E, Ohyama S, et al. Anti-IL-31 receptor antibody is shown to be a potential therapeutic option for treating itch and dermatitis in mice. Br J Pharmacol. 2014;171(22):5049–58. doi:10.1111/bph.12823.

14. Hanifin JM, Irvine AD, McLean WH, et al. Commentary: new drugs for atopic dermatitis may provide clues to basic mechanisms of itch and inflammation. J Am Acad Dermatol. 2016;75(3):504–5. doi:10.1016/j.jaad.2016.06.013.
15. McKnight W. Conference coverage: nemolizumab improved most common symptoms in moderate, severe atopic dermatitis | Dermatology News. Dermatology News. http://www.mdedge.com/edermatologynews/article/107327/atopic-dermatitis/nemolizumab-improved-most-common-symptoms-moderate. Published 2016. Accessed 12 Feb 2017.
16. Nograles KE, Zaba LC, Shemer A, et al. IL-22–producing "T22" T cells account for upregulated IL-22 in atopic dermatitis despite reduced IL-17–producing TH17 T cells. J Allergy Clin Immunol. 2009;123(6):1244–1252.e2. doi:10.1016/j.jaci.2009.03.041.
17. Guttman-Yassky E, Dhingra N, Leung DY. New era of biologic therapeutics in atopic dermatitis. Expert Opin Biol Ther. 2013;13(4):549–61. doi:10.1517/14712598.2013.758708.
18. Fujita H. The role of IL-22 and Th22 cells in human skin diseases. J Dermatol Sci. 2013;72(1):3–8. doi:10.1016/j.jdermsci.2013.04.028.
19. Auriemma M, Vianale G, Amerio P, Reale M. Cytokines and T cells in atopic dermatitis. Eur Cytokine Netw. 2013;24(1):37–44. doi:10.1684/ecn.2013.0333.
20. Guttman E. A Study of ILV-94 (Anti-22 Antibody) Administered via IV in Atopic Dermatitis. http://grantome.com/grant/NIH/UM1-AR063917-01A1.
21. Krueger JG, Fretzin S, Suárez-Fariñas M, et al. IL-17A is essential for cell activation and inflammatory gene circuits in subjects with psoriasis. J Allergy Clin Immunol. 2012;130(1):145–154.e9. doi:10.1016/j.jaci.2012.04.024.
22. Papp KA, Reid C, Foley P, et al. Anti-IL-17 receptor antibody AMG 827 leads to rapid clinical response in subjects with moderate to severe psoriasis: results from a phase I, randomized, placebo-controlled trial. J Invest Dermatol. 2012;132(10):2466–9. doi:10.1038/jid.2012.163.
23. Griffiths CEM, Strober BE, van de Kerkhof P, et al. Comparison of ustekinumab and etanercept for moderate-to-severe psoriasis. N Engl J Med. 2010;362(2):118–28. doi:10.1056/NEJMoa0810652.
24. C-Y W, Chang Y-T, Juan C-K, et al. Depression and insomnia in patients with psoriasis and psoriatic arthritis taking tumor necrosis factor antagonists. Medicine (Baltimore). 2016;95(22):e3816. doi:10.1097/MD.0000000000003816.
25. Koutruba N, Emer J, Lebwohl M. Review of ustekinumab, an interleukin-12 and interleukin-23 inhibitor used for the treatment of plaque psoriasis. Ther Clin Risk Manag. 2010;6:123–41. http://www.ncbi.nlm.nih.gov/pubmed/20421912. Accessed 13 Feb 2017.
26. Suárez-Fariñas M, Ungar B, Noda S, et al. Alopecia areata profiling shows TH1, TH2, and IL-23 cytokine activation without parallel TH17/TH22 skewing. J Allergy Clin Immunol. 2015;136(5):1277–87. doi:10.1016/j.jaci.2015.06.032.
27. Khattri S, Brunner PM, Garcet S, et al. Efficacy and safety of ustekinumab treatment in adults with moderate-to-severe atopic dermatitis. Exp Dermatol. 2017;26(1):28–35. doi:10.1111/exd.13112.
28. Tamagawa-Mineoka R, Okuzawa Y, Masuda K, Katoh N. Increased serum levels of interleukin 33 in patients with atopic dermatitis. J Am Acad Dermatol. 2014;70(5):882–8. doi:10.1016/j.jaad.2014.01.867.
29. Savinko T, Matikainen S, Saarialho-Kere U, et al. IL-33 and ST2 in atopic dermatitis: expression profiles and modulation by triggering factors. J Invest Dermatol. 2012;132(5):1392–400. doi:10.1038/jid.2011.446.
30. Xencor Reports XmAb®7195 Top-line Interim Phase 1a Results Showing Rapid Reduction of Serum IgE in. http://www.prnewswire.com/news-releases/xencor-reports-xmab7195-top-line-interim-phase-1a-results-showing-rapid-reduction-of-serum-ige-in-healthy-volunteers-300027621.html. Accessed 13 Feb 2017.
31. Arm JP, Bottoli I, Skerjanec A, et al. Pharmacokinetics, pharmacodynamics and safety of QGE031 (ligelizumab), a novel high-affinity anti-IgE antibody, in atopic subjects. Clin Exp Allergy. 2014;44(11):1371–85. doi:10.1111/cea.12400.

32. Soumelis V, Reche PA, Kanzler H, et al. Human epithelial cells trigger dendritic cell–mediated allergic inflammation by producing TSLP. Nat Immunol. 2002;3(7):673–80. doi:10.1038/ni805.
33. Schwartz SD, Regillo CD, Lam BL, et al. Human embryonic stem cell-derived retinal pigment epithelium in patients with age-related macular degeneration and Stargardt's macular dystrophy: follow-up of two open-label phase 1/2 studies. Lancet. 2015;385(9967):509–16. doi:10.1016/S0140-6736(14)61376-3.
34. Hawkey CJ, Allez M, Clark MM, et al. Autologous hematopoetic stem cell transplantation for refractory crohn disease. JAMA. 2015;314(23):2524. doi:10.1001/jama.2015.16700.
35. Petrou P, Gothelf Y, Argov Z, et al. Safety and clinical effects of mesenchymal stem cells secreting neurotrophic factor transplantation in patients with amyotrophic lateral sclerosis. JAMA Neurol. 2016;73(3):337. doi:10.1001/jamaneurol.2015.4321.
36. Connick P, Kolappan M, Crawley C, et al. Autologous mesenchymal stem cells for the treatment of secondary progressive multiple sclerosis: an open-label phase 2a proof-of-concept study. Lancet Neurol. 2012;11(2):150–6. doi:10.1016/S1474-4422(11)70305-2.
37. Sun L, Akiyama K, Zhang H, et al. Mesenchymal stem cell transplantation reverses multiorgan dysfunction in systemic lupus erythematosus mice and humans. Stem Cells. 2009;27(6):1421–32. doi:10.1002/stem.68.
38. Le Blanc K, Frassoni F, Ball L, et al. Mesenchymal stem cells for treatment of steroid-resistant, severe, acute graft-versus-host disease: a phase II study. Lancet. 2008;371(9624):1579–86. doi:10.1016/S0140-6736(08)60690-X.
39. Kim H-S, Yun J-W, Shin T-H, et al. Human umbilical cord blood mesenchymal stem cell-derived PGE $_2$ and TGF-β1 alleviate atopic dermatitis by reducing mast cell degranulation. Stem Cells. 2015;33(4):1254–66. doi:10.1002/stem.1913.
40. Na K, Yoo HS, Zhang YX, et al. Bone marrow-derived clonal mesenchymal stem cells inhibit ovalbumin-induced atopic dermatitis. Cell Death Dis. 2014;5(7):e1345. doi:10.1038/cddis.2014.299.
41. Kim H-S, Lee JH, Roh K-H, Jun HJ, Kang K-S, Kim T-Y. Clinical trial of human umbilical cord blood-derived stem cells for the treatment of moderate-to-severe atopic dermatitis: phase I/IIa studies. Stem Cells. 2017;35(1):248–55. doi:10.1002/stem.2401.
42. Dastidar SG, Rajagopal D, Ray A. Therapeutic benefit of PDE4 inhibitors in inflammatory diseases. Curr Opin Investig Drugs. 2007;8(5):364–72. http://www.ncbi.nlm.nih.gov/pubmed/17520865. Accessed 13 Feb 2017.
43. Megna M, Napolitano M, Patruno C, et al. Systemic treatment of adult atopic dermatitis: a review. Dermatol Ther (Heidelb). 2016;7(1):1–23. doi:10.1007/s13555-016-0170-1.
44. Souness JE, Aldous D, Sargent C. Immunosuppressive and anti-inflammatory effects of cyclic AMP phosphodiesterase (PDE) type 4 inhibitors. Immunopharmacology. 2000;47(2–3):127–62. http://www.ncbi.nlm.nih.gov/pubmed/10878287. Accessed 13 Feb 2017.
45. Samrao A, Berry TM, Goreshi R, Simpson ELA. pilot study of an oral phosphodiesterase inhibitor (apremilast) for atopic dermatitis in adults. Arch Dermatol. 2012;148(8):890–7. doi:10.1001/archdermatol.2012.812.
46. Griffiths CEM, Van Leent EJM, Gilbert M, Traulsen J. Cipamyflline Study Group. Randomized comparison of the type 4 phosphodiesterase inhibitor cipamfylline cream, cream vehicle and hydrocortisone 17-butyrate cream for the treatment of atopic dermatitis. Br J Dermatol. 2002;147(2):299–307. http://www.ncbi.nlm.nih.gov/pubmed/12174103. Accessed 13 Feb 2017.
47. Hanifin JM, Chan SC, Cheng JB, et al. Type 4 phosphodiesterase inhibitors have clinical and in vitro anti-inflammatory effects in atopic dermatitis. J Invest Dermatol. 1996;107(1):51–6. http://www.ncbi.nlm.nih.gov/pubmed/8752839. Accessed 13 Feb 2017.
48. Hoppmann J, Galetzka C, Höfgen N, Rundfeldt C, Bämer W, Kietzmann M. The phosphodiesterase 4 inhibitor AWD 12-281 is active in a new guinea-pig model of allergic skin inflammation predictive of human skin penetration and suppresses both Th1 and Th2 cytokines in mice. J Pharm Pharmacol. 2005;57(12):1609–17. doi:10.1211/jpp.57.12.0011.

49. Mease PJ. Apremilast: a phosphodiesterase 4 inhibitor for the treatment of psoriatic arthritis. Rheumatol Ther. 2014;1(1):1–20. doi:10.1007/s40744-014-0005-4.
50. Fala L. Otezla (Apremilast), an oral PDE-4 inhibitor, receives FDA approval for the treatment of patients with active psoriatic arthritis and plaque psoriasis. Am Health Drug Benefits. 2015;8(Spec Feature):105–10. http://www.ncbi.nlm.nih.gov/pubmed/26629274. Accessed 13 Feb 2017.
51. Volf EM, S-C A, Dumont N, Scheinman P, Gottlieb ABA. phase 2, open-label, investigator-initiated study to evaluate the safety and efficacy of apremilast in subjects with recalcitrant allergic contact or atopic dermatitis. J Drugs Dermatol. 2012;11(3):341–6. http://www.ncbi.nlm.nih.gov/pubmed/22395585. Accessed 13 Feb 2017.
52. Ghoreschi K, Gadina M. Jakpot! New small molecules in autoimmune and inflammatory diseases. Exp Dermatol. 2014;23(1):7–11. doi:10.1111/exd.12265.
53. Levy LL, Urban J, King BA. Treatment of recalcitrant atopic dermatitis with the oral Janus kinase inhibitor tofacitinib citrate. J Am Acad Dermatol. 2015;73(3):395–9. doi:10.1016/j.jaad.2015.06.045.
54. Keystone EC, Taylor PC, Drescher E, et al. Safety and efficacy of baricitinib at 24 weeks in patients with rheumatoid arthritis who have had an inadequate response to methotrexate. Annals of the Rheumatic Diseases. 2015;74(2):333–340. doi:10.1136/annrheumdis-2014-206478.
55. Jabbari A, Dai Z, Xing L, et al. Reversal of Alopecia Areata Following Treatment With the JAK1/2 Inhibitor Baricitinib. EBioMedicine. 2015;2(4):351–355. doi:10.1016/j.ebiom.2015.02.015.
56. Bowton DL, Dmitrienko AA, Israel E, Zeiher BG, Sides GD. Impact of a soluble phospholipase A2 inhibitor on inhaled allergen challenge in subjects with asthma. J Asthma. 2005;42(1):65–71. http://www.ncbi.nlm.nih.gov/pubmed/15801331. Accessed 14 Feb 2017.
57. Leaker BR, Barnes PJ, O'Connor BJ, et al. The effects of the novel SHIP1 activator AQX-1125 on allergen-induced responses in mild-to-moderate asthma. Clin Exp Allergy. 2014;44(9):1146–53. doi:10.1111/cea.12370.
58. Pettipher R, Hansel TT, Armer R. Antagonism of the prostaglandin D2 receptors DP1 and CRTH2 as an approach to treat allergic diseases. Nat Rev Drug Discov. 2007;6(4):313–25. doi:10.1038/nrd2266.
59. Jarnagin K, Chanda S, Coronado D, et al. Crisaborole topical ointment, 2%: a nonsteroidal, topical, anti-inflammatory phosphodiesterase 4 inhibitor in clinical development for the treatment of atopic dermatitis. J Drugs Dermatol. 2016;15(4):390–6. http://www.ncbi.nlm.nih.gov/pubmed/27050693. Accessed 5 Dec 2016.
60. Stein Gold LF, Spelman L, Spellman MC, Hughes MH, Zane LTA. Phase 2, randomized, controlled, dose-ranging study evaluating crisaborole topical ointment, 0.5% and 2% in adolescents with mild to moderate atopic dermatitis. J Drugs Dermatol. 2015;14(12):1394–9. http://www.ncbi.nlm.nih.gov/pubmed/26659931. Accessed 16 Feb 2017.
61. Paller AS, Tom WL, Lebwohl MG, et al. Efficacy and safety of crisaborole ointment, a novel, nonsteroidal phosphodiesterase 4 (PDE4) inhibitor for the topical treatment of atopic dermatitis (AD) in children and adults. J Am Acad Dermatol. 2016;75(3):494–503.e4. doi:10.1016/j.jaad.2016.05.046.
62. Furue M, Kitahara Y, Akama H, et al. Safety and efficacy of topical E6005, a phosphodiesterase 4 inhibitor, in Japanese adult patients with atopic dermatitis: results of a randomized, vehicle-controlled, multicenter clinical trial. J Dermatol. 2014;41(7):577–85. doi:10.1111/1346-8138.12534.
63. Ohba F, Matsuki S, Imayama S, et al. Efficacy of a novel phosphodiesterase inhibitor, E6005, in patients with atopic dermatitis: an investigator-blinded, vehicle-controlled study. J Dermatolog Treat. 2016;27(5):467–72. doi:10.3109/09546634.2016.1157257.
64. Hanifin JM, Ellis CN, Frieden IJ, et al. OPA-15406, a novel, topical, nonsteroidal, selective phosphodiesterase-4 (PDE4) inhibitor, in the treatment of adult and adolescent patients with mild to moderate atopic dermatitis (AD): a phase-II randomized, double-blind, placebo-controlled study. J Am Acad Dermatol. 2016;75(2):297–305. doi:10.1016/j.jaad.2016.04.001.

65. Quintas-Cardama A, Vaddi K, Liu P, et al. Preclinical characterization of the selective JAK1/2 inhibitor INCB018424: therapeutic implications for the treatment of myeloproliferative neoplasms. Blood. 2010;115(15):3109–17. doi:10.1182/blood-2009-04-214957.
66. Slominski A, Pisarchik A, Zbytek B, Tobin DJ, Kauser S, Wortsman J. Functional activity of serotoninergic and melatoninergic systems expressed in the skin. J Cell Physiol. 2003;196(1):144–53. doi:10.1002/jcp.10287.
67. Palmqvist N, Siller M, Klint C, Sjödin AA. human and animal model-based approach to investigating the anti-inflammatory profile and potential of the 5-HT2B receptor antagonist AM1030. J Inflamm. 2016;13(1):20. doi:10.1186/s12950-016-0127-2.
68. Kanhere A, Hertweck A, Bhatia U, et al. T-bet and GATA3 orchestrate Th1 and Th2 differentiation through lineage-specific targeting of distal regulatory elements. Nat Commun. 2012;3:1268. doi:10.1038/ncomms2260.
69. Peltonen J, Pylkkänen L, Jansén C, et al. Three randomised phase I/IIa trials of 5% Cis-urocanic acid emulsion cream in healthy adult subjects and in patients with atopic dermatitis. Acta Derm Venereol. 2014;94(4):415–20. doi:10.2340/00015555-1735.
70. Kezic S, O'Regan GM, Yau N, et al. Levels of filaggrin degradation products are influenced by both filaggrin genotype and atopic dermatitis severity. Allergy. 2011;66(7):934–40. doi:10.1111/j.1398-9995.2010.02540.x.
71. Bissonnette R, Poulin Y, Zhou Y, et al. Efficacy and safety of topical WBI-1001 in patients with mild to severe atopic dermatitis: results from a 12-week, multicentre, randomized, placebo-controlled double-blind trial. Br J Dermatol. 2012;166(4):853–60. doi:10.1111/j.1365-2133.2011.10775.x.
72. Zhao Y, Meng S, Noto PB, et al. The LXR ligand VTP-38543 represents a new class of therapeutic agents for the treatment of atopic dermatitis. (Poster presented at Society for Investigative Dermatology; May 2015; Atlanta, Georgia).
73. Friedman A, Agnihothri R. Eczema Drugs in Development I National Eczema Association. https://nationaleczema.org/research/phases-drug-development/. Published 2015. Accessed 27 Feb 2017.
74. Battersby AJ, Khara J, Wright VJ, Levy O, Kampmann B. Antimicrobial proteins and peptides in early life: ontogeny and translational opportunities. Front Immunol. 2016;7:309. doi:10.3389/fimmu.2016.00309.
75. Arias CA, Murray BE. Antibiotic-resistant bugs in the 21st century—a clinical super-challenge. N Engl J Med. 2009;360(5):439–43. doi:10.1056/NEJMp0804651.
76. Pintér E, Pozsgai G, Hajna Z, Helyes Z, Szolcsányi J. Neuropeptide receptors as potential drug targets in the treatment of inflammatory conditions. Br J Clin Pharmacol. 2014;77(1):5–20. doi:10.1111/bcp.12097.
77. Maggi CA. Tachykinins and calcitonin gene-related peptide (CGRP) as co-transmitters released from peripheral endings of sensory nerves. Prog Neurobiol. 1995;45(1):1–98. http://www.ncbi.nlm.nih.gov/pubmed/7716258. Accessed 16 Feb 2017.
78. Joos GF, Vincken W, Louis R, et al. Dual tachykinin NK1/NK2 antagonist DNK333 inhibits neurokinin A-induced bronchoconstriction in asthma patients. Eur Respir J. 2004;23(1):76–81. http://www.ncbi.nlm.nih.gov/pubmed/14738235. Accessed 16 Feb 2017.
79. Werfel T. Overview of ZPL-3893787 (ZPL-389) clinical trial for atopic dermatitis. Eur Med J. 2016. http://emjreviews.com/videos/overview-of-zpl-3893787-zpl-389-clinical-trial-for-atopic-dermatitis/. Accessed 16 Feb 2017.
80. Machelska H, Pflüger M, Weber W, et al. Peripheral effects of the kappa-opioid agonist EMD 61753 on pain and inflammation in rats and humans. J Pharmacol Exp Ther. 1999;290(1):354–61. http://www.ncbi.nlm.nih.gov/pubmed/10381799. Accessed 16 Feb 2017.
81. Millan MJ, Członkowski A, Morris B, et al. Inflammation of the hind limb as a model of unilateral, localized pain: influence on multiple opioid systems in the spinal cord of the rat. Pain. 1988;35(3):299–312. http://www.ncbi.nlm.nih.gov/pubmed/2906425. Accessed 16 Feb 2017.
82. Tominaga M, Ogawa H, Takamori K. Possible roles of epidermal opioid systems in pruritus of atopic dermatitis. J Invest Dermatol. 2007;127(9):2228–35. doi:10.1038/sj.jid.5700942.

83. Inan S, Cowan A. Kappa opioid agonists suppress chloroquine-induced scratching in mice. Eur J Pharmacol. 2004;502(3):233–7. doi:10.1016/j.ejphar.2004.09.010.
84. Roblin D, Yosipovitch G, Boyce B, et al. Topical TrkA kinase inhibitor CT327 is an effective, novel therapy for the treatment of pruritus due to psoriasis: results from experimental studies, and efficacy and safety of CT327 in a phase 2b clinical trial in patients with psoriasis. Acta Derm Venereol. 2015;95(5):542–8. doi:10.2340/00015555-2047.
85. Lim K-M, Park Y-H. Development of PAC-14028, a novel transient receptor potential vanilloid type 1 (TRPV1) channel antagonist as a new drug for refractory skin diseases. Arch Pharm Res. 2012;35(3):393–6. doi:10.1007/s12272-012-0321-6.
86. Yun J-W, Seo JA, Jeong YS, et al. TRPV1 antagonist can suppress the atopic dermatitis-like symptoms by accelerating skin barrier recovery. J Dermatol Sci. 2010;62(1):8–15. doi:10.1016/j.jdermsci.2010.10.014.
87. Cheon C, Park S, Park J-S, et al. KM110329 in adult patients with atopic dermatitis: a randomised, double-blind, placebo-controlled, multicentre trial—study protocol. BMC Complement Altern Med. 2013;13(1):335. doi:10.1186/1472-6882-13-335.

FSC
www.fsc.org
MIX
Papier | Fördert gute Waldnutzung
FSC® C083411

Kolibri 360 GmbH
Ferdinand-Jühlke-Straße 7
99095 Erfurt, Deutschland
produktsicherheit@kolibri360.de